Fifty Years of Practice

The Case Studies of Shudō Denmei

Fifty Years of Practice

THE CASE STUDIES OF SHUDŌ DENMEI

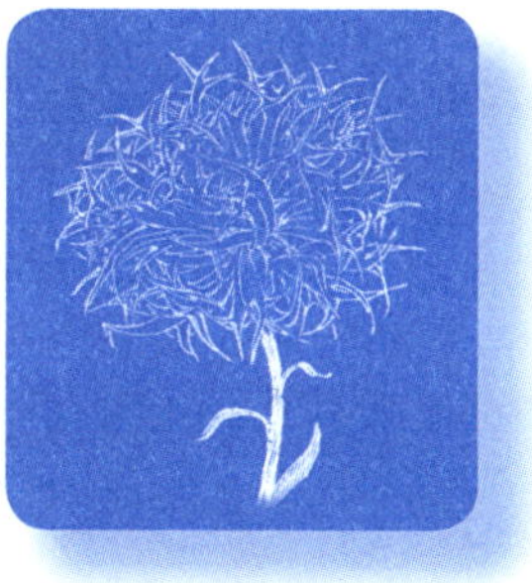

Shudō Denmei

TRANSLATED BY

Stephen Brown

EASTLAND PRESS ▸ SEATTLE

Originally published in Japanese as *Shudo Denmei Shorei-shu*
by Ido No Nippon Sha, Inc. (Tokyo), 2013

English language edition published by Eastland Press, Inc.
P.O. Box 99749
Seattle, WA 98139, USA
www.eastlandpress.com

Library of Congress Catalog Card Number: 2022934621
ISBN: 978-0-939616-98-5

2 4 6 8 10 9 7 5 3 1

Illustrations by Bruce Wang
Book design by Gary Niemeier

Cover illustration of the feathery crane chrysanthemum by Keika Hasegawa
from the series "One Hundred Chrysanthemums by Keika" (1893).

TABLE OF CONTENTS

TRANSLATOR'S FOREWORD

I am very pleased that Shudo Denmei's third English text has finally become available. His first text explains his approach to Meridian Therapy, and his second explains how he palpates and needles his favorite points. This text completes a series by offering a wealth of case studies. In these pages Shudo Denmei offers us clinical insights and wisdom gleaned from over half a century of practice. This is a rare and honest reflection of one man's lifelong quest to apply acupuncture and moxibustion to cure all manner of diseases—his own as well as those of his patients. Shudo Denmei demonstrates how an acupuncture practice can be a lifelong process of continuous learning and innovation.

One of the hallmarks of the Shudo style is self-treatment, and through ceaseless practice on himself, Shudo Denmei developed his signature needling technique, SRT or super-rotation technique. This discovery (although it could be a rediscovery of what ancient practitioners already knew) that a needle need not be inserted to be effective, came in modern times from practitioners of Meridian Therapy in Japan. In the case of Shudo Denmei, this is a hard-won conviction from using SRT over and over on himself and his patients. Along with his quest to make his acupuncture more effective, Shudo Denmei has made a parallel effort to make his acupuncture easier to receive for patients. I find it surprising how seldom we acupuncturists take "our own medicine." This could change once more acupuncturists learn about the patient-friendly Shudo style.

Even if you haven't had the opportunity, as I have, to observe Shudo Denmei in the clinic over the last twenty-five years, it is evident from reading his texts that his acupuncture treatments have shifted away from retaining needles (as recommended in his first book) to very superficial and non-retaining techniques. He doesn't justify or explain this change except to say that, "I keep working to make my acupuncture simpler and more effective." Even though he has become one of the most senior practitioners among all Japanese acupuncturists, Shudo Denmei continues to look for ways to improve his treatments. This is refreshing in a field where other, far less experienced, practitioners argue for their methods with smug certainty.

I have done my best to convey the unique voice of this spokesperson for Meridian Therapy as well as all traditional Japanese styles of acupuncture. In presenting his case histories, Shudo sensei used a narrative style in order to create a more personable and readable account of his clinical work.[1] Coming from the "prewar generation," his depth and breadth of knowledge in the field of acupuncture and everything Japanese posed not just some linguistic challenges, but cultural ones as well. If there are any errors or inconsistencies in the text, the fault is entirely mine.

What I appreciate most about my eminent teacher is his humor and disarming honesty. He intentionally included some cases to illustrate how his acupuncture isn't "almighty" and falls short of his own ideal. I am sure that I'm not the only one who appreciates his sharing of his mistakes and questions as much as he does his successes. And it is this attitude of questioning and continuously studying and seeking a better way that is the hallmark of what, over the years, has evolved into the Shudo style. Rather than adhering to classical concepts or fixed ideas about treatment, he has remained a student of clinical experience and invites us to have the courage to continually deepen our knowledge and skill.

Even with an honest and detailed account of clinical experiences as recounted in this text, there is still a wide gap between the author and reader. One cannot fully grasp Shudo style treatments without visiting his clinic or watching him give a treatment in a seminar. Fortunately, technology is catching up to fill the gap left by even a good text such as this one. An abundance of video footage has been made available on YouTube, although most of it is in Japanese without subtitles. You can watch the video of Shudo Denmei giving treatments in his clinic. Search for the video titled "Shudo Denmei Clinical Acupuncture Cases Vol. 1." There are also DVDs available of Shudo Denmei teaching. They can be ordered from najom.org as well as from lhasaoms.com.

Finally, I would like to express my gratitude to Dan Bensky and John O'Connor of Eastland Press who have tirelessly supported my efforts to make Shudo Denmei's remarkable work known in the West. I am glad to see that Shudo Denmei's spirit of selfless service is alive and well outside of our profession.

—Stephen Brown
Bainbridge Island, Washington

---

1. Note that some of these cases are from a time before Dr. Shudo was established in the practice of Meridian Therapy. Some lack consistency or are missing some information. These cases are primarily presented as a narrative to illustrate the progress of Dr. Shudo's practice and his approach to treatment.

PREFACE
TO ENGLISH LANGUAGE EDITION

For 15 years after I first opened my practice, I practiced the Sawada style which I had learned from my teacher. After that I started to adopt various other methods, and finally Meridian Therapy became the center of my practice. I get really good results and sometimes I wonder if this is due to my own ability. But the truth is that I am simply riding on a treatment system called Meridian Therapy. It is just that wonderful and one of the best treatment systems in the world. There are, however, some difficulties awaiting those who want to learn Meridian Therapy. I wrote *Introduction to Meridian Therapy* to share the tricks I learned to overcome these difficulties. So I simplified Meridian Therapy in my own way. It is a very convenient approach for clinical practice. Those who are dissatisfied with it can make it more complex. It is not as hard to make something complex as it is to simplify it. This text presents the outcome of how I developed and applied my approach. I listed all the conditions that I have treated without regard to the results. I wanted to show how my approach can be applied to any condition.

Recently, treating special effect points is popular among acupuncturists in Japan. The problem with special effect points is that there is a limit. There is no rule in how points are used together. Unless one treats with a focus on the meridians, there is danger of ending up at a dead end.

This text came into being with the help of the famous translator Stephen Brown, as well as the support of Dan Bensky and John O'Connor of Eastland Press. The good will of Tobe Shinichiro of Ido-no-Nippon, the Japanese publisher, was also indispensable. It is an honor and I am deeply grateful.

I tell my students that "heart is above knowledge and skill." Even if one has great knowledge and skill, an acupuncturist without "heart" cannot be called great. What do I mean by heart? Acupuncture and moxibustion are founded on the ideology of Daoism and Confucianism. These are great for upright conduct and providing treatment, but fall a bit short when it comes to concern for others. In this sense, Christianity and Buddhism have a stronger altruistic sensibility. The maxim from the Tendai sect of Buddhism, "Forget oneself and serve others," is, I believe, ideal. This maxim is my motto in life. With this philosophy, work that seems difficult is successfully completed and every day is fulfilling. So when I say "heart," I am talking about the spirit of selfless service. I hope that you work diligently at your acupuncture practice for the sake of your patients. If you do so, I am sure everything will work out well and you will enjoy success.

Occasionally people from America and Europe show up at my clinic. When I ask them where they learned about me, they tell me that they read *Introduction to Meridian Therapy.* I would be gratified if this text also served to create this kind of connection.

INTRODUCTION

HOW DO WE EXAMINE and treat our patients? Even if one is well trained, lack of experience and anxiety often make it hard to perform well. This is like athletes losing in the first rounds of Olympic competition even though they are top performers. This problem is even greater for acupuncturists with inadequate training and lack of experience. When I opened my practice, this was exactly my situation, so patients didn't get better, and I had few patients. This created a vicious cycle. How I overcame this obstacle and adjusted my trajectory to become successful is a story in itself. Sharing the haphazard course of my practice development may be of some help to those on this path.

My teacher, Miura Nagahiko (1897-1975), practiced his own style based on his own understanding of the Sawada style. He had amazing sensitivity in his fingers to detect and treat tender and hard points, and with his sharp mind he even applied Western medical concepts. This was a difficult approach for a clumsy guy with a slow brain like myself. So I studied other methods of diagnosis and treatment beside my teacher's and tried them out in my practice, and I kept whatever worked. This is a process that is still in progress. After fifty years, the way I practice has changed dramatically, but the desire to get my patients better as fast as I can remains unchanged.

I was attracted to Meridian Therapy, a system by which one can determine the treatment from the pulse. There was no teacher in my area, and I couldn't often travel to Tokyo for instruction, so mostly I had to study this on my own.

In contrast, Ryodoraku, a system using a machine to measure electric resistance on the skin, could tell you the condition of the body and there was someone right in Ohita where I live who was willing to teach me. I used the Neurometer for one year but couldn't get the hang of it.

The pulse diagnosis system of Hashimoto Masa, described in serial form in the *Journal of Japanese Acupuncture and Moxibustion* around that time, was similar to that of Meridian Therapy. It was also quite simple, so I practiced it quite a bit, but this too didn't work out. This was due to my misfortune of only being able to study on my own.

The auricular acupuncture of Paul Nogier was also introduced in the *Journal of Japanese Acupuncture* around 1958 by Nagatomo Tsugio. He even came to Ohita to teach this system, and I received some instruction from Ohta Rinsai in Kumamoto who had learned the system. It is one microsystem in which the part reflects the whole. It worked quite well, and I still often use it today.

The Fukaya moxibustion method, developed by Fukaya Isaburo (1900-1974), was another moxibustion method I learned that was based on different principles than Sawada style moxibustion, which I had learned from my teacher. It has great value and I use this system daily.

I also learned micropuncture, or blood-letting, but it takes time to bleed vascular spiders, and there are issues in terms of effect and hygiene. Now I only use it to bleed a few drops from LI-1 in cases of tonsillitis.

Needle-head moxibustion, called *kyutoshin* in Japan, is another method I tried out, but I abandoned it because it requires too much time and attention.

In the beginning I wasn't able to understand Meridian Therapy by studying it on my own. I began to get some idea of it at the Kyushu (Southern Island) Meridian Therapy Seminar in the mid-1960s taught by Dr. Ohta, and this imprecise understanding has continued to this day. At first, I adopted Okabe Sodo's approach of retaining needles. I transitioned gradually to using this approach so that my patients wouldn't notice, and it seems that most of them never did. Regular patients started to comment that my treatments were having a better effect. Over a period of many years I transitioned from retaining needles to simple insertion (non-retaining). Since the early part of this century my treatment system primarily consists of super-rotation technique, or SRT, with insertion at a few key points, and three to five needles retained in the abdomen or back associated points. This is my solution to the question of how to treat many patients by myself quickly and effectively. In this way, my style today has settled into Meridian Therapy as my primary approach, with Sawada style moxibustion, auricular acupuncture, and the Fukaya moxibustion method thrown into the mix.

Summary

Treatment methods that are part of the Shudo style: Meridian Therapy, Fukaya moxibustion method, and auricular acupuncture.

One of the policies of the local study group, which is called *Gensai Juku* (*'Gensai'* is another reading of my name and *'juku'* means study group), that I began with colleagues thirty years ago, is to study both Eastern and Western medicine without bias. After I began studying Meridian Therapy, I started to read the classics. In the beginning, I found it more difficult than English. In addition, due perhaps to the lack of essence and purpose, I can't continue for long. I hit the wall after a while. It's an unfortunate character flaw, but I have another character trait that saved me: perseverance.

Sometime after hitting the wall, I would go back and give it another try. As long as I kept this up, I wouldn't stop completely. I gradually became able to read the Chinese without Japanese notations. Yet the classics of acupuncture are vast in number, and I haven't read everything, or even given a cursory review of some important books. I have read *Basic Questions (Su wen)* and *Vital Axis (Ling shu)*, *Classic of Difficulties (Nan jing)*, and *Compilation of Acupuncture and Moxibustion (Zhen jiu jia yi jing)* over and over again. I take what I understand and test it clinically and apply what I can. This is a very difficult undertaking, but it will probably continue until I die. This is really challenging, but it is also my joy.

In chapter 10 of *Vital Axis*, in the section about disease of the arm greater yin Lung meridian, there is a part that is normally thought in Japan to say, "Urine is frequent with yawning." This is interpreted in many commentaries in Japan to mean urinary frequency and yawning. Somehow this didn't make sense to me. When I asked Kodera Toshiko, who is well read in the medical classics, about this, she told me that yawning helped the function of the Lungs. This made some sense but it still didn't really fit in my mind.

So I went in search of the source of this interpretation and finally found it in Okamoto Ippo's interpretation of the medical classics. Since it was the view of a venerable classical scholar from the Edo period, it seems that scholars of subsequent times just went along with it. When you look up the character that is translated as 'yawning' in this passage, 欠 *jie*, in a dictionary of Chinese characters, you find a few different meanings: yawning of course, but also 'open' or 'lacking.' So one may suggest the above passage could be saying "urination is frequent and insufficient." This is the interpretation that makes sense clinically. The sense of incomplete urination is a symptom that appears with Lung deficiency, and needling LU-9 makes urination more complete.

I found a commentary in an eleventh-century Chinese text, *Illustrated Classic of Acupuncture and Moxibustion Holes on the Bronze Man*, on this same passage stating, "[The character] 數 *shu* means frequency; 欠 *jie* means scanty. So it is saying urination is frequent but scanty." So my interpretation of frequent but insufficient was validated by this text as well as in my own experience.

On the other hand, when one becomes erudite in the classics of medicine, there is a tendency to make light of modern medicine, and this is a problem. We must apply the amazing knowledge of modern medicine for the benefit of our patients. I learned manual orthopedic tests at clinical skills seminars of the Japanese Acupuncture Association. These tests are very useful, and I make use of them every day. There are things that cannot be learned from just the classics. What causes the symptom of claudication? Is the back pain caused by a disc herniation or spinal stenosis? Or could it be caused by occlusive arteriosclerosis? You are far more likely to find the right answers to such questions with orthopedic tests.

I had a recent case, a woman over 80 who came in for low back pain. I suspected occlusive arteriosclerosis, so I needed to refer her to a vascular specialist. It just so happened that she had received a coronary stent at a large local hospital. So I referred her back to this hospital. It is tricky writing the referral letter to the doctor. I would like to see the younger generation of acupuncturists learn how to communicate better with doctors. Anyway, I wrote, "I can't feel the pulse in the artery of the right lower limb, so please examine and treat." I did not mention the symptoms or which artery exactly.

I received a reply soon thereafter. "As you have pointed out, it seems to be a case of occlusive arteriosclerosis of the right lower limb. But this patient has a chronic kidney dysfunction, and aggressive treatments using contrast agents cannot be recommended. I have decided to use drug therapy for the time being. I will decide the course of treatment based on the outcomes." So this patient couldn't simply be treated with balloon dilation therapy. Whether the patient is to be treated at the hospital or in conjunction with acu-moxa, you will be able to provide a better treatment if you know about Western medical treatments.

This case did not involve orthopedic tests, but I had another recent patient, a woman in her 70s with low back pain. Her movements seemed a bit slow. Her speech was also a bit hesitant. There was no cogwheel motion in movements of her wrist and elbow joints, but there seemed to be some stiffness. There were no tremors in the fingers. I asked in a whisper close to her ear, "Are you sure you don't have Parkinson's?" She replied, "Wow, how did you know? My husband told me I shouldn't tell you about that." This made her trust me completely. I explained to her that acu-moxa treatments can prevent the progression of Parkinson's symptoms. If things go well, they may even reduce them a little. This brought a change to her expression.

Summary | Don't be biased; learn from both Eastern and Western medicine.

My Clinical Practice from Diagnosis to Treatment

In our treatments, we have to face each patient, one on one. It is a moment of truth. Depending on the outcome, we either gain their trust or lose it. This can be a terrifying moment. We really must focus our heart and mind for best results. I would like to explain the process of how I examine and treat my patients.

Intake 1: Medical history and symptoms chart

The moment a patient walks into my clinic the examination (looking exam) has already started. We greet each other for the first time and in that moment we each make some judgments. We note each other's appearance, dress, voice, movements, and facial expression.

For first office calls, patients have filled out their medical history and symptoms chart. The key question is, "What is your problem now?" My chart has 44 items starting with headache. Patients circle the ones they have. This gives me a general idea, but sometimes they just circle "low back" or "knee" and give no details. Others don't even bother to circle a symptom. They either don't like to write or would rather explain about it in person. When that's the case I usually ask a series of questions, as follows:

> "How long have you had this?"
> "Is this the first incident of this?"
> "What movements increase the pain?"
> "Does the pain get worse at night?"
> "Is there pain without movement?" (spontaneous pain)
> "Is there any numbness?"
> "Have you been examined by a doctor for this? If so, what was the diagnosis?"

If it seems warranted, I ask about their medical history in greater detail.

> "Have you had any surgery?"
> "What diseases are you being treated for by a doctor now? What drugs are you on?"
> "Do you have diabetes? Do you know your blood sugar count?"

In contrast to patients who don't write down much, there are those who fill in every space in great detail. I suspect such patients have a psychosomatic condition.

Intake 2: Orthopedic tests: The points to use for symptomatic treatment

I get the general picture from questioning and the history and symptoms chart. When it is a musculoskeletal disorder, I perform orthopedic tests. The results will provide more information about the treatment method and prognosis. The points to use for symptomatic treatment come to mind as I do the tests. There are many good texts on how to do manual orthopedic tests. You must practice them repeatedly to make them routine. If you are not used to doing them, you can't do them well when you need to. This is true for needle insertion as well. It is important to get together with colleagues and practice needling techniques on each other to get good feedback.

Summary | Perform orthopedic tests for musculoskeletal disorders.

Intake 3: The Four Examinations

After the orthopedic tests I continue to examine and treat the patient, but I want to step back here and explain how I go about the Four Examinations in my practice. I must warn you that this is my own approach and does not necessarily represent the standard practice. There are many methods of examination in East Asian medicine, but the Four Examinations are the cornerstones. They are looking, listening, questioning, and palpating. I will start again with the looking exam.

LOOKING

This refers to visual observation, but there is a slight difference. First, I observe the patient as a whole. How do they move? Is it quick or slow? Do they seem to have spirit? Spirit refers to the strength to live; it is also called Stomach qi. One look and you can tell something is wrong, the person doesn't have long to go. This is not easy to tell without experience, but it is very important. In time you will learn to recognize this.

Next I look at the complexion. The original meaning of the looking examination was to discriminate the five colors or complexions. They are green, red, yellow, white, and black. So we try to discern the color of the face. If the complexion is bluish for example, that would mean it is a disease of the Liver (organ or meridian). Reddish would be the Heart. Yellowish would be the Spleen. Pale would be the Lung. Blackish would be the Kidney.

In real practice, however, you rarely see a bluish face. A slight blue/greenish hue is enough. The most important thing is whether the complexion has luster. If the greenish complexion has luster, the patient is fine; this is true for the other colors as well. So look for whether there is a healthy shine under the skin.

In addition, the color and luster of certain parts of the face are examined (Fig. Intro-1). On the midline between the eyebrows is the Liver area. Two finger-widths above that is the Heart area. The lowest part of the bridge of the nose, just below the Liver area, is the Lung area. The end of the nose is the Spleen area. The center of the jaw is the Kidney area. When the skin in any of these areas is dark or pale, it means there is a problem in the corresponding organ or meridian. For example, if there is a different color in the center of the forehead, there is a Heart imbalance.

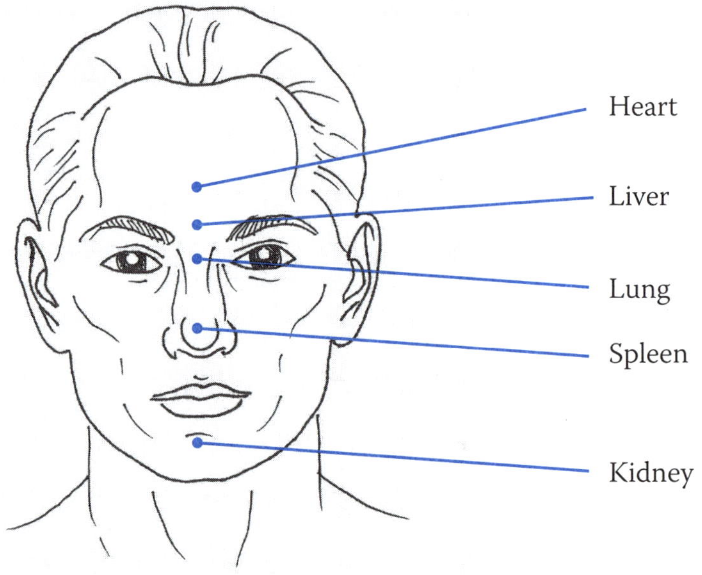

Fig. Intro-1 Organ correspondences on the face

Even if you are unable to find any detailed difference like this, look for complexions that are ashen, or dull eyes without spirit. The character for 'looking' (望 *bō/wàng)* in the looking examination means to gaze from a distance, so it is important to watch from a slight distance.

It is also said that thin and small ears indicate weak Kidneys. Those with thick and large earlobes have strong Kidneys. Those with narrow eyes have a weak Liver. Those with thin noses have weak Lungs. Those with thin lips have a weak Spleen. These features are hereditary and there's nothing that can be done about it, but you can make note of congenitally weak organs.

Those with vertical creases between their eyebrows, narrowed eyes, few words, and tendency to look down have depression. If they continue treatment, the creases disappear and their eyes open wider. They begin to speak more. Their face starts to brighten. Tracking changes in expression is also part of the looking examination.

Summary | Key points in looking examination: Does the complexion have luster? Are the eyes bright?

LISTENING & SMELLING

This is determining which of the five organs are involved in the voice, manner of speech, and odor of the patient. In practice this is difficult. One is supposed to discriminate the traditional five notes in this examination. There are also the five voices: the low groaning voice for the Kidneys, a higher shouting voice for the Liver, a sonorous singing voice for the Spleen, a sighing voice as if about to cry for the Lung. The important thing, regardless of the tone, is that the voice is clear and strong. Be careful about patients with a tinny voice, or speech that is weak or unclear even with effort. They are certain to have a serious problem. Question them in detail and refer them for a medical examination if you have trouble getting clear information.

Judging the patient's mouth and body odor is also part of the listening examination. When patients have bad breath, I examine their tongue. Most often they have a tongue coating. A white coating is fine, but not a yellow or brown one. The thicker the coating, the more serious the problem in the Spleen and Stomach. Those with gum disease also have bad breath. Often a patient is unaware of their own bad breath. Many young people have bad breath too. One might hesitate to bring this up even to family members, but it is no use to beat around the bush. In recent medical opinion, periodontal disease can lead to diabetes and arteriosclerosis. So explain this to the patient and suggest dental treatment and encourage proper dental hygiene. It's a good idea to get dental calculus removed three or four times a year. This will improve treatment results, in contrast to receiving just acu-moxa treatments. It is important to realize that we will be treating more internal organ disorders and lifestyle diseases in the future, so we must be ready to look at the big picture.

Some patients have strong body odor. The classics say that those with a Liver problem smell rancid, those with a Heart problem smell scorched, those with a Spleen problem smell fragrant, those with a Lung problem smell fishy, and those with a Kidney problem smell putrid. This is worth keeping in mind.

Summary | Key points in listening examination: Be careful about patients with a thin voice. Refer those with periodontal disease to a dentist.

QUESTIONING

The purpose of the questioning examination is to determine which yin organ is out of balance. What do we question the patients about? In the classics, questions about taste preferences are important. Those who crave sweet things and those who can't stand sweet things have a Spleen imbalance. Preference for sour foods is associated with a Liver imbalance. Preference for salty foods is associated with a Kidney imbalance. Preference for hot or spicy foods is associated with a Lung imbalance. Preference for bitter foods is associated with a Heart imbalance. In my experience these associations have some merit. We must eat a variety of foods with all of these five tastes. It is abnormal to suddenly crave just one flavor.

The additional questions needed are about likely symptoms. Each organ and meridian has its own symptomatology. This is based on chapter 10 of *Vital Axis.*[1] For example, when you think the patient has Liver deficiency, ask if they have low back pain, knee pain, headache, dizziness, irritability, and vision problems. If any of these symptoms exist, that means your guess is right and the accuracy of your diagnosis increases. In my practice these days I find out about diabetes by inquiring about the blood sugar and the HbA1c levels. Of course, you must not forget the essential questions such as urination, bowel movements, and sleep. Constipation is quite common.

Summary | Key points in questioning: Ask about taste preferences. Inquire about symptoms associated with affected organs and meridians.

PALPATION

Finally, I come to palpation, in which the body is examined. Examining the body thoroughly is one of the key features of Japanese styles of acupuncture. In recent years, styles of inserting needles without touching the skin have become popular, especially outside of Japan, but this is not in alignment with the original intention and practice of acupuncture. I don't recommend it.

1. For detailed symptomatology of each organ and meridian, see Chapter 4 of my text, *Introduction to Meridian Therapy.*

There are many types of palpation, but let me begin with abdominal palpation. Our hands must be warm and one hand should be slightly cupped before placing it gently over the navel. Gently stroke above and below, right and left, of the navel. Then stroke the subclavicular areas around LU-1. Look for deficient areas. The Spleen area is halfway between the xiphoid process and the navel. The Kidney area is below the navel. The Liver area is to the left of the navel. The Lung areas are the subclavicular areas around LU-1.

Next, press around the navel, above and below, right and left. If there is a pulsation when pressing over the navel gently, it is a Spleen imbalance. If a pulsation is found to the left of the navel, it is a Liver imbalance. If it is to the right of the navel, it is a Lung imbalance. If it is below the navel, it is a Kidney imbalance. Abdominal palpation is helpful especially when pulse diagnosis does not yield clear information. These two methods of abdominal palpation may be enough for a beginner.

I palpate a bit deeper than the surface in my practice. Pinching diagnosis is a good way to find abnormalities in the deeper level. I pinch the skin over points on the abdomen to look for tender or abnormal points. I pinch with my thumb and index finger and add a slight twist. An abnormal point will feel a bit thicker and swollen. The tenderness is unpleasant. I find most abnormalities from pinching in the upper abdomen (above the navel). Remember to be careful because strong pinching is painful, and those with allergic skin conditions may get subcutaneous bleeding. Keep it gentle.

Next, I press gently to look for indurations (hard points). I find nodules between 5mm and 1cm in size. Usually they are also tender. They are easy to find once you have some experience, and you can track changes in them with treatment. It does, however, take some time before one becomes proficient in locating them. Accurately locating points is important on every part of the body, and it just takes practice and more practice. This is the fate of anyone who wants to become a professional. The more the effort, the greater the reward of expertise.

Points with pinching abnormalities or indurations indicate some abnormality in underlying organs. I will go over this again in Chapter 10 (digestive disorders), but the simple correspondence is as follows:

CV-14	→	Heart
CV-12	→	Stomach
Left ST-21	→	Pancreas
Right ST-24	→	Duodenum
Left ST-19	→	Stomach
Right ST-19	→	Gallbladder
Right LR-14	→	Liver

These correspondences are a simplification, of course, but they have clinical utility. I suggest you study the connection of these points to underlying organs and use them in your practice. In some cases, I press a bit harder than usual. Tenderness or hardness serves as reference when I suspect there is pathology in internal organs. For example, when I suspect gallbladder disease, I stand to the right of the patient and press right ST-19 diagonally (laterally) upward with the right middle finger. If there is a problem, the point will feel different from the surrounding area, and it is often tender or indurated.

Summary

Key points in abdominal palpation: Palpate the surface of the abdomen to find imbalances in the five yin organs. Detect abnormality in underlying organs by pressing specific points.

—Pulse Palpation

Pulse diagnosis is the principal palpation technique in Meridian Therapy, but sometimes it is difficult even when you have experience. I have sought instruction over the years and learned through repeated trial and error. For details on pulse diagnosis technique I would refer you to my text, *Introduction to Meridian Therapy*. I will limit myself to a brief explanation here.

Place your fingers on the three positions (distal, middle, and proximal) on both sides. Press the fingers over the pulse on the surface (light pressure) and deeper (heavy pressure) to find the level at which the pulse is the strongest. This may seem simple, but it takes some experience to find the middle level. This is the level at which I check the quality of the pulse. The ideal quality at the middle level is smooth, soft, and large with some resilience. This is known as a pulse with "good Stomach qi." It means the function of the digestive system is good and this ideal pulse is found in healthy athletes and children. In elderly people like myself, the pulse is harder. Taking the pulses of younger people, I often feel how enviably soft theirs are. Having said that, the pulse must not be too soft, lack resilience, or collapse under pressure.

After examining the pulse at the middle level, relax the pressure and then press deeper to the deepest level. Find the weakest position at the bottom of the pulse. It takes some experience to find the deficient position, but keep practicing until you get it. Pay special attention to the positions at the deep and superficial level that are different from others at the same level. The position that is strong at the superficial level and weak at the deep level is often related to the primary pattern. For example, when the Gallbladder position is strong and the Liver position is weak, it is Liver deficiency.

Determine the pattern of imbalance (證 *shō/zhèng)* based on the pulse, and then recheck the pulse after some treatment, or at the end of treatment. This is called rechecking the pulse. The aim of treatment is to get the pulse closer to the ideal pulse with good Stomach qi. The classics say that it cannot be adequately described. So the pulse feels so good it's beyond description. In any case, there is some mistake when the pulse becomes faster or harder with treatment.

Summary | Key point in pulse diagnosis: Excess at superficial level and deficient at the deep level in the same position often determines the pattern.

—Meridian Palpation

Palpation along the distal course of the meridian is useful for confirming the diagnosis and finding the best points to treat. For a Spleen deficiency patient, Spleen meridian points such as SP-2 (tonification point) and SP-3 (source point) tend to be depressed. With some practice you will get a feel for which points are good for treatment and which ones aren't.

While it isn't strictly speaking meridian palpation, it is important to check the front alarm points associated with the diagnosis. It is also important at times to palpate the affected joint to find which meridians are involved. As you continue treatment over time, it will aid in monitoring changes and determining which meridians need more work.

INTEGRATING THE FOUR EXAMINATIONS

Integration of the Four Examinations means putting all the different findings from the different examinations together to determine the pattern. This serves to prevent the danger of jumping to conclusions from one notable finding. If one is not careful, there is a tendency to identify the pattern just from the pulse. Although the pulse is central to Meridian Therapy, it is best to keep the big picture in view.

If I think a patient has Spleen deficiency from looking, listening, and palpation, I ask the patient some questions to find out if he has any Spleen deficiency symptoms. "Does food taste good? Do you eat on schedule even though you are not hungry? Otherwise does your body feel heavy, do you have difficulty sleeping, bad moods, and pain or heat in a joint? Do you crave sweets, and do you have stomach or abdominal pain?" So I ask about symptoms of both the Spleen and Stomach. When the patient doesn't have any of these symptoms and has low back pain or coughing instead, it conflicts with what you have found. This means that you must start over and reconsider your diagnosis. I am relieved when things match up with the integration of the Four Examinations. It is important to determine the pattern, but this is not always easy. It takes a great deal of practice.

Summary | Put together all the information from the Four Examinations to determine the diagnosis.

Treatment

Let's say that the primary pattern has been determined to be Spleen deficiency. We start the treatment by palpating the five-phase points. Check for depressions at SP-2, SP-3, and SP-9 on both sides. Also check for indurations at SP-4 and SP-8. I palpate points with the tip of my middle finger with the index and ring fingers together behind it. You can stroke the point upward (following the course of the meridian) or you can stroke back and forth. When there is a depressed point, it is one that should be tonified. Conversely, when the skin is thick and firm, that point is not used.

In any case, SP-3 can be selected as the basic tonification point. Stroke it gently. Points on the hands and feet, including most of the five-phase points, are sensitive and unskillful insertion can be painful. For tonification, one must be able to insert the needle painlessly. I routinely use super-rotation technique. I start with SP-3 on the left side and take a little more time. I rotate the needle for about 20 seconds. If I feel the arrival of qi, I remove the needle right after that. If I don't feel anything, I still remove the needle after 20 seconds.

Then I recheck the pulse. If the pulse has changed, and the weak pulse becomes stronger, or the pulse becomes more full or floating overall, it means the tonification of SP-3 has had an effect. If the pulse becomes amazingly balanced and even, the treatment of right SP-3 and PC-7 on both sides can be done in only a few seconds each. When the first needle does not bring any change, tonify the next point with more careful attention. Also check the abdomen. If the differences felt earlier change with the above treatment, that means the root treatment was a success.

Of course, the ability to detect changes in the pulse and abdomen after tonifying a few points indicates an advanced level of skill. It is not something one can accomplish without practice. After tonifying four root treatment points, one can disperse LR-1 and SP-1, as done by Yanagiya Sorei (1906-1959: the founder of the Meridian Therapy movement). This is fine, although it is not something I do. I generally recheck the pulse for excesses at the yang level, and do some dispersion if there are any excessive yang meridians. Regardless of excess in the yang, I needle CV-12, left ST-21, and CV-6 on the abdomen. In cases of reflux syndrome, I might needle CV-14 or CV-17 if there is a reaction.

Next, I apply five rice-grain-size cones of direct moxa on CV-12 and ST-36. As long as the cones are small—between sesame and rice-grain size—patients are able to bear the heat. And sometimes they say it even feels good. Larger cones are too painful. When it's too hot, if you let the cones burn down only to about 80%, then patients will say that the heat feels good. No matter how effective direct moxibustion may be, it is of no use if patients don't like it and stop coming. So mild heat is enough.

Next, the patient lies face down. I check for reactions and differences over the Governing vessel and the back associated points, but beginners can't do this quickly. So, in cases of Spleen deficiency, look for depressions at BL-14, BL-15, and BL-20. Treat the deficient points either by simple insertion or retained needle. Check for tension in the neck and shoulders and tenderness on the upper Governing vessel points. If there is any reactive point, needle it lightly. Needling too deeply or too intensely will affect their sleep, so be sure to be gentle.

Let's say this patient's primary complaint is low back pain. I will examine the condition of the back in detail. If it is a myofascial back strain, I needle the Iliac point (Fig.

Intro-2), BL-27, or BL-52. When I find an obvious induration, things are simple, but when it's not so clear I ask the patient. I have him move his waist around and point to the most painful spot. It is usually around BL-52 or lower, around BL-27. Ask with your hands on the patient's back. Usually they point to the lower end. Palpate the Iliac point carefully. I press with my right middle finger with a small circular motion downward toward the foot. Find an induration, and then try needling right into that point.

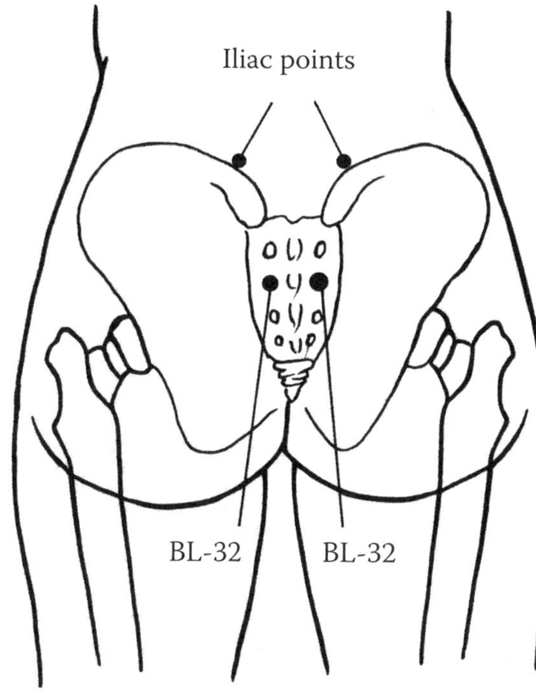

Fig. Intro-2 Iliac points

I start out using SRT with slightly faster rotations. I do this for about 20 seconds and then ask the patient to move his waist again. If the pain is better, the effect is good. If there is no change in the pain, or if the patient is used to acupuncture, I insert the needle. I start the needle the same way as in SRT, without tapping the needle in. I just rotate the needle in, slowly and carefully. I use a 30mm, 02 gauge (0.12mm) needle.

I usually run into a hard place at about 5mm deep when I insert slowly while rotating. I stop inserting the needle further and continue just rotating. It starts to feel pretty good. Here I am referring to *my* sensation. Sometimes the patient says "that's it!" And sometimes the patient feels nothing. The sensation felt by the practitioner is called "the arrival of qi." The brain is what registers the arrival of qi, so if the patient is unable to feel anything, it is because the ability to register stimulation is diminished. If I reinsert a needle again in the same point, patients always say that they feel it the second time. So the arrival of qi is something felt first by the practitioner; the patient doesn't have to feel anything. When the qi arrives, usually the pain has eased when the patient moves his waist.

Sometimes I can't find an induration at the Iliac point. In these cases I needle the most depressed and deficient point. The arrival of qi is hard to feel in such cases. It isn't such a clear response. It feels like something changes but it's very subtle.

After treating the Iliac points, I look for reactions in other points and apply SRT. If it's a point on the yang meridian, I disperse by not closing the point after removing the needle. I spend only a second or two on each point. Points palpated for the above low back pain case would include BL-20, BL-27, BL-40, BL-58, BL-59, and the Gluteal point (Fig. Intro-3). I would conclude the treatment with five cones of direct moxa on the Gluteal point and BL-59. When the back pain is severe, I would apply 10 cones on the Gluteal point. If the pain has diminished with movement, that is good. It is fine if the pain is not all gone. It will go away in time. I recheck the pulse and conclude the treatment.

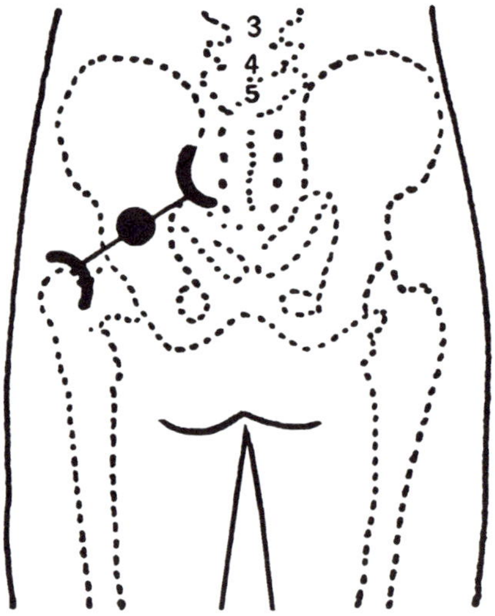

Fig. Intro-3 Gluteal point

Summary

- I use SRT (super-rotation technique) on most points.
- SRT for 20 seconds on key points, 1-2 seconds on other points.
- Feel for the arrival of qi on key points.

Prognosis and Treatment Frequency

In cases of paralysis when there is a limited window during which recovery is possible, I explain this to the patient and have them come in as often as possible, even every day. Acute pain also should be treated every day until it begins to ease. With acute pain, I ask patients to refrain from drinking alcohol and taking baths. Pain does diminish with a bath, but later it becomes even worse.

In chronic cases, treatment once a week is best. If there are reasons that weekly treatment is difficult, I see them once every other week or once a month, but patients must make an extra effort, such as doing moxibustion at home. When I know about how long it takes to recover from a condition, I inform the patient. For example, most cases of vertigo resolve in three to five treatments. Benign positional vertigo takes longer, from one to three months. Myofascial back pain usually resolves with several treatments. If there is disk herniation, it takes three months. I don't tell patients when to come for treatment. When they ask me when they should come, I suggest dates and times of open appointments. In either case, I don't compel patients to come on my schedule. There are many patients who want treatment but can't come for various reasons. Not everyone has the means. I had one senior colleague who used to say, "Make them come every day for three months. In three months most patients get better. We don't have to worry about the financial status of patients." But I wonder...

Summary | Treat once a day for acute conditions, once a week for chronic conditions. Don't push your treatment regimen on your patients.

About Super-Rotation Technique (SRT)

Here I would like to explain about by needling technique, super-rotation technique or SRT. It was briefly described in Chapter 3 of my previous text, *Finding Effective Acupuncture Points,* under the name "super-superficial insertion." I changed the name to describe its most distinctive feature: minute and rapid rotations of the needle. Also, since the needle is never inserted more than half a millimeter, "technique" is a more appropriate term.

Many needling techniques have been developed in the long history of acupuncture. It may be due to my lack of knowledge, but I have never heard of another technique resembling SRT. It is defined by very superficial needling with high-speed rotations. This is the primary technique I use in my practice today. SRT is starting to become known in the United States but is still not that well known in Japan. This technique did not come from any theoretical consideration. It emerged naturally from my practice from my desire to improve results.

Let me list the effects of SRT.

1. When you receive SRT, your mood lifts. Your spirit becomes bright. So your expression becomes cheerful, you look younger, and women look more beautiful.

2. SRT is effective for pain. The painful places can be treated directly without any danger of aggravation.

3. Fatigue diminishes right away. The conclusion of the Labor and Welfare Department of Japan is that there is no effective treatment for fatigue, but SRT brings immediate relief from fatigue.

❹ SRT on hard points sometimes softens it. Since there is little needle sensation, patients who dislike it, like children, prefer SRT.

❺ Elderly patients usually have many symptoms, but treating many points with SRT does not cause fatigue from over-treatment.

❻ The practitioner giving SRT does not get tired. I am over 80 years old, but I believe one of the reasons I can still maintain a full-time practice is because of self-administering brief SRT treatments a few times daily.

So, I recommend that you try SRT instead of inserting needles and see how it works for yourself.

How to perform SRT

When you are using a needle with a tube, place the needle and tube on the point. The needle tip should just come in contact with the skin. You may touch the head of the needle protruding from the tube, but you must not hit it. Even if you tap it lightly, it can go in a few millimeters, so do not apply any force.

After the needle tip has firmly (and painlessly) contacted the skin, remove the tube as you hold the needle securely in place with the thumb and index finger of your left (or non-dominant) hand. Hold the needle handle between the thumb and index finger of your right (or dominant) hand. Keep the index finger fixed as you move the thumb back and forth across it to make small rotations. (Please see the YouTube video: https://www.youtube.com/watch?v=LLEU4eqde6g.)

These "rotations" are very minute, even 90 degrees is too much. It doesn't feel good. Aim for a rotation of about 20 degrees. The speed of the back-and-forth movement should be as quick as possible. In the beginning, aim for about five times a second. With some practice, you will be able to increase it to about eight times a second. When the rotations are very minute, it looks like the thumb is not moving—just vibrating.

As you continue to rotate the needle, it becomes a little heavy, or harder to rotate. This is the arrival of qi, but it's not the same as that felt when the needle is inserted as mentioned earlier. It is very subtle. For beginners, it is difficult to feel. Once the arrival of qi is felt, the needle can be removed. For tonification, the point is closed or pressed after removing the needle. For dispersion, the point is not closed or touched after removal. I continue applying SRT on the point for 20 seconds on the most important root treatment point, and also on one most important local point. For all other points, 2-3 seconds is enough for me; each practitioner can decide this for themself.

SRT is easiest to apply with the needle vertical to the skin, but, when you are treating tonification points, it is even better to angle the needle 45 to 30 degrees with the flow of the meridian. Often if you let go of the needle after applying SRT, it has been inserted very slightly without trying. If you want to retain the needle that way, take the handle of the needle and gently lay it against the skin.

Needles to use for SRT

Any needle that you like should work, but I find the longer needles over 40mm hard to use. It is difficult to rotate the needle rapidly. I find 30mm needles the easiest to use. The needle thickness is between Japanese 02 and 1 gauge (0.12-0.16mm). I use stainless steel needles in my practice, but silver may have a softer feel.

When to use SRT

In general, I perform the root treatment with SRT. Nowadays I also use SRT most of the time for branch or symptomatic treatments. I insert the needle in 3-5 local points with indurations. Balance in treatment, or proper emphasis of insertion (light to heavy), can be obtained in this way. This applies to life in general. Strong emphasis on everything does not work very well. Superficial needling relaxes the body. Adding a few inserted points into the mix puts appropriate tension into the system for balance.

Summary

Super-rotation technique (SRT) is defined by superficial needling with high-speed rotation. SRT is effective for fatigue and pain. Use inserted needles here and there for balance.

Secrets to Success

An acupuncturist must be healthy to be effective. If our health is delicate, we must take steps to improve it. We must be sure not to accumulate worries or stress. We must cultivate a harmonious relationship with our partner and good relationships in our practice. Even placing just one needle, if there is something that worries us, we can't insert the needle to good effect. We need to be cheery and even a bit hyper. Of course, we don't want to be manic, but being depressed is no good either. We must use acupuncture to keep our five organs and spirits in balance. This is why I recommend self-treatment every morning.

My secrets to success are as follows:

- Love your work.
- Love your partner.
- Love the place you live.

This is known as the "principle of the three loves." It dispels unhappiness.

So, I cultivate optimal health, and my attitude in my work is to "forget oneself and serve others." This principle of putting others first resolves all problems.

Summary

The secret to success is the "principle of the three loves." Cultivate optimal health yourself; then forget about yourself and serve others.

CHAPTER 1

Diseases of the Cranium and Face

1. Headache overview

Sometimes a distant forgotten memory is suddenly revived. It gets triggered in me by the word "headache." I experienced sinister headaches in my youth. When my headaches got bad, I could not even read books, which was my favorite thing. I would darken my room and just sit still. I would have my mother push on the crown of my head. It was probably around GV-20 to GV-22.

Once I began practicing acupuncture, I realized that it had a wonderful effect on headaches and heaviness of the head. In Western medicine, anti-inflammatory and analgesic medications are administered and sometimes, if the headache is really severe, triptans. I don't have any experience with these drugs, but I hear that even if the pain stops, it doesn't feel so good. I have written before about the time I had a headache from a hangover and needled LR-1, and *the pain just subsided like water draining out*. The experience of pain going out like the tide with nothing left behind is hard to replicate.

The treatment of headaches overlaps quite a bit with treatment of vertigo, so please also refer to that section in Chapter 14. The point to keep in mind about treating headaches is that in some cases Western medicine is far more effective and there is no reason to continue attempting to cure it with acupuncture. So it is best to refer unresponsive cases to a neurologist or specialist for a medical diagnosis.

In the classics, it says true headaches (真頭痛 *zhēn tóu tòng)* cannot be cured and that reversal headaches (厥頭痛 *jué tóu tòng*) can be cured. True headaches may refer to headaches from lesions like brain tumors or subarachnoid hemorrhages. In the *Classic of Difficulties* (ch. 60) it says that reversal headaches are caused by the wind-cold pathogen stagnating in yang meridians of the arm, and further that the pathogen enters the brain in true headaches. This may be so, but it's hard to verify. The point is to confirm whether it is a headache that can be treated with acupuncture, but this is important even from the perspective of modern medicine. I will list the varieties of headaches I have treated in my career.

1.1 Headaches from neck and shoulder tension (tension headaches)

This type of headache is associated with strong tension in the muscles of the neck and shoulder, commonly known as *katakori* in Japan. In Western medicine they are called tension headaches. Acupuncture and moxibustion are indicated for headaches that come from neck and shoulder tension. It is ideal when the exact focus of tension can be pin pointed, but there are times when it cannot. Many such patients complain of tension and pain in the occipital region. Sometimes there is nausea, but they rarely vomit. This is what distinguishes it from migraines, because migraine patients often vomit. The main points to palpate for tension of the trapezius muscle are GB-21, BL-10, and Upper BL-10 (Fig. 1-1) and BL-43. For tension in the scalene muscles, palpate ST-12 or the tight point above it in the scalenes (Scalene point). For tension in the SCM muscles, palpate Yanagiya's GB-20 (Fig. 1-2) and TB-16. Otherwise I choose among BL-2, GV-22, GB-5, and the auricular vertigo point (Fig. 1-3). As for the root treatment, most cases have Liver deficiency. Pay attention to dispersion of the Gallbladder meridian. For more detail, refer to the section on neck and shoulder tension in Chapter 3 (p. 87).

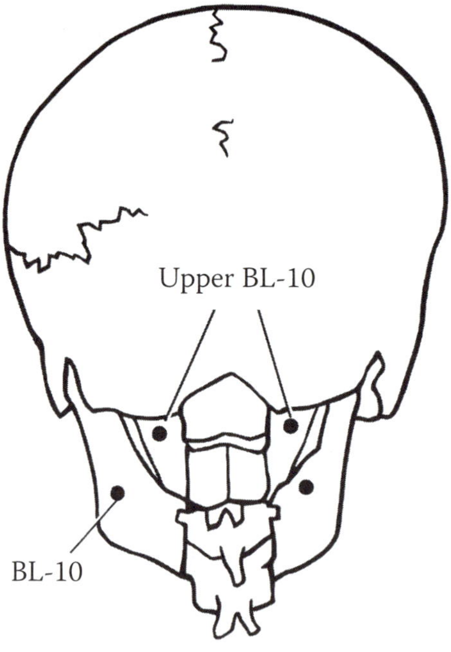

Fig. 1-1 Upper BL-10

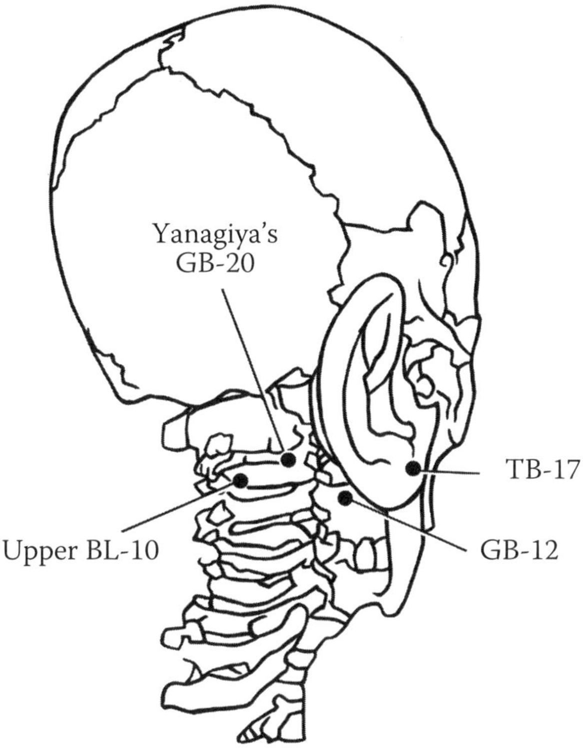

Fig. 1-2 Yanagiya's GB-20

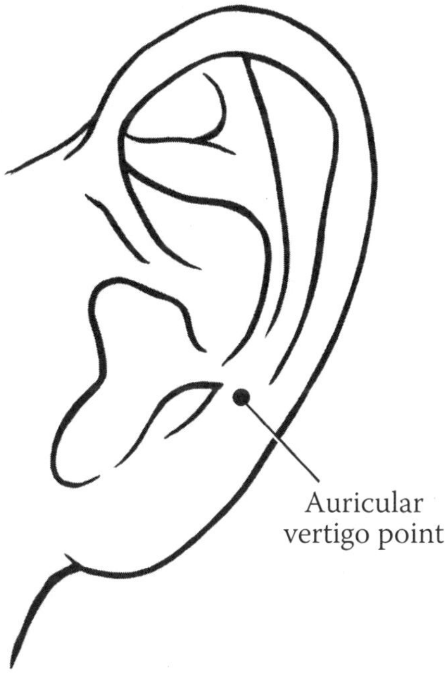

Fig. 1-3 Auricular vertigo point

1.2 Occipital neuralgia

Sometimes the occipital region begins to throb all of a sudden. The pain radiates up and forward along the Bladder and Gallbladder meridians, so many patients rush to get an exam from a neurologist. The examination comes up with nothing. Doctors explain the situation to patients in one of three ways:

"There is nothing wrong. Don't worry about it."

"It comes from tension in your neck and shoulders."

"It might be good to get some acupuncture or massage."

The last two explanations usually come from experienced doctors.

When it comes to treating occipital neuralgia, the key point is whether it is related to the cervical vertebrae. If there is a connection, look for reactive points and they will guide us toward which points to treat. The reaction in the case of cervical vertebrae involvement, more than tenderness at Upper BL-10, which is common, is a broad area of hardness at the attachment of the trapezius onto the occiput. Obviously, this obstructs circulation to the occipital nerves. If the tightest point can be accurately located and treated, the pain will go away instantly. As for depth of insertion, superficial or super-rotation (SRT) is most effective. Insertion deeper than 5mm is not recommended.

Refer to the case history of occipital neuralgia at the end of this chapter (see p. 65 below).

1.3 Chickenpox and herpes zoster (shingles)

The headache is similar to occipital neuralgia, but it doesn't respond immediately to acu-moxa treatment. Usually when there is no change at all and the pain persists in cases of occipital pain that should resolve in just one treatment, suspect chickenpox or shingles. If there are vesicles, you can find them by looking through the hair, but it's difficult to be certain if it's still in the pre-vesicle stage. Anyway, it is best to refer to a doctor those cases that have an acute onset or in cases that don't respond to treatment or become even worse. When there is a herpes outbreak on the face it can cause visual impairment, and when it's on the head there is risk of contracting encephalitis or meningitis. For more detail, refer to the section on chickenpox and shingles in Chapter 14, p. 338.

1.4 Trigeminal neuralgia

This is primarily facial pain, rather than a headache, and it takes some skill to treat trigeminal neuralgia. To put it simply, inserting needles in painful places can aggravate the pain. Even pressing lightly on the face to find tender points can aggravate the pain. Often even gently stroking over the face causes pain. In such cases, have the patient point out the painful places. If you use SRT, the painful points can be treated directly. The points that are often reactive include BL-2, LI-20, and GB-5. The key points for treatment are GB-20, GB-21, and LI-11. On GB-21 especially, I use multiple cones of direct moxibustion (about 30 cones). This often relieves the pain.

Refer to case history 21 below in the trigeminal neuralgia section of this chapter (p. 38).

1.5 Glaucoma

As ocular pressure increases with glaucoma, neck and shoulder tension and headaches increase. The headaches, especially, can get bad. The dire outcome of loss of vision is rare these days, but even for the young and middle aged, in many cases the cause of chronic headaches turns out to be glaucoma. That is why I always press over the eyes gently and advise seeing an ophthalmologist when they seem a bit hard. Acupuncture and moxibustion are particularly effective for glaucoma. For details, refer to the section on glaucoma in Chapter 2.

1.6 Nasal diseases

If the eyes can cause headaches, what about the nose? When there is sinusitis, often there is also tension and pain in the occipital area. I treat points around the nose like M-HN-3 *(indo/yìn táng)*, LI-20, BL-2, and GV-23, along with LI-10 on the arm. Sinusitis is associated with the *yang ming* (Stomach and Large Intestine) meridians. For details, refer to the section on glaucoma in the next chapter (p. 70).

1.7 Migraines

Migraines are most commonly seen in women of menstruating age. Often the pain is one sided in the frontal to temporal region. The pain is said to occur with the dilation of blood vessels, so it is often not good when migraine patients are in warm places. If the complaint is always getting a headache when going to department stores or places with many people, you can be sure it's a migraine. It seems to be closely associated with the menstrual cycle, and often the worst pain is just before or during the period. So patients tend to get bad migraines every month, and I tend to see such patients several times a month.

For local treatment you can palpate indurations in the affected temporal muscle (around GB-5) and insert needles superficially. These needles can be retained. Also treat points that are very reactive among GB-20, Yanagiya's GB-20, and BL-10. It is also important to check for reactions and treat points related to menstruation including SP-6, ST-27, and BL-27. If the patient is also experiencing menstrual pain, I place three cones of stick-on moxibustion on both BL-52.

Case Study 1

Patient: Female, 58 years old

First Office Call (hereafter FOC): March 30, 2011

Main Symptoms: Left sided migraine headaches

Pulse Diagnosis: Liver deficiency

Assessment: Tenderness and induration at left GB-5. Also indurations at GB-20 and Yanagiya's GB-20.

Branch Treatment: Needles inserted at above points (GB-5, GB-20, and Yanagiya's GB-20) followed by direct moxibustion. Also direct moxibustion at GB-21 and LI-11. All points were treated bilaterally.

Comments: Rather than migraine headaches as the patient claimed, they were probably temporal headaches caused by stiffness in the neck. Since she had Liver deficiency, probably the reactive excess of the Gallbladder meridian manifested as excess symptoms in her shoulder, neck, and head.

1.8 Chronic (non-specific) headaches

There are headaches that don't fit into any of the above categories. These are the called "habitual headaches" in Japan. In bad cases, patients have headaches every day and take medicine three times daily. Usually these are over the counter medications containing aspirin. This type of headache is quite common.

I treat chronic headaches like this as Liver deficiency. The root treatment points are LR-8 and KI-10, and LR-1 is also good. For the branch treatment I include GV-22, auricular vertigo point, GB-21, and LI-11. The headaches go away when these treatments are continued. It is natural pain relief that is different from taking medications. There is a good possibility that these patients will become regular patients after the headache resolves.

Summary

- Identify the type of headache and refer to a physician if necessary.
- Liver deficiency is the most common pattern.
- Use LR-1 and auricular points.

2. Stroke overview

Back when I was starting out my practice, the terms "brain congestion" (cerebral hemorrhage) and "encephalomalacia" (cerebral infarction) were still in use. Cases with high blood pressure with a flushed face were labeled "brain congestion," and cases with low blood pressure and pale face were labeled "encephalomalacia." The treatment was enforced bed rest, and to begin physical therapy after three weeks if the condition was stable. So treatment was still very primitive. It reminds me of the early tuberculosis treatment regimen of fresh air, rest, nutrition. Today, 50 years later, there have been dramatic advances with brain scans, surgery, and powerful thrombolytic agents.

I had my doubts about keeping the patient in bed and not doing anything, and also felt that something could be done with acu-moxa, so I took on stroke patients. This was before treatment protocol for strokes existed, and I had no clue how to treat such patients. I searched for literature, but unlike today, there was very little. Particularly when it came to treatment soon after the stroke, there was almost nothing. So I was groping but carefully started to treat stroke patients. Eventually the word must have spread because I began to get more and more calls to treat stroke victims. (In the early days I used to do house calls.) As I continued my trial and error, I figured out what worked and what didn't. I discovered my bag of tricks for treating stroke victims. I decided this information must be made available, so I submitted an article to the *Journal of Japanese Acupuncture and Moxibustion (Ido-no-Nippon).* This article was my starting point with my long relationship with that publishing company. My article was published in 1972, issues 333 and 334. The main points were as follows:

- The outcomes are better the sooner treatment is initiated.
- Recovery is best within the first month. After 3 months, 6 months, and a year, recovery is poor.
- Keep insertions shallow, and do not cause needle sensation. (*Note:* Now I recommend contact needling or SRT.)
- Root treatment: Liver deficiency is most common. There is some Lung and Spleen deficiency cases, but these are mostly cases with loss of appetite (cerebral infarction).
- Branch treatment: LI-10, LI-11, ST-36, GB-34, M-UE-22 *(bā xié)* web of fingers (Fig. 1-4) and M-LE-8 *(bā fēng)* web of toes (Fig. 1-5).

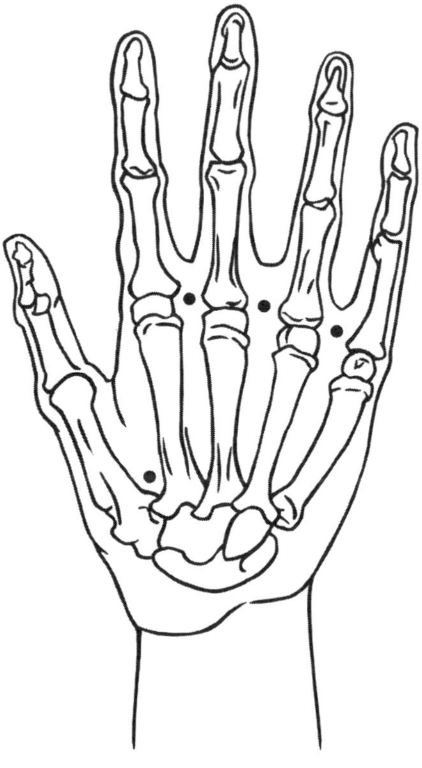

Fig. 1-4 M-UE-22 *(bā xié)*

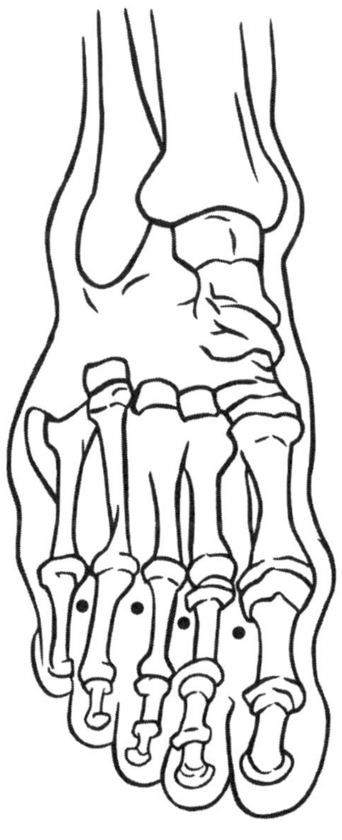

Fig. 1-5 M-LE-8 *(bā fēng)*

- Treat both sides, not just the affected side, and needle only the four limbs. Do not use any moxibustion.
- Do some gentle passive exercise of the four limbs. (Passive exercise involves no effort on the part of the patient.) Massage is also good. In mild cases, have the patient do gentle movements.
- Do the above treatment quickly (within 10 minutes). Treat patient frequently—twice a day if possible.
- If the patient is responding well, begin adding points on the torso after a week. Shallow insertion on the affected side at SI-11, SI-9, GB-21, Onodera's point (Fig. 1-6), BL-58, and BL-59.

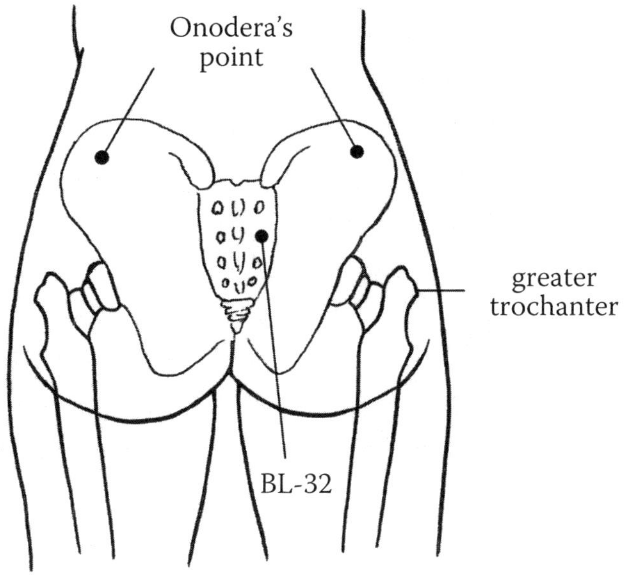

Fig. 1-6 Onodera's Point

- After a week, some moxibustion can be added. Don't let the cone burn down more than 80%. Start with three cones each on LI-10 and ST-36. At this stage, avoid treatment of occipital and posterior neck region. Do not needle or apply moxa on points like BL-10 and GB-20.
- When the patient complains of stiffness in the posterior neck region, place an intradermal needle in the ear (auricular vertigo point). An intradermal needle can also be placed safely in GB-20.
- Treating the posterior neck region in the early stage sometimes makes the patient worse.
- A patient's condition can deteriorate as a matter of course a few days after a stroke. If you commence treatment early, just to avoid a misunderstanding, explain that this is possible and that it is not caused by acupuncture.

- The patient must not get up for a few days after a stroke. Urination and bowel movements must be taken care of in bed. It is fine to move around in bed, and the patient can lie on his side.
- If the patient's condition is stable, they can start practicing getting out of bed in a week to 10 days.
- Next, patients must practice walking. Some patients lack motivation, but they must be encouraged to start walking.
- The goal is to attain recovery within one month in mild cases, and within three months for medium cases.[1] In mild cases, aim for complete recovery so the patient is back to normal. For medium cases, aim for about 80% recovery because 100% recovery is difficult to attain. In serious cases, aim for 50% recovery. When treatments are continued month after month, you will reach a point where there is no more improvement.
- If there are speech impediments, retain a needle in the auricular vertigo point and have the patient practice vocalizing as you perform passive movements with their limbs. Start with vowel sounds and gradually progress to consonants. Remove the ear needle when done, or an intradermal needle can be retained.
- When the blood pressure is extremely high, and it doesn't go down even after treatment, needle the points in the web of the fingers and toes as an emergency measure. Remove needles and check the blood pressure again, and if it is still high, repeat the same treatment. It is thought that these points serve to open up peripheral arterioles. It is an excellent emergency measure.
- Just as it is said "the danger past and God forgotten," even when patients recover from a stroke, many go back to the same lifestyle and have a recurrence. Even if there are no symptoms, it is desirable to get a few, or at least one, acupuncture treatment a month. Preventative treatments to prevent recurrence are important.

Reviewing this article on strokes that I wrote more than 40 years ago, I think it still stands the test of time. It even seems like modern medicine has come closer to my approach. Does it still have some value today? Surgery and thrombolytic agents work wonderfully, and stroke patients in Japan are put on a physical therapy regimen called "rehab." This English term gives the public the impression that it's an advanced form of treatment. "Rehab" primarily consists of massage and passive exercise. Acupuncture and moxibustion can actually have a greater effect. Even if acupuncture were provided in hospitals, I believe it would create a more effective form of "rehab." When surgery is called for, by all means this should be performed first. Once the patient returns home, acupuncture treatments can be done at home, if house calls can be arranged. I don't think good "rehab" should be limited to hospitals and medical facilities.

---

1. My understanding of the severity of stroke: Mild cases have slight aphasia and loss of grip strength, and these issues are easy to miss without paying attention. Serious cases cannot speak, have serious paralysis like hemiplegia. Those between mild and serious are medium cases.

Summary

- Treatment should begin as soon as possible. Recovery is best when treatment begins in the first month.
- Contact needling or SRT is recommended.
- Treat only the four limbs in the beginning.

2.1 Types of strokes and response

Strokes (cerebrovascular accidents) are classified into four main categories in Japan. Cerebral hemorrhage and subarachnoid hemorrhage are caused by hemorrhaging. Cerebral infarction (thrombosis or embolism) and TIA (transient cerebral ischemia) are due to heart and vascular disease. Cerebral embolism tends to occur with heart disease, and often murmurs can be heard when listening to the heart sound. Cerebral thrombosis comes from arteriosclerosis. Both of these conditions can be treated in the same way, but cerebral embolism tends to recur so closer attention needs to be paid.

TIAs are often a precursor to cerebral infarctions. Even if the symptoms quickly resolve, there is danger that a real cerebral infarction could occur soon. So I strongly recommend the involvement of a specialist before commencing treatment. The acupuncture treatment for TIA can be the same as for strokes. Cases of subarachnoid hemorrhage usually go straight to the hospital because the headache is severe. The problem is when the headache is mild, because while they may be due to neck and shoulder tension, they could be a precursor of a shingles attack or part of a TIA. If a questionable headache doesn't improve at all after one treatment, refer the patient to a neurologist. Some patients have a congenital cerebral aneurysm. If you suspect a stroke, perform tests that acupuncturists can do but send the patient to a specialist if there is any doubt.

- Measure the blood pressure.
- Check tendon reflexes. Look for pathological reflexes like the Babinski's reflex.
- One way I check reflexes is to apply direct moxibustion (half rice-grain size) on ST-36 on both sides. Make the patient bear the heat. In some strokes the heat is unbearable on the affected side and the leg begins to shake.
- Have the patient squeeze both your hands at once. The affected side will be weaker.
- Have the patient alternately raise each leg. The affected side will be hard to raise. With the patient seated on the treatment table, place your palm under the heel and have them press down: the weaker leg is the affected side.
- Check the movement of fingers. Have the patient flex each finger starting with the thumb, and look for smooth movement. Have them move fingers of both hands at once. Also check more complex movements like opening and closing between the thumbs and middle fingers, as well as opening and closing between the ring and little fingers.
- Listen for speech impediments. Speech problems often occur with right-sided hemiplegia.

- Look for problems with walking.
- Ask about urination and bowel movements. What about their sleep? Any headaches? Any diabetes? Have they seen a doctor about this? As you question them in detail, it should become clear whether it is something that can be treated with acu-moxa. As I treat very elderly patients on a regular basis, it's very important to know how to identify strokes and other serious conditions, because patients sometimes see me first before consulting a doctor.

Summary

- Pay attention to symptoms and identify the type of stroke.
- Examine carefully to determine if the patient needs medical attention.
- When in doubt, play it safe and refer to a specialist first.

2.2 Needling points between fingers and toes

Things don't always go the way they should. I will mention a case in which acu-moxa had to be used to treat a stroke. I don't have much to add, however, to the treatment protocol outlined above. I just want to relate my experience with the points between the fingers and toes, M-UE-22 *(hachija/bā xié)* and M-LE-8 *(hachifū/bā fēng)*.

In my early days, I was asked to make a house call and the patient's main symptom was numbness in his right hand. I took his blood pressure and it was extremely high. I was young and inexperienced, and scared, so I had him get a doctor to make a house call. The doctor was able to come right away, and after a brief examination, he drew some blood from a vein in the upper arm. That brought the blood pressure down, and the doctor said he would be all right. But the next day I was asked to make another house call, and found the patient had hemiplegia. Since there was no useful medical treatment at the time, I started treating the patient with acu-moxa, and he eventually recovered completely.

In about a year's time, he again complained of numbness on the right side along with high blood pressure. This time I had more confidence and needled the points in the web of his fingers and toes. After two rounds of quickly inserting and withdrawing needles, his blood pressure became normal and his numbness was gone. When I did another house call the next day he was fine. The points between the fingers and toes are just that effective. This kind of experience is rare today. In those days I inserted the needle a few millimeters. Sometimes the needle slips right in and other times the point is hard and it is difficult for the needle to get in. I imagine that the harder the point is, the more advanced the arteriosclerosis. Nowadays I use super-rotation (SRT) for my elderly patients with arteriosclerosis.

One of the members of our local study group had an experience of treating a relative who had inoperable cerebral hemorrhage. I was told that, as he continued treating this patient doing a root treatment and treating the points between the fingers and toes with SRT, there was unexpected improvement according to the brain scans.

2.3 Keys to treating the sequelae of strokes

❶ Treat for Liver deficiency: SRT on LR-8, KI-10, ST-36, LI-10 and LI-11, points in the web of his fingers and toes (affected side only). Three cones of moxa burnt down only 80% on ST-36 and LI-11.

❷ Give above treatment of only distal points daily for about five days. If the symptoms do not get worse, then add points like SI-9, SI-11, Onodera's point, BL-58 and 59. Continue this treatment for about five days and if the symptoms get worse, revert to the original treatment. When symptoms don't get worse, add more points like GB-21, BL-18, and BL-23. The main thing in monitoring the patient's progress is that the symptoms, such as speech problems or paralysis, do not get worse.

❸ When the hardness at GB-20 doesn't soften, retain an intradermal needle in the auricular vertigo point or directly in GB-20. Remember: acupuncture in the occipital region is the last stage of treatment, which only comes after the patient has shown steady improvement, as it is a local treatment and more risky. Play it safe and use SRT in the beginning.

❹ Among these are cases with severe numbness and deep pain, known as thalamic pain because it is caused by lesions in the thalamus. There is unbearable pain deep inside the body. These patients resist acu-moxa, and inserting needles in the painful areas will make things even worse. It is best to use SRT or contact needling at distal points only. Also treat GV-20, GV-22, and the auricular vertigo point.

❺ When the patient is on antihypertensive drugs, make it very clear that they must not stop taking them without their doctor's consent. It is fine if their blood pressure is stable, but it is sure to rise. If they were taking drugs before the stroke and they stop taking them, there is a chance of having another stroke.

Case Studies

I rarely treat strokes these days. All cases below except for Case Study 2 are from back in the days when I used to make house calls.

Case Study 2

Patient: Male, 73 years old (Buddhist priest)

First Office Call (FOC): October 22, 2010

Main Symptoms: Paralysis in right arm

History: Cerebral contusion, diabetes, left-sided facial paralysis, diplopia

Pulse Diagnosis: Slightly rapid, Liver deficiency

Assessment: Blood pressure: 155/95, temperature: 97.9°F.

Grip strength in right hand is almost absent. He has some speech impediment. Checking strength of feet, the right foot has less strength in flexion.

Treatment: I judged this to be a case of cerebral infarction that had caused hemiplegia. I performed the standard stroke treatment: SRT on LR-8, KI-10, ST-36, LI-11, and GB-21, and the following points just on the right: between the fingers and toes at M-UE-22 *(hachija/bā xié)* and M-LE-8 *(hachifū/bā fēng)*, SI-11, Onodera's point, BL-58 and BL-59.

This was followed by direct moxibustion on LI-11, ST-36, SI-11, and Onodera's point on the right.

An intradermal needle was retained at the auricular vertigo point on the right. I decided against treating the neck and occipital area.

Comments: After the treatment I told the patient he needed to be examined by a neurologist, and referred him to a doctor I knew. His expression betrayed some misgiving, and later I became worried about him so I called his home, but I couldn't get ahold of him. I contacted his close relatives and explained what was happening and told them that he needed to be taken to a hospital. Shortly after that I got a call back from his family. The patient hadn't returned home and they couldn't find him. I had an idea, and I went to the neighborhood karaoke joint, and he was singing all by himself. He was examined by a neurosurgeon soon thereafter, and a cerebral infarction was confirmed. He was hospitalized right away.

The patient was discharged after one month, and he returned to me for low back pain treatment and thanked me for rescuing him. He said it was really a close call. Acupuncture and moxibustion treatments are usually enough for such cases, but when we think of the condition of the brain, the need for rest, thrombolytic agents, and possibly surgery, not to mention rehabilitation, the wisest course is to let specialists handle the case. When I think about it, however, just 50 years ago, all they had in these cases was bed rest. What a long way medicine has come!

Case Study 3

Patient: Male, 65 years old (farmer)

FOC: June 13, 1970

Symptoms: Had difficulty moving left leg after work last evening. Could not walk to the bathroom this morning, was surprised and requested a house call. Recently developed a loss of appetite, leg fatigue, and insomnia. He smokes 40 cigarettes a day.

Pulse Diagnosis: Tight, excess, Liver deficiency

Assessment: Blood pressure: 185/100. Strength in raising left leg was slightly diminished, but otherwise his mobility was fine.

Treatment:

(1st)[2] Standard acupuncture for this problem on the four limbs: LR-8, KI-10, ST-36, LI-11 and LI-10, points between the fingers and toes at M-UE-22 *(hachija/bā xié)*

2. The same basic point combination of the first treatment was used in subsequent treatments. All the case studies that follow were the same in this regard, except where noted.

and M-LE-8 *(hachifū/bā fēng)* on the left, followed by light passive exercises. Blood pressure following treatment was down to 170/90.

(2ND) Jun 14 – Blood pressure: 130/80. Also treated tender points on the shoulder and low back. Also needled GB-21, SI-11, SI-9, Onodera's point, BL-25, BL-58 and BL-59.

(3RD) Jun 15 – Blood pressure: 120/80. Some numbness in arms and low back pain. Treatment similar to above.

(6TH) Jun 19 – Blood pressure: 155/80. Direct moxibustion applied on left SI-11, LI-11, and Onodera's point.

(7TH) Jun 20 – One week after the onset, the patient can walk without difficulty.

I added acupuncture on GB-20 and stopped doing the passive exercises.

(8TH) Blood pressure: 155/??. Has extreme numbness from fingers to back of left hand.

(11TH) Blood pressure: 180/80. Patient is able to leave his house.

(20TH) Jul 29 – Patient comes to my clinic for treatment. Blood pressure: 132/85. Just some numbness remains at the tips of the thumb and index finger of the left hand. The paralysis is completely gone, and he is able to engage in farm work.

COMMENTS: The points effective for the numbness in the hand and foot were at the tips of the fingers at M-UE-1 *(shí xuān)* and toes. I inserted the needles just 1mm. I believe the well points would work just as well.

Case Study 4

PATIENT: Male, 65 years old

FOC: March 31, 1970

SYMPTOMS: Right-sided hemiplegia started two days ago

PULSE DIAGNOSIS: Floating, tight, slow, Liver deficiency

ASSESSMENT: Blood pressure: 155/90. Grip strength weak on right. When he sticks his tongue out, it deviates to the left. Severe speech impediment.

TREATMENT: Standard acupuncture for this problem at LR-8, KI-10, ST-36, LI-11 and LI-10, points between the fingers and toes at M-UE-22 *(hachija/bā xié)* and M-LE-8 *(hachifū/bā fēng)* on both sides, SI-11, and Onodera's point. This was followed by passive exercises.

(2ND) Blood pressure: 150/78. Paralysis is a little worse.

(4TH) Blood pressure: 145/75. Paralysis is a little better. Speech is clearer.

(6TH) Apr 10 – Added direct moxibustion to the acupuncture on LI-10, TB-4, ST-36, and ST-41.

(7TH) Apr 11 – Grip strength in right hand increases slightly.

(8TH) Apr 14 – Discomfort in occipital region. Simple insertion[3] in GB-20.

---

3. Simple insertion: Technique of inserting a needle to depth but not retaining (non-retained needle).

(9TH) Apr 16 – Blood pressure: 130/80. Needle inserted into auricular vertigo point and retained for 5 minutes.

(10TH) Woke up with heavy head and crawled to bathroom. Cannot walk.

(11TH) Can touch thumb and index finger, but not the other fingers. Can flex and extend ankles but cannot move toes.

(13TH) Can touch thumb and middle finger.

(14TH) Apr 26 – Can move first and second toes well. Pain in the mid-back. Inserted needle in BL-17.

(15TH) Able to walk without a cane, but his movements are slow.

(24TH) May 24 – Blood pressure: 150/??. Heaviness in head. Direct moxibustion on GV-20.

(26TH) Treatment frequency reduced to once every 5 days.

(31ST) Jun 27 – It has been 3 months since onset. Treatment frequency once a week. He can do light work.

Subsequently this patient recovered completely and resumed farm work.

Comments: When I saw this patient the second time, his symptoms had become worse than the first time. This is something we need to pay close attention to. The symptoms of a stroke can become worse either gradually or quickly. Even if the symptoms are mild, lesions close to the brainstem can be life-threatening. We can relax and just do our work when the patient is in the care of a physician.

Case Study 5

Patient: Female, 60 years old

FOC: December 15, 1969

Symptoms: She had a stroke on November 21. Her blood pressure at that time was 190/120. She felt faint. She was hospitalized with left-sided hemiplegia. She cannot move her left side at all.

Assessment: Blood pressure is 120/80. It is difficult to say how much recovery is possible, but it has been 25 days from onset, which is within one month. I decided this was a case worth trying and began treating her in the hospital.

Treatment: Superficial, simple insertion at LR-8, KI-10, LI-11, ST-36 and LI-10, as well as the points between the fingers and toes at M-UE-22 *(hachija/bā xié)* and M-LE-8 *(hachifū/bā fēng)*. This was followed by passive exercises.

(2ND) Dec 16 – Patient had shoulder pain on the affected side due to laxity. Simple insertion at M-UE-48 *(mae kengū/jiān qián)* (Fig. 1-7) and SI-11 on the left.

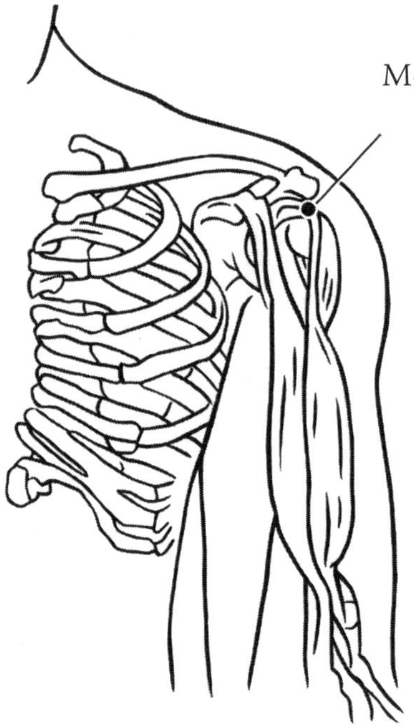

Fig. 1-7 M-UE-48 *(mae kengū/jiān qián)*

(**6th**) Dec 20 – Treating patient every day. She can move her toes a little. She can also move her leg a bit.

(**9th**) Dec 23 – She can move her fingers a little. Direct moxibustion at ST-41, ST-36, Onodera's point, and LI-10.

(**10th**) Treatment reduced to every other day.

(**14th**) Blood pressure: 145/80. She is able to raise both her arm and her leg, and strength is returning.

(**19th**) She begins practicing walking with a walker.

(**20th**) Her fingers reach her palm when gripping.

(**25th**) She can raise her arm all the way up when lying face up.

(**28th**) She begins practicing sitting. She has low back pain.

(**30th**) Discharged from hospital. Blood pressure: 130/80. She can walk on her own.

(**44th**) March 30, the following year. Blood pressure: 125/78. Pulse floating and tight; Spleen deficiency. I recommended home treatments with direct moxibustion at ST-41, ST-36, LI 11, LI-10, and TB-4. Patient is able to get through her daily routine on her own.

Comments: When I concluded treatments, the patient had recovered to the point of being able to take walks on her own. She continues to exercise so that she will be able to engage in light work. Her wish was to be able to do things for herself, so the outcome is not bad. Let me review the possible reasons that this patient, who was completely paralyzed in half of her body, recovered to this point.

❶ Treatments were started within one month (25 days) of onset of the stroke.

❷ Once some movement was restored, the patient made diligent effort to do exercises on her own.

This reason is especially important because good results cannot be expected unless patients have the will to do everything possible to cure themselves. As for the first reason, there is an inclination toward natural recovery within the first two months, as noted earlier. It is clear from this case, however, that far better outcomes can be obtained by adding acu-moxa treatments instead of leaving things to nature alone. The fact that this patient's arm and leg, which could not move at all, started to be able to move after the sixth day can be viewed as an effect of acupuncture.

Case Study 6

Patient: Female, 74 years old

FOC: March 22

Symptoms: She had a stroke causing right-sided hemiplegia one week ago. She has a poor appetite and is constipated. Speech impediment is serious and she cannot form words. Mental disturbance is also evident.

Assessment: Tendon reflexes are abnormally strong on the right side. She has a thick white tongue coating. Right arm is cold to touch and cannot be moved at all. Able to move right leg some.

Pulse Diagnosis: Floating, tight, rapid. Pulse rate: 84

Treatment: Simple insertion at LR-8, KI-10, LI-11, ST-36 and LI-10, points between the fingers and toes at M-UE-22 *(hachija/bā xié)* and M-LE-8 *(hachifū/bā fēng)* on both sides. This was followed by passive exercises.

(2nd) Mar 24 – Blood pressure: 172/84. Coldness in arm and tongue coating are both gone.

(3rd) Mar 26 – Blood pressure: 160/70. In addition, needled GB-21, SI-11, SI-9, Onodera's point, BL-25, BL-58 and BL-59 on the affected side.

(4th) Blood pressure: 172/78. She is able to lift arm 90 degrees. The leg can be raised about 10cm. Knee flexion of 90 degrees.

(5th) Speech impediment is improving.

(7th) Opening and closing of hand is normal.

(9th) Apr 10 – Blood pressure: 188/90. Direct moxibustion applied to LI-10, LI-11, TB-4, ST-36, and ST-41 on affected side.

(10th) Apr 13 – Direct moxibustion applied to SI-11, Onodera's point, and GV-20.

(11th) Able to sit up on her own. Able to crawl.

(**17TH**) Blood pressure: 230/90. She crawls to go to the bathroom.

(**21ST**) Blood pressure: 220/90. She is able to walk without a cane.

(**22ND**) May 26 – Blood pressure: 220/85. Treatments concluded.

COMMENTS: I had my doubts about her prognosis because of her advanced age and mental disturbance, but her recovery picked up in the last half of her course of treatments. She lived a long way away, and I figured it was fine if she could just get back to her daily life, so I discontinued treatment (house calls). Two years later I learned that she went to visit friends in the neighborhood and experienced no constraints in her life. So even with elderly patients, good results can be obtained by beginning treatments soon after the stroke. In this case, if the blood pressure is not managed better there will be a recurrence.

3. Dementia

Dementia is a disease that is seen quite often these days. It is inescapable when the elderly population is growing, but can something be done with acu-moxa? Also is there any way we can prevent dementia?

Case Study 7

PATIENT: Male, 57 years old

FOC: November 20, 2006

SYMPTOMS: Early onset Alzheimer's disease

HISTORY: Surgery for prostate cancer three years ago. Another prostate surgery a year ago. The reduction of PSA was not adequate, so he began hormone shots.

PULSE DIAGNOSIS: Liver deficiency

TREATMENT: SRT on LR-8, KI-10, ST-36, CV-12, CV-6, CV-3, BL-2, GB-5, Yanagiya's GB-20, GB-21, BL-15, BL-18, BL-23, and BL-23. Direct moxibustion on LI-11, ST-36, BL-18, BL-52, and BL-32.

COMMENTS: I treated this patient 34 times from November 20 to October 12 the following year. Even though I gave regular treatments for almost 11 months, no clear result was obtained. It is difficult to determine if there was any benefit. Even though his pulse would improve, it did not translate to an improvement in his condition. So it may be necessary to work with doctors to monitor results of brain imaging.

I am presenting only one case study of Alzheimer's, but I have experience with a case of vascular dementia. Back in the days when I was doing house calls, I treated an elderly woman with hemiplegia who was incoherent. I gave her several treatments, and one time she suddenly said, "Oh, what happened to me!" Her consciousness had become clear all at once. I explained to her what had had transpired, and once she understood that she had had a change in consciousness after a stroke, she settled down.

4. Mental illness

I have arrived at the discussion of mental problems or psychological issues, which was one of my aims in writing this text. Up until this time, it seems like the acupuncture profession in Japan has been preoccupied with the treatment of musculoskeletal conditions like back pain, neck and shoulder stiffness (*katakori*), and knee pain. I say "it seems," but this tendency is evident if you survey the papers submitted to acupuncture associations, especially the Japan Society of Acupuncture and Moxibustion. This tendency exists even in the Japan Traditional Acupuncture Society, which espouses the classical approach to treatment. Of course, acupuncture is indicated for the above conditions, and certainly good results can be obtained. Yet I think it's an insult to our medicine to focus only on these and not take on other diseases. My experience is that acu-moxa is effective for a wide variety of conditions.

It can be said in general that those diseases that are hard to treat in Western medicine are usually difficult to treat with acu-moxa. Sometimes, however, we can get unexpected results. There may have been a belief in Japan that acu-moxa is not effective for internal or psychological conditions. I think we must take on all kinds of diseases to see if we can help. It's not good if the condition gets worse, but it's worth trying even if there is no effect. Even if there is no effect with one acupuncturist, there could be an effect with another acupuncturist. There are few other professions where the results vary so much according to the practitioner. It just means that there is that much difference in technical expertise.

This is something I am always saying, but acupuncture is more of an art than a science. One improves with daily practice. As Yanagiya Sorei (1906-1959, the founder of the Meridian Therapy movement) stated, "If one needle—a piece of wire—can be used to resolve all manner of disease, then it is only natural that one's technique needs to be perfected."

This also relates to the statement, "The practice of medicine is an art based on science,"[4] so let's all work to improve our technique until we die. The improvement of our technique ultimately becomes an issue of our mind. There is a story in the third chapter of *Zhuangzi* in which a butcher displays his skill to the king of the state of Liang. The king is greatly impressed at his skill and compliments him. The butcher replies that his aim is the Way, beyond skill. This means that when we take technique to its limit, we go beyond skill to the Way. The Way is the realm of the heart/mind.

So let's consider the heart/mind. In East Asia, the character for heart (心) generally includes mental, emotional, and spiritual aspects of our psyche. When this character for mind is used, it usually refers to our mental functions, but it has broader implications. There are many sayings in Japan about the elusive yet essential nature of the heart/mind. To mention just a few: "The mind is vital." "The mind confuses the mind." "The

---

4. Hinohara Shige-aki and William Osler, "Art of Medicine East and West," *Journal of the Japan Meridian-Flow Society,* Vol. 23, No. 1.

mind has its own mind." "Keep the mind tethered."

Dealing with our mind is a really difficult issue whether in religion, philosophy, psychology, or medicine. Can one who cannot even control his own mind hope to stabilize the mind of others? Can we be so arrogant as to claim to help others with their minds?

My method of balancing the mind is not something that I devised from learning or theory. It is an actual experience I discovered through my own practice. I read the classics of East Asian medicine and got some vague idea about the mind, and over the years this idea gradually coalesced into an understanding from clinical experience. So my approach is very pragmatic and clinical.

4.1 The discovery of SRT

What it took for me to be able to balance the mind was the discovery of the super-rotation technique (SRT). About ten years ago, I officially named my method the super-rotation technique, as I had originally called it super-superficial insertion. I created this term SRT because it's a technique that never existed before. It is defined by very superficial insertion and high-speed rotations.

I found by using SRT that it treated not only physical problems, but psychological problems as well. That is, with SRT the spirit brightens and one begins to feel optimistic. I am not sure why this is so. In terms of Western medicine, I believe it would be said that the right neurochemicals are secreted in the right amounts, but this is just conjecture and there is no evidence. In terms of classical acupuncture, it can be explained as the balancing of the five yin organs bringing harmony to the spirits. The *Systematic Classic of Acupuncture and Moxibustion (針灸甲乙經 Zhēn jiǔ jiǎ yǐ jīng)* is a classic that concisely explains the earlier classics. The first chapter of the first volume of this text is titled "Discussion of the Essence and Spirits of the Five Yin Organs." It explains how the heart/mind is housed in the five yin organs. A spirit called the etheric soul (魂 *hún*) resides in the Liver; spirit (神 *shén*) resides in the Heart; intention (意 *yì*) resides in the Spleen, corporeal soul (魄 *pò*) resides in the Lung, and purpose (志 *zhì*) resides in the Kidneys. These aspects of the heart/mind are collectively called the five spirits (五神 *wǔ shén*) or sometimes the five essences (五精 *wǔ jīng*).

These five spirits are held to govern all the activities of the heart/mind. Even though the spirits housed in each of the five yin organs have different names, they can all be called "motivation" or "will to do" when viewed from a clinical perspective. It is true, however, that the nature of these spirits are slightly different from each other. The term etheric and corporeal souls (魂魄 *hún pò*) are used together to mean courage and vitality in Japan, but they are each different. Nevertheless, they are both aspects of motivation: the willingness or ability to perform a function.

When the five spirits in the five yin organs are all functioning evenly, our state of heart/mind is ideal. When there is irregularity in their functions, or more or less of one aspect, there is instability in the heart/mind and this causes mental or psychological issues. How then can we detect those imbalances that cause instability in the heart/mind?

The answer is differential diagnosis of the yin and yang organs. But this seems cumbersome. I have also chosen to use the contraction acu-moxa in the text because the term acupuncture and moxibustion, though accurate, is just too clumsy and repetitive. My understanding is that the yin and yang organs and meridians are an interconnected whole, so it also involves a diagnosis of the meridians. In other words, all we have to do is find out which meridians are deficient and which are excessive. I rely on the identification of the pattern (証 *shō/zhèng*) used in Meridian Therapy. Based on the four examinations, I determine which meridians are deficient and excessive. Thus I know which yin and yang organs are deficient and excessive. The heart/mind is not balanced because the five yin organs are not in harmony. If a person has mental or psychological problems, does harmonizing the five yin organs actually bring balance to the mind? Yes, it really does. It is a very simple principle. Why then do most acupuncturists never realize this? The answer seems to be in the type of acupuncture treatment used to tonify or disperse the deficiencies and excesses.

4.2 Harmonizing the five yin organs

I will explain my method of balancing the five yin organs. For example, when the *hún* of the Liver declines, this is labeled Liver deficiency in Meridian Therapy. The standard treatment for Liver deficiency is tonification of LR-8 and KI-10. Sometimes LR-8 and KI-10 are tonified and the low back pain improves, but irritability remains. Why is this? Is there a problem with the needling technique? The tonification method I learned in Meridian Therapy was to insert the needle 1 to 3mm and withdraw or retain for a while.

These days I use SRT. I rapidly rotate the needle with its tip resting on the skin for 10 to 20 seconds, and I begin to feel the needle become heavy. This is the arrival of qi. I remove the needle. I take the pulses again and confirm that the pulses have become balanced. I look for improvements not only in the weak positions, but also in the overall quality of the pulse. The pulse becomes soft and smooth, what is called good Stomach qi in the pulse. After the root treatment, I continue using mostly SRT for the branch or symptomatic treatment as well, and this lifts the mood of the patient. This means the five yin organs have become balanced. The patient gains energy and motivation. SRT is the needling technique I have devised from many years of clinical experience, and I believe this is precisely what was being talked about in the first chapter of the *Systematic Classic of Acupuncture and Moxibustion,* entitled "Discussion of the Essence and Spirits of the Five Yin Organs."

4.3 Scope of mental illness

The general term mental illness refers to a broad category of symptoms and diseases including schizophrenia, depression, panic disorder, hyperventilation syndrome, and psychosomatic conditions that used to be called "autonomic dysregulation" in Japan. If we include depressive symptoms that are not full-blown clinical depression, it may be said that we are literally surrounded by mental illness. When I reflect on my own mental state, I am not always that happy. I have days with inexplicable moodiness, dissatisfaction, and irritability for no reason. This is a common experience. In times like this I use SRT on myself to balance the five yin organs and this invariably helps relieve my angst.

4.4 How to detect mental or psychological issues

The two things that indicate mental issues more than anything else are:

1. Difficulty sleeping, or serious insomnia
2. Lack of appetite

One must treat patients with care when they have these two signs and also complain of being out of balance mentally or emotionally. Giving treatment to alleviate these symptoms becomes an important aim.

1. Easy to fatigue, the body feels heavy
2. Sense of energy and well-being is poor in the morning, but improves in the afternoon
3. Lack of libido
4. Loss of interest in things
5. Worrying over small things
6. Palpitations

The objective signs are as follows:

1. Laconic with a reluctance to speak: Sometimes they don't even answer questions.
2. No smile. Wrinkles between the eyebrows. Eyes narrow and become slanted down.
3. Stooping forward
4. Lack of attention to make-up and appearance
5. Filling in the intake questionnaire with many complaints and in great detail

On my intake form there is a long list of symptoms and new patients are asked to put a circle next to the symptoms they presently have or occasionally have. When the form is full of circles, I suspect depression right away.

There are practitioners who say that acupuncturists should stay away from the treatment of depression. That's because there is a danger of suicide. In serious cases, this is indeed an issue. I have maintained that acu-moxa, especially SRT, is effective for mental illness. I have had good results with depression, especially mild cases with depressive symptoms. I would like to see acupuncture become a treatment of choice. Having said this, in many cases the results are not immediate. It can be a long process. So the key is how to get patients to come in for treatments regularly for long enough to get good results.

4.5 Case studies of depressive syndrome

Case Study 8

Patient: Female, 56 years old

FOC: May 7, 2005

Main Symptoms: Many symptoms including headaches, anxiety (medicated), neck and shoulder stiffness, palpitations, low back pain, and easily fatigued. She has been suffering for two years. The medical diagnosis is "chronic pain." Injections for depression helped temporarily. She does have an appetite.

Previous Diagnosis: Uterine fibroids, chronic pain, autonomic dysregulation

Pulse Diagnosis: Sunken, slow, and deficient. The left positions are especially sunken. Lung deficiency.

Assessment: Tenderness at SP-6, BL-52, GV-9, GV-11, and GV-22

Treatment: SRT on LU-9, SP-9, CV-12, BL-2, LI-11, GV-9, GV-10, GV-11, BL-13, BL-20, BL-58, BL-52, GB-20, GB-21. Direct moxibustion on GV-22, SP-6, GV-9, GV-10, GV-11, BL-52.

(2nd) May 14 – Liver deficiency. This pattern continued in subsequent treatments.

(5th) Can sleep without medication.

(7th) Worries about marriage of her child causes insomnia again.

(13th) Aug 12 – She is doing better. Reduce treatments to every other week.

(14th) Pulse becomes more floating for the first time.

Comments: I could tell this patient was depressed with just one look. Her neighbor became worried and brought her in, almost against her wishes. As we repeated treatments, she began to show her smile and her face became rounder. She began to gain weight and even started to worry about her appearance. Chronic pain is a relatively new concept in Japan, but treating such patients for mental illness makes the pain go away as well.

Case Study 9

Patient: Female, 47 years old (business owner)

FOC: June 16, c. 2000

Main Symptoms: Loss of motivation

This patient has been coming to me for treatment several times a year. Her main complaint was that she was running out of energy and wanted a recharge. Her physical symptoms included occasional bladder discomfort, urticaria (hives), and heaviness in her head. She always feels better after a couple of treatments. Recently she has come in more frequently, probably because she got a divorce and took over as the president of a company.

Pulse Diagnosis: Liver deficiency

Treatment: SRT on CV-12, CV-6, CV-3, SP-6, LR-8, LI-11, BL-2, BL-52, BL-23, BL-18, BL-43, BL-58, GB-20, GB-21. Intradermal needle retained in right ST-19. This patient dislikes moxibustion, so recently I have been retaining the needles in the abdomen and the back for 5 minutes each side. She improved after first treatment and still comes in for occasional treatments. After each treatment she does well for quite a while. Since the main complaint is simply a loss of motivation, the effect of SRT is quick.

Case Study 10

Patient: Female, 18 years old

FOC: November 29, 2004

Main Symptoms: She is facing college entrance examinations and is feeling anxious and a little depressed. Her physical symptoms include neck and shoulder stiffness, headaches, heaviness in head, anxiety, numbness in her arms and legs, constipation, chapped lips, flushing, upper back pain, swelling, and menstrual pain.

Pulse Diagnosis: Lung deficiency

Treatment: SRT on LU-9, SP-3, ST-36, LI-11, CV-12, CV-6, BL-2, GB-20, GB-21, BL-13, BL-20, BL-52, GV-10. Direct moxibustion on GV-10, BL-52, SP-6 (tender).

Progress: She received 15 weekly treatments until March 23 of the following year. She was in an auto accident during this time and had neck pain, but she was accepted into college without a problem and became vivacious.

Comments: Acupuncture and moxibustion gave her a boost when she was feeling down, and she passed her college entrance examinations. This was probably the first experience she had of depression, but she will probably remember acupuncture when she faces any challenges in the future.

Case Study 11

Patient: Female, 61 years old

FOC: May 8, c. 2002

Situation: Three months ago she had a temperature of 37.2°C (her normal is 35°C), along with diarrhea and loss of appetite. She lost 5kg and was admitted to a public hospital for examination. She was told the cause of the low grade fever was unknown and 37°C was in the normal range.

Current condition: She is in low spirits, wakes in the middle of the night, and gets about four hours of sleep every night. She has little appetite, and soft stools. Her temperature is 36.3°C.

Pulse Diagnosis: Sunken and slow; Spleen deficiency

Tongue: Thick white coating

Assessment: Sensitivity to pinching at left ST-21. The paraspinal musculature was softer from left BL-17 down to BL-21, and pleasurable tenderness with pressure. I believe it began with a viral infection from the symptoms of the onset, but this is contradicted by the examination at the hospital. Sensitivity to pinching at left ST-21 and the slight tightness and tenderness indicate an abnormality in the pancreas or the stomach. The lack of appetite and soft stools make me suspect a chronic pancreatic disease. The primary indicators of treatment outcome for this patient are appetite and temperature (reducing slight fever).

Treatment: SRT on SP-3, PC-7, ST-36, CV-12, left ST-21, CV-6, BL-20, BL-15, GB-20, GB-21, and Onodera's point and on the left side only BL-17, BL-18, and BL-19. Direct moxibustion on both ST-36 and BL-17, 18, 19 and 20 on the left side. Intradermal needle retained in left ST-21.

Progress: She only came in for three treatments in the first year. Starting March 31, 2003, however, she began to come in regularly. She went to a university hospital for an exam and got the diagnosis of a possible pancreatic cyst and pancreatitis, as well as depression. She was prescribed antidepressants and tranquilizers. Later on, pancreatic disease was ruled out. Then she came for 36 treatments in 2004. During this period she received diagnoses such as multiple gastric polyps and gastric reflux, but her lack of appetite continued. Her pulse usually indicated Spleen deficiency, but sometimes it was Lung or Kidney deficiency. In 2005, she received seven treatments up until March 12.

On March 22 she experienced spontaneous pain in her sciatic nerve, that is, she experienced pain at rest. Her pulse pattern was Liver deficiency. Her appetite increased and by June 7 she had gained 2kg. By June 15 she had gained 3kg, and by June 29 she had gained a total of 4kg. She received a total of 36 treatments in 2005. During this period her appetite went up and down and she also developed a mild case of anal prolapse. In 2006 she received 16 treatments up until August 1. During this time her appetite and sleep improved and her tongue coating became normal. Her lower abdomen became firm, her waist and hips increased in size, and she had ample physical strength. On May 30 she complained of diarrhea and abdominal pain. Her amylase values increased for a short period at this time. Her primary physician admitted then that her earlier symptoms may have been related to her pancreas after all.

Comments: When there is even a little improvement, patients tend to continue treatments, but when there has been no improvement, patients will drop out after a while. This patient hung in there for a whole year without much improvement. She was friends with two other patients, one from outside our prefecture and another who lived in our prefecture but far away. They were all about the same age and seemed to enjoy each other's company. They were always on the phone exchanging information. The woman from outside our prefecture was the first to improve—her rheumatic joint pain began to go away. Along with the alleviation of pain she started to gain weight and her mood became brighter. Having watched this process, the above patient must have kept her hope that this was also possible for her. Also, later on, her first grandchild was born, and this had a good effect on her. Even though she sometimes complained that it was a long distance to travel for treatment, she seemed joyful. It might be her persistence that really made the difference.

Case Study 12

Patient: Female, 37 years old

FOC: April 19, 2005

Symptoms: Hay fever, low back pain, migraine headaches. She wrote down autonomic nervous dysregulation in her intake form. She has no appetite and her sleep is poor.

Pulse Diagnosis: Lung deficiency

Treatment: SRT on LU-9, SP-3, CV-12, LI-11, ST-36, GB-20, GB-21, GV-10, GV-11, BL-23, Iliac point, BL-32, BL-40, BL-59. Needles retained superficially in LI-20 and Upper BL-10. Direct moxibustion on GV-23, Iliac point, GV-10 and GV-11.

Progress:

(2nd) April 26 – Lung deficiency. She got dizzy when she had her shoulders massaged.

(5th) May 20 – Lung deficiency. She feels down.

(7th) June 6 – Dizziness and palpitations. She has been feeling really depressed.

(8th) June 14 – She felt better for 4 days after the last treatment. She sneezes. Temperature: 36.9°C. Lung deficiency. She got dizzy during the treatment, but it stopped after retaining needles in LR-1.

(9th) June 21 – She has been doing great since her last treatment. People at home told her she's like a different person when she comes back from acupuncture. She likes to clean and has gotten so into it that she has tired herself out.

(10th) July 5 – She has been having headaches and feeling down. The exam at the neurologist showed no abnormalities.

(13th) Aug 2 – She started working at a pickling factory.

(14th) Aug 16 – She is able to work somehow.

Comments: This patient was smiling, but I suspected depression from her symptoms. After coming for treatment a few times, she began to talk about being treated for depression at a hospital. She did not improve immediately, but in time her strength increased and she developed the desire to work. Patients like this need to be treated with care and be prepared for long-term treatment.

Case Study 13

Patient: Female, 51 years old

FOC: September 25, 2007

Symptoms: Her primary complaint is left shoulder pain that began two months ago. Otherwise she has low back pain and knee pain.

Assessment: Movement is restricted in her shoulder, abduction is only 80 degrees, slight heat can be palpated on the shoulder, but there is no spontaneous pain. Even though there is localized inflammation, I view this as a case of frozen shoulder (adhesive capsulitis).

Pulse Diagnosis: Sunken, slow, deficient; Lung deficiency. The primary pulse quality was sunken.

Root Treatment: SRT on LU-9, LI-11, BL-13

Branch Treatment: Shoulder (left only) – SRT on M-UE-48 *(mae kengū/jiān qián)*, SI-9, SI-11.

Other – SRT on BL-52, M-LE-16 (the inner 'eye' of the knee), ST-36, BL-40, CV-12, GB-20, GB-21, BL-58. Direct moxibustion on M-UE-48 *(mae kengū/jiān qián)*, SI-9, SI-11 (left side) and M-LE-16 and ST-36.

Comments: In this case the first treatment was September 25 and the second was October 3, with a week between treatments. The pulse presented with Liver deficiency at the second treatment. The patient told me then that she had been suffering from depression for a year, but that she felt much better after the first treatment. She claimed that the depressive symptoms had completely lifted in one treatment without my ever having known about it. This means that treating the body had healed her mind. This is understandable because the needling technique was primarily SRT. Even so, it's amazing that one year of depressive symptoms would resolve in just one treatment. It's interesting also that her pulse pattern changed from Lung deficiency to Liver deficiency.

Over the course of about ten treatments, she occasionally complained about the return of depressive symptoms. Here is a brief sketch:

(1st) Sept 25 – Lung deficiency.

(2nd) Oct 3 – Liver deficiency, much improved.

(6th) Jan 16 – Lung deficiency; her child and grandchild came to stay for a period and depression (working too hard to please) returned.

(7th) Jan 22 – Liver deficiency, doing better.

(8th) Jan 28 – Lung deficiency; has insomnia.

(11th) Feb 22 – Liver deficiency, doing well.

When patients have Lung deficiency, I always find they have some symptom of mental problems such as insomnia, loss of appetite, or bad mood. Furthermore, their expression tends to be dark. They frown; their smile is gone. When they feel good, they brighten up and talk more openly.

I don't think inserting needles will heal mental problems. With superficial needling or SRT the symptoms can sometimes lift in just one treatment. But this patient's shoulder is not completely healed. Yet she has almost forgotten about it. Sometimes I don't even treat her shoulder. There is no spontaneous pain, and she's not worried about it. So it is clear that mental stability is her real desire.

Summary

- Suspect mental issues in cases with a sunken pulse and Lung deficiency.
- Observe patient's expression and inquire about sleep and appetite.
- Use only SRT in treatment.

Case Study 14

Patient: Female, 60 years old

FOC: May 17, 2006

Situation: The patient lives alone. She was a kindergarten teacher until she retired. Once she didn't have work to do, she became anxious and started to have insomnia and loss of appetite. She received the diagnosis of depression and was prescribed medications. She feels really uncomfortable from time to time.

Assessment: She points to the pit of her stomach as the focus of her discomfort. She has glaucoma in her left eye. She has daily bowel movements.

Pulse Diagnosis: Sunken; Lung deficiency

Root Treatment: SRT on LU-9, SP-3, LI-11, ST-36, BL-13, BL-20 and CV-12

Branch Treatment: SRT on CV-6, PC-7, GB-20, Yanagiya's GB-20, GB-21, BL-11, BL-17, BL-52. Direct moxibustion on CV-12, LI-11, ST-36, BL-13, BL-17, BL-20, BL-52, and M-LE-5 *(shitsumin/shī mián)* (Fig. 1-8).

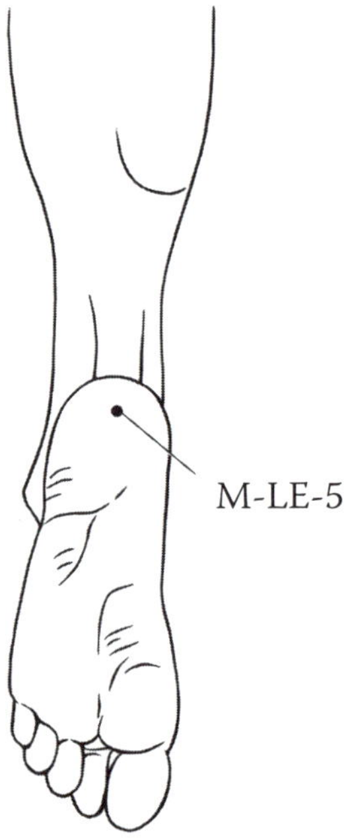

Fig. 1-8 M-LE-5 *(shitsumin/shī mián)*

Comment on Point Selection: Reflecting on my point selection back then, I was using many points unrelated to the pattern. PC-7 in the above case, for example. I was aiming to improve appetite, but LU-9 and SP-3 are sufficient for that purpose. BL-11 was also unnecessary. BL-17 was for poor appetite and especially a stuck feeling in the stomach. BL-52 was for the back pain. M-LE-5 *(shitsumin/shī mián)* is effective for insomnia. GB-20 and Yanagiya's GB-20 was for the glaucoma, but Yanagiya's GB-20 by itself is sufficient. Points on the occiput, however, I use on everyone, not just those with mental issues. They are indispensable acupuncture points for modern people.

Progress: This patient received 51 treatments from May to December. During October, especially, she came 15 times, sometimes coming in every day.

(7th) Lung deficiency. She begins to talk.

(8th) Liver deficiency. She starts to alternate between Lung and Liver deficiency from about this time.

(12th) Sept. 11 – Lung deficiency. Discomfort in the center of her chest. Added SRT and moxibustion on CV-17.

The following year she received 82 treatments. When she wasn't feeling good she came in every day. When she felt better she came in twice a week. Eventually she started to come in once a week, but she didn't feel comfortable going without treatment longer. She continued to take her medications.

(52nd) Lung deficiency. Appetite and sleep are good.

(65th) Tests at a hospital reveal abnormalities in liver function.

(78th) She gets deep sleep for three hours and then drifts in and out of sleep.

(97th) Appetite is great. She has gained weight and is worried about her appearance.

The second year after she started treatments, she came in once a week without fail. She continues to alternate between Lung and Liver deficiency.

Comments: The key to treating this case was the use of SRT and Lung deficiency. Nevertheless, it has been a very long process. I would like her to get by with one treatment a month, but she still needs weekly treatments. I leave the frequency of treatment up to the patient, so if she is suffering, the frequency increases. I ask her if she wants to back off to every ten days, but she doesn't reply. The desire of her body for acu-moxa is the reason she has kept coming so long. People don't keep coming just because I tell them to. She is doing well when her appetite and sleep are good. I always question her before every treatment, and I know she's doing well when she is talkative, her makeup is on right, and her facial expression is soft and relatively relaxed. She is not doing well when she complains that her head is heavy or painful and there is discomfort from her chest (around CV-17) down to her stomach.

Her physical symptoms are relatively few including headaches, low back pain, and fatigue in her legs. Her weight has increased compared to the time she started getting treatments. It is a problem to gain too much weight, but it's also not good to have poor appetite and lose weight. It is difficult to strike a balance. This patient continues taking the medications prescribed at the hospital and survives on one acupuncture treatment a week. I'm sure she will come around when she finds more purpose in her life. She usually doesn't say much, but now and then she asks me: "Doctor, will I get better?" I reply, "You will be fine. Certainly you'll get better."

When I am taking her pulse she sometimes asks, "How is my condition today?" When she has Liver deficiency I say, "Your pulse is very good." When she has Lung deficiency I say, "Your condition is a little low. Are you having trouble sleeping? I will give you some get up and go energy." Both the treatment and dealing with such patients is difficult. Our words carry a lot of weight. We must choose our words carefully.

■ CLINICAL STORY: Young Person in Bad Mood

I have a patient in middle school who likes to do comedy routines, who comes in for treatment from time to time. This time his main complaint was, "I don't feel good." When I am treating someone primarily for mental issues, I don't concern myself with individual symptoms. He had Liver deficiency. I just did the standard treatment using only SRT. I found indurations at GB-21 and Yanagiya's GB-20 and treated these. There was silence all through the treatment.

He came in three days later for another treatment. It seems he has decided to try a different path from being a comedian. "How are you feeling?" I asked. "He's doing great. When he came in last time he had nausea and diarrhea," his grandmother who accompanied him explained. Then he spoke up: "Dr. Shudo's acupuncture really works! He knows what's inside your mind." What can you say to that?

4.6 Concluding remarks on managing mental illness

Assessment: One eventually learns to tell depressive patients just by their demeanor. There are cases of depression known as smiley depression in Japan, however, so you can't be sure. Depressed patients have a characteristic way of talking. Instead of being laconic, they sometimes leave out even important things. So we have to use the other examinations of the Four Exams of East Asian medicine to figure out what is going on.

Treatment: As I have stated already, it's better not to insert needles. There is some tolerance of superficial needling like SRT, but even this can cause fatigue if too many points are treated. The less needle stimulation, the shallower the depth, and the shorter time the needles are retained, the better in the beginning. If you get the sense that it's a complicated or difficult case, refer them to a psychologist. The finding of specialists are useful for us acupuncturists. There are very effective drugs like SSRI, which has been called a miracle drug. It saves a lot of people. It has been pointed out, however, that long-term use of antidepressants changes one's personality. It would be ideal if the use of drugs could be reduced or eliminated with acu-moxa.

Having said that, it is not wise for acupuncturists to direct patients concerning drugs. It can lead to big mistakes. Also, don't speak encouraging words. All you have to do is express understanding. They say that when one speaks to depressed patients, one should merely repeat their words. When a patient is really depressed, it is very difficult to say just enough and no more. It is something that takes study and experience. I said "really depressed," but is there "fake depression"? I hear there is. Some doctors call it "fabricated depression." When times are tough, many things don't go according to our wishes. It is said there has been a growing "infantilization" in Japan, where many children are raised without discipline and few demands. For the most part children get things their way all through school and join the adult world without major challenges. Then they run into an obstacle in the real world and they can't handle the frustration and become depressed.

Obstacles are part of life. It never occurs to immature adults that this is the way things are, and that they were born to overcome their unique challenges. They think, "This must be depression that I have heard so much about." They go to a doctor and say I am sure I have depression. Even if the doctor doesn't really think so, there are plenty who will prescribe a mild antidepressant just in case. Of course, the drugs don't work. These patients don't have the will to overcome obstacles. Underneath all of this is an imbalance in the five yin organs. If this imbalance is corrected with SRT, they can build up the strength and will that they need to overcome challenges.

What can those that don't practice Meridian Therapy and don't discern the pulse and patterns do? There must be a good way to give treatment. The Sawada style[5] for example. This style has a protocol using standard points for moxibustion. They are CV-12, left TB-4, CV-6, LI-11, ST-36, KI-6, GV-12, TB-15, BL-17, BL-18, BL-20, BL-23, and BL-32. My teacher who practiced a form of Sawada style said there was no need to treat these points unless they were tender and did not select them for the most part. Anyway, one could use needles on these standard points instead of moxibustion. As my teacher said, usually these points are not tender. So instead, select the points that are depressed and deficient. It could add up to quite a few points. You may add a few points for psychological issues like GV-20 and GV-9. Whatever the points, the needle technique must be SRT. So what I am suggesting is that you keep your point selection system, but just change the technique to SRT.

4.7 What is true health?

Human beings consist of mind and body. Balance in both mind and body is health. If this is the case, it is amazing how many people are unhealthy. When a person receives acupuncture for physical problems, not only do the mental issues resolve, but the spirit brightens. When a person receives acupuncture when their spirits are down, not only does the spirit lift, but physical problems are resolved as well. This is the ideal, and to achieve this we must *harmonize the five yin organs.* SRT is a method to achieve this end. I am convinced that we can get as close as possible to an ideal state of health this way.

In general, it is believed that health is having no problems in both mind and body, but there are slightly different views. The preamble to the constitution of the World

---

5. Sawada style: A treatment style primarily using direct moxibustion developed by Ken Sawada (1877-1938) and made popular by his student, a medical doctor, Shirota Bushi (1900-1974) in the mid-20th century.

Health Organization begins with the following definition of health: "Health is a state of complete physical, mental and social well-being and not merely the absence of disease or infirmity." So this definition holds that beyond physical and mental health, one can be considered truly healthy only when willing to contribute to society. It is cruel to point this out to those who are suffering from mental illness, but given that forgetting about yourself and serving others is the secret to solving all manner of problems, I would like everyone to realize this truth.

5. Parkinson's disease

The line-up of diseases changes with the times. Tuberculosis was king in Japan right after World War II. It was even called "the disease that would destroy our country." My family too lost four members, and I was almost among them. Now, almost 70 years after the war, cancer is the top killer, and competes with heart disease. Parkinson's disease is also seen to be on the rise in recent years. Why is this? The aging of our population, our increasingly complex society, and the increase of pollutants and chemicals in our environment come to mind, but the cause is a mystery. Another name for this disease is paralysis agitans, which is just the Latin translation of "shaking palsy." As this name reflects, Parkinson's causes tremors and gradually one's movements become uncoordinated. This "shaking" is actually a form of clonus, a series of involuntary, rhythmic, muscular contractions and relaxations. This is different from the tremors seen in the elderly, as they are a "pill-rolling" motion between the index finger and the thumb. Clonus is easy to recognize once you see it. Also movements are impaired and there is intermittent resistance or a ratcheting feeling when gently mobilizing the elbow and wrist joints. This is also called "cog-wheel rigidity." These impairments in movement become worse the more this disease progresses. Parkinson's patients trip easily, tend to be constipated, suffer from depression, have tension in the neck, pain in the back, and a generalized stiffness. They suffer with mental and physical impediments. There must be a way we can relieve these symptoms with acu-moxa. No matter how hard I try to treat them, however, it seems like the symptoms improve only to get worse later. The sense of futility is inescapable.

One day I was greatly encouraged by the words of one physician. He is quite knowledgeable about East Asian medicine and I heard his lecture. He had been treating a Parkinson's patients for ten years and complained to a colleague that the patients had not improved at all. His colleague exclaimed, "The symptoms have not progressed for ten years? That's fantastic!" That's right. It's a valuable treatment to keep a progressive neuro-degenerative disease from progressing. This encounter changed that doctor's perspective completely. As a practitioner using acu-moxa to treat Parkinson's disease, I also gained a great deal of confidence from this story. Even though I was encouraged to learn that just maintaining the current status is good for a progressive neurological disease, it is only human nature to desire even incremental improvement. When treatments are continued with this intention, there can be some improvement—in some cases even dramatic improvement.

In the 12th-century work *Mysterious Mechanism at the Origin of Pathology in Basic Questions* (玄機原病式) by Liu Wan-Su, there is a commentary on the passage in chapter 74 of *Basic Questions* that states, "All [disorders] of wind with swaying and dizziness relate to the Liver." In this classic, any type of tremors or loss of coordination and balance was attributed to the pathogen of wind. So the tremors in Parkinson's disease belong in this category. The pathogen of wind is, of course, related to the wood phase or Liver and Gallbladder. Thus treatment of the Liver and Gallbladder meridians is indicated. In fact, I find that most Parkinson's patients present with Liver deficiency.

5.1 Treatment of Parkinson's disease

Pulse diagnosis: Many have Liver deficiency. Those with Lung or Spleen deficiency tend to be depressed.

Root treatment: Use SRT only. LR-8 and KI-10 for Liver deficiency, LU-9 and SP-3 for Lung deficiency.

Other points: Use SRT on GV-22 (or 20), Yanagiya's GB-20 (or standard GB-20), LI-11, PC-8 (see discussion above), ST-36, LR-3, Onodera's point, and SI-11.

Intradermal needles: Use auricular vertigo point. Pinch both antitraguses and retain in the harder side. Make sure the needle stays in until next treatment. Next time, retain in the opposite ear.

Moxibustion: GV-22, LI-11, PC-8, ST-36, Yanagiya's GB-20, SI-11, GV-21, BL-18, Onodera's point

Caution about treatment: Increase or decrease the number of points treated based on the symptoms. Judge the amount of treatment based on the severity of symptoms, the pulse, and the reactions palpated at the points. Many points can be tolerated with SRT, but sometimes even this is too much and it's better to use a needle-like tool, such as a teishin.

Summary

- Parkinson's disease can be treated with acu-moxa.
- It requires regular treatments. It will stop the progress of the disease and alleviate symptoms.
- Liver deficiency is common.
- Use SRT or teishin for treatment.

Case Study 15

Patient: Male, 67 years old

FOC: September 8, 2006

Symptoms and Condition: He was diagnosed with Parkinson's disease seven years ago. Tremors are greater on his left side. He has impairment in fine motor skills. He also has constipation, coughing, night sweats, and stiffness in his neck and shoulders. His appetite is good.

Pulse Diagnosis: Liver deficiency

Treatment: SRT on LR-8, KI-10, LI-11, ST-36, CV-12, CV-6, GB-20, GB-21, SI-11, BL-18, BL-23, BL-25, BL-58, Onodera's point, and all of the well points of the left hand and foot. Needle retained after SRT at CV-22 and auricular vertigo points. Intradermal needle retained in left auricular vertigo point. Direct moxibustion on LI-11, ST-36, SI-11, and Onodera's point.

Progress: I have been treating this patient once a week for six years. His posture has become slightly stooped and he has insomnia and depressive tendencies from time to time, but other than that his symptoms have not progressed. He no longer has tremors or coughing. He is a poet and his poems are published in a national newspaper column. He has written about boosting his body with moxibustion.

Case Study 16

Patient: Male, 72 years old

FOC: March 9, 2011

Main Complaints: Tremors are mainly on his right side. He has difficulty keeping balance when walking and also has urinary frequency.

Pulse Diagnosis: Lung deficiency

Treatment: Teishin used on LU-9, SP-3, CV-12, LI-11, ST-36, BL-2, Yanagiya's GB-20, GB-21, BL-13, BL-43, BL-20, BL-58. Direct moxibustion on Yanagiya's GB-20, BL-13, LI-11, and ST-36.

Progress:

(2nd) His tremors were much improved. I switched from teishin to a needle and applied SRT.

(3rd) The tremors have stopped.

(4th) Patient has Liver deficiency. Tremors have not returned.

(6th) Patient has Liver deficiency. Since he was doing so well, we reduced the treatments to once every 10 days from April onward.

Comments: The tremors were pretty bad in this patient at his first treatment. At the second treatment you had to watch closely to notice. It was really an amazing change. He had no more tremors after the third treatment. He rode his bicycle 3km with no difficulty to my clinic. A year later now, he comes in for treatment every other week. He continues to do very well.

I used teishin on this patient because he was especially sensitive to needles. When a patient is sensitive or deficient, and I sense that a teishin will be more effective than inserted needles or SRT, I use teishin from the start. I gradually switch over to SRT as the patient becomes accustomed to stimulation.

For those patients who seem to be weak or sensitive, in the first treatment I use a teishin on one of the root treatment points to see if it balances the pulses. When this is all it takes to balance the pulses, I do the rest of the treatment with teishin. When the pulses do not balance with teishin, I use SRT. If I need to use needle insertion on a local point for a symptom, I limit myself to just one point. From the second treatment onward I try to use SRT where possible, if the patient can tolerate it and the results justify it.

Case Study 17

Patient: Female, 72 years old

FOC: January 16, 2007

Main Complaint: Tremors that are greater in her right arm

Pulse Diagnosis: Liver deficiency

Treatment: SRT on LR-8, KI-10, LI-11, PC-8, ST-36, GB-20, GB-21, SI-11, BL-43, Onodera's point, and BL-58. Needle retained after SRT at CV-22, auricular vertigo points, BL-18, and BL-23. Direct moxibustion on CV-22, LI-11, ST-36, SI-11, BL-18, and Onodera's point.

Progress: This patient had a slight tremor, but it got much worse on the night after he received his diagnosis from a doctor. His right arm was the worst. It was alleviated with SRT on PC-8. His movements also became more nimble.

Case Study 18

Patient: Male, 50 years old

FOC: May 26, 2007

Occupation: He mostly edits on a computer for a newspaper.

Symptoms and Condition: Tremors on the left side. They are worse in his arm than in his leg. He experiences stiffness and difficulty in movement. His head feels heavy, he also has anxiety, difficulty swallowing, neck and shoulder tension, shoulder pain, as well as numbness in his hands and feet. He also complains of cold feet, upper back pain, discomfort in chest, palpitations, abdominal distention, low back pain, fatigue, loss of motivation, and insomnia. His appetite and bowel movements are fine. He doesn't smoke or drink alcohol.

Pulse Diagnosis: Liver deficiency

Treatment: SRT on LR-8, KI-10, CV-22, Yanagiya's GB-20, LI-11, PC-8, ST-36, LR-3, Onodera's point

Progress: **(4th)** June 13: In addition to the standard treatment, I inserted needles in CV-12 and left PC-6 for stomach discomfort and poor appetite. Intradermal needle retained in left auricular vertigo point. Direct moxibustion on left ST-21.

(9th) Sept 12: Needle inserted in PC-8, followed by direct moxibustion.

(**13TH**) Nov 7: Lung deficiency. His father just died, and he's exhausted. Intradermal needle retained in CV-12.

(**14TH**) He got hemorrhoids.

(**18TH**) Lung deficiency. His tremors are usually minimal, but they get worse when he gets tense.

COMMENTS: Because this patient lives in another prefecture and the demands of his work schedule, he can't come often. He has many symptoms and appears to be really suffering. Recently I have been using a teishin on some points.

Case Study 19

PATIENT: Male, 67 years old

FOC: November 17, 2004

SYMPTOMS AND CONDITION: He has tremors in his right arm and leg. He took some drugs for it when it was still mild, but he felt sick and the tremors just got worse, so he stopped taking them (with the doctor's agreement). He was referred to me by his doctor. He has anxiety, hip joint pain, low back pain, and weight loss. His sleep and appetite are fine. His stools are hard, and he wakes up about twice a night to urinate.

PULSE DIAGNOSIS: Flooding; Liver deficiency

TREATMENT: SRT on LR-8, KI-10, ST-36, LR-3, LR-1, LI-11, CV-12, CV-6, GB-20, GB-21, right SI-11, BL-18, BL-23, BL-58, right Onodera's point

Direct moxibustion on CV-22, GB-21, LI-11, ST-36, LR-3, right SI-11, and right Onodera's point

PROGRESS: I treated him seven times in the year he first came. The following year I treated him 46 times. He came faithfully almost every week.

(**42ND**) Oct 8 – Tremors in the leg have subsided.

Two years after the first year I treated him 37 times.

(**83RD**) Oct 16 – facial herpes zoster on the right side.

In the third year of treatment I treated him 30 times for a total of 120 treatments up to that point. Initially his tremors were alleviated by SRT on points near the ends of the affected digits, but the effect didn't last. I started treating PC-8 instead and there was some improvement.

He has been coming for treatment more than eight years now, and it is obvious it is wearing on him. His symptoms are slowly progressing, but he is still able to come for treatments on his own.

Case Study 20

PATIENT: Female, 70 years old

FOC: April 20, 2007

Symptoms and Condition: She has major tremors in her right arm and leg. The tremors in her arm especially are so great she almost has to hold it still with her other arm. Curiously, her doctor insists, "It's not Parkinson's disease. It's autonomic dysregulation." She has no other symptoms.

Pulse Diagnosis: Liver deficiency

Treatment & Progress: I treated her 25 times in the first year (2007). I used PC-8 using both SRT and direct moxibustion. Patient also did moxibustion at home. This reduced the tremors to some extent but it was still not satisfactory. The tremors in her leg, however, were almost gone. Now in 2011, after four years of treatment, her tremors on the right side get worse from time to time, but they are better in general when compared to when she first came for treatment. She has no tremors on the left side.

Observations

Acupuncture and moxibustion have a definite effect on the three main symptoms of Parkinson's disease: reduced movement, muscle rigidity, and tremors. They not only stop the progress of the disease, but bring a degree of recovery. Furthermore, treatment of PC-8 can alleviate or eliminate tremors in many cases. Parkinson's disease is designated as an intractable disease, and it is indeed difficult to treat. So it is no small thing if the symptoms can be ameliorated even a little.

The location of PC-8

In the 2010 Meeting for the International Standardization of Point Locations, the point locations that had been proposed in previous meetings by representatives from Japan, China, and Korea were officially ratified. Listening to the explanation by the representative of the Second Japan Acupoint Committee, I learned that they had discussed my "Parkinson's" point. In reviewing the location of PC-8, it was explained that a difference had been found between the location used by the Japanese and that proposed by China and Korea. The first location is at the center of the palm between the metacarpals of the third and fourth digits. The latter location is in the palm just proximal to the metacarpal-phalangeal joint of the third digit, on the ulnar side of the space between the second and third metacarpals. (*Note:* The point is on the palm where the tip of the middle finger lands when making a fist.)

Since I started using PC-8 for tremors, however, the reaction for PC-8 seems to show up in a different place from both these locations. I now locate PC-8 on the ulnar side of the second metacarpal. More precisely, it is found on the induration (hardness) or tender point on the tendon of the flexor digitorum of the index finger. The greater the induration or tenderness, the greater the effect.

So my location is right on the tendon of the flexor digitorum of the index finger or slightly toward the middle finger. When I palpate my own PC-8, I flex the tip of my other thumb and press on the tendon and between the fingers. There is usually marked tenderness when there is a hardening in the tendon.

I decided to try PC-8 out for tremors in Parkinson's cases. The results weren't fantastic, but it seemed like it had some effect. The results improved as I continued to gain clinical experience and fine-tuned the location of this point. The effect is such that now I am starting to think that PC-8 works not only for tremors, but also for Parkinson's disease itself.

6. Trigeminal neuralgia

Pain is really hard to deal with and can become unbearable when it becomes intense. You even start thinking thoughts like it would be better to die if only you could get rid of the pain. For me, my first real experience of pain was during an operation for an inguinal hernia. I was in the sixth grade, and this was back when surgical anesthesia was nowhere nearly as advanced as today. They told me I cried for two hours straight. Something like this would be unthinkable today.

My second encounter with severe pain was with appendicitis. It started to hurt in the middle of the night and the pain continued until my parents took me to the hospital the next morning. These days, they would call an ambulance and operate right away. My third experience of pain was after I contracted tuberculosis. Dry pleurisy caused labored breathing and a sharp stabbing pain in the chest. I also endured days of terrible headaches for unknown causes.

Even after I recovered from tuberculosis and opened my practice, I continued to experience pain all over. I had every kind of pain including temporal headaches, neck pain, chest pain, iliocecal pain, low back pain, leg pain, to knee pain. Oh the sense of relief when the pain subsided! When I managed to get some relief from acupuncture, I even felt a sense of pleasure.

There is a wide variety in pain sensations. Sharp pain and dull pain. Pain as if you've been hit by a bat and pain as if you've been stabbed. Pain accompanied by numbness, deep organ pain, throbbing pain, stinging pain, and burning pain. Acupuncture works well for pain in general. On the other hand, it can also make the pain worse. Even if we leave the issue of pulse diagnosis to the side, I believe the outcome depends on the approach to treatment, especially the needle insertion technique.

Among nerve pain, trigeminal neuralgia is the worst. That is why it is known as unbearable pain. They say it even hurts when someone passes by. The slightest of drafts can set it off. So this means that just touching the face to find which points to treat aggravates the pain. Thus point palpation, stroking, as well as pressing are all out.

Back in the days when I used to make house calls, I inserted needles in the face of a young man who had facial pain. His pain got even worse and I still remember that bitter experience. Ever since then I have refrained from using the direct method for facial pain. I ask the patient to tell me where the pain is and then determine which branch of the trigeminal nerve is involved. Further, I have the patient point to the places that hurt the most. In cases of severe pain, just have them point at it, and whatever you do, don't touch these places. Touching the skin can trigger the pain. I had trouble treating such cases back when the direct method, that is, local treatment, was my main approach. In desperation I started needling the points on the exact opposite side of the pain. This is known as contralateral needling, but I arrived at it by chance.

6.1 Reflections on treating *katakori* (neck and shoulder stiffness)

The condition called *katakori* in Japanese is well known, and many Japanese have this complaint. I have found that any symptom above the shoulders is always connected to the neck and shoulder stiffness of *katakori* to a greater or lesser extent.

Another story from my house call days. I was treating the grandpa of the house when the junior high boy came home early from school with his teacher. The teacher told us that the boy seemed to have bad facial pain, and he brought him home to rest. The grandpa asked me to treat the boy so I gave it a go. This was when I was just learning Meridian Therapy, and I gave the boy my acupuncture treatment but the boy was no better off. So I decided to give him direct moxibustion on GB-21 on the painful side, even though he would have to endure some more pain. The boy was lying on his side covering his face. I began to apply multiple cones of direct moxa. I don't remember how many cones I applied, but the boy's pain went away completely. He came to my clinic the next day, but the pain hadn't returned. He was cured with two treatments. This was good experience for me; ever since then I always use direct moxibustion on GB-21 on the affected side whenever there is difficult pain in the cranium. This even works for toothaches.

It is said that GB-21, named "the well on the shoulder," works for anything to do with the shoulders. What then about the neck—the lateral and posterior aspects? From my experience I can say that points like GB-20 and TB-16 are effective when some reaction or difference can be palpated. Almost always you will find an induration on the affected side. Patients can even handle insertion at these points as long as it's shallow.

The above are stories from before I came up with SRT, so how do I treat these cases now that I primarily use SRT?

6.2 Shift towards an indirect method

It works really well to use SRT on patients that feel pain even just with touch. Of course you have to be careful not to press the point. The pain resolves fairly quickly. Does this mean that the direct method is enough as long as the needling is delicate? Not always. There are patients who cannot tolerate even SRT, and sometimes only teishin is indicated. It seems to me that more and more patients these days are suited to teishin. How delicate can human beings become? If things keep going the way they are going, it may be that indirect methods will rule.

When it comes to indirect methods, Meridian Therapy is one of the best. Things go well if you identify the pattern and give a treatment according to the basic principles. At least, it is supposed to. When the result is not so good, that's when we have to resort to direct methods or an entirely different approach.

What I do is to examine the painful area. The first branch of the trigeminal nerve (ophthalmic nerve) is along the course of the Bladder, Gallbladder, and Stomach meridians. The second branch of the trigeminal nerve (maxillary nerve) is along the course of the Stomach, Large Intestine, Gallbladder, and Triple Burner meridians. The third branch of the trigeminal nerve (mandibular nerve) is along the course of the Stomach and Large Intestine meridians. This applies to the treatment of facial paralysis also, but we notice that the *yáng míng* meridians cover a large area of the face. That is why we often use points on the Stomach and Large Intestine meridians. My favorite points are LI-4, LI-10, LI-11, and ST-36.

I find in cases of trigeminal neuralgia that the pattern is often Liver deficiency. Sometimes it is Lung deficiency. The treatment in cases of Liver deficiency would look like this: SRT on LR-8, KI-10, CV-12, CV-6, LI-11, ST-36, GB-20, BL-18, BL-23, GB-21, and BL-58; direct moxibustion on LI-11, ST-36, and GB-21.

6.3 The mystery of pain

It is said in medicine recently that there is no such thing as idiopathic nerve pain. There is always some cause for nerve pain to occur. In the case of trigeminal neuralgia, the cause is said to be contact between nerves and blood vessels. The nerve wears with age and the insulating myelin sheath becomes damaged so that the blood vessels come into contact with the nerve. That's what they say, but this was the same explanation given for facial nerve spasms.

Pain cannot be measured by any machine. It is a subjective sensation of each individual. The Pain Scale (PS: gradations of pain) is a subjective measure or pain. There are those who have pain tolerance and people like me who are very sensitive to pain. This must be an inborn tendency. Even though they say that strong people can withstand pain, it seems to be related to an innate tendency of high pain thresholds.

My mother had mysterious powers. A long time ago a young man in our neighborhood suffered from pain of unknown origin. No cause could be found, but he was bedridden. His pain would ease only when my mother stroked him. So she was called to his bedside all the time to help ease his pain. What was strange is that other people stroking him didn't have the same effect. This man eventually recovered and moved north to Tokyo, but in his later years he came back south to visit me at my clinic and reminisced about his healing. He seemed so grateful to have received my mother's healing touch.

In Japan the common word for treatment is *te-ate*, or "placing hands on." So there must something in the hand that has the power to relieve pain. Practitioners who continue practicing for many years seem to increase this ability. It is said that sometimes being touched by spiritual people can cure diseases. Legends like sick people just touching the clothes of spiritual masters being instantly cured also occur, as rare as this may be.

Case Study 21

Patient: Male, 78 years old

FOC: November 17, 2003

Main Complaint: Pain over the whole right side of his face. It is especially strong around the maxilla (the second branch of the trigeminal nerve)

Pulse Diagnosis: Liver deficiency

Treatment: SRT on LR-8, KI-10, ST-36, LI-11, GB-20, GB-21, BL-43, BL-18, BL-20

Local Treatment: SRT on right side only: BL-2, GB-14, ST-7

Direct moxibustion on right side only: LI-11 and GB-21

Progress:

(2nd) Pain is gone. No need for medications.

(13th) There is a little pain. Kidney deficiency.

(17th) Pain has returned. Lung deficiency.

(18th) Pain went away after last treatment.

This patient has come faithfully for weekly treatments for nine years and his facial pain has not returned.

Comments: This patient received medication and a variety of treatments before he came to me for treatment, but nothing worked. His pain resolving so quickly may have been because his case was not serious.

7. Facial paralysis (Bell's Palsy) overview

When people first meet, where do they look? In some special cases it may be the shoes, sox, or the bust, but most always we first look at the face, especially the eyes. Even a shy person like me who finds it difficult to look someone in the eye takes a quick look at the face and makes various judgments. If the person is a patient, I am "discriminating." I might think, "she lacks vitality," or "he's trying too hard," or even "he looks depressed; I wonder what he's worried about?" Sometimes people try various things to hide what's going on inside. They will change their make-up, hair style, or dress up. But there is no way to hide deformity in one's face. Deformity in the face is tragic, especially when it is on a young woman.

My elder sister had an episode of facial paralysis when she was in the sixth grade. My parents were very concerned and took her to doctors and acupuncturists but her face never returned to normal. Her face was obviously lopsided until she died at the age of 68. She and my parents must have carried a burden all of their lives. My sister did have a good prospect for marriage, but she wasn't counting on it because he was handsome. But the world doesn't always go according to what we expect, as this man came through and married my sister. His mother was the kind of person who liked to help the weak and disadvantaged, and perhaps he took after her. Anyway they had six good looking boys and girls and spent a happy life together.

As they say in Japan, "Disease is in the blood." Even if a disease is not inherited, since most of our genes come from our ancestors, we can't say that there is no connection at all. In some cases there is a big connection. The disease manifests when the conditions are bad, or when we are unlucky. Facial paralysis seems to be hereditary to some extent. These patients are susceptible to problems in the nerves. Not only paralysis, but they also tend to get neuralgia, neuritis and herpes, which is seen quite often these days.

7.1 Cases where acupuncture was effective

Just a while back my own wife contracted facial paralysis on the left side. I had just completed a video shoot with my publisher and called my wife, and she said, "I'm sorry to have to tell you this ..." Her face on the left side was distorted and tea leaked out of the left side of her mouth. I asked if she could make movements in her left forehead, and she said she couldn't. In that case, I said, there's no need to go to a neurologist, you will get completely better with my treatments starting tomorrow. I wasn't just overconfident because I had been drinking. There was experience and a track record behind my words.

Starting the next day, I began to treat her every day. From about the fourth day my wife started to show signs of improvement, and in about 10 days her symptoms completely resolved. The recent medical opinion is that facial paralysis is caused by a virus, and it occurs when one's immunity is low or stress has been high. I don't think my wife is under that much stress, but this year has been full of momentous events for me that might happen once in a lifetime. I became ill myself, so it appears that I made my "better half" worry.

In the very first year of my practice a young man in our neighborhood came to see me. He had facial paralysis. It was my very first experience with this disorder and I had no confidence that I could help him. Twenty days after beginning treatment, there was no sign that he was getting any better. I decided that I would return his treatment fees if he didn't get better, but thankfully he eventually completely recovered. This patient was 25 years old at the time, but later on he became the president of a big company. Fifty years later his mother contracted facial paralysis at the age of 90. She said that it didn't matter if it didn't get better at her age, but her son became angry at her passivity and insisted that she come in to see me. Her face did recuperate beautifully. In the end, the mother and son both agreed that it was better to correct problems even in advanced age.

Back in the days when I used to make house calls, I went to treat a patient hospitalized for hemiplegia from cerebral infarction. One of her grandchildren visiting her at the time had facial paralysis. She was a little girl about two years old. I gave her pediatric acupuncture (no insertion) all over her body, and then inserted just one needle around ST-2 on the affected side. My insertion technique wasn't so good and the point bled one drop, and the girl began to cry. Anyway, she was there the next day when I went again to treat her grandmother and her symptoms were gone. Her condition was thus cured in two treatments. This incident is still fresh in my memory.

Even though facial paralysis is easy to cure, it is rare for it to resolve in just one treatment. Nevertheless, sometimes it happens. There have been times when I haven't been able to treat a patient the second time until several days later because of extended New Year's holidays. In one case the facial paralysis completely resolved in that time. It can resolve that easily. There are many ways to treat facial paralysis, but acu-moxa is among the most effective. Just the other day an orthopedic doctor referred a facial paralysis patient to me, saying that acupuncture worked better than the methods he used. So times are changing and acupuncture is becoming more accepted.

Even though facial paralysis is easy to cure, not much can be done for cases in which several years have passed. The sooner treatment is started after the onset, the easier it is to cure. It becomes more and more difficult as time passes. Ideally it should be treated within one month, and at the very most within three months. There is still some hope within one year, and even after a year has passed some cases improve little by little. I don't know of any other effective treatment. If time and money are not an issue, it is wise to continue treatment.

7.2 The causes of facial paralysis

❶ Various injuries

❷ Exposure to cold or wind. Being affected by a cold draft after going to sleep with the window open or riding in a car with the window open. This is the pathogen of wind-cold in the classics.

❸ Oitis media, neurinoma (nerve sheath tumor) of the auditory nerve, or swelling in the parotid gland can spread to or compress the facial nerve.

❹ Sometimes pathology at the base of the cranium or brainstem impacts the facial nerve.

❺ Sometimes it occurs with pathology in the brain or medulla oblongata and polyneuritis or Guillain Barre Syndrome.

❻ Certain infectious disease like diphtheria and Weil's disease can cause paralysis in the facial nerve.

❼ It can also occur with poisoning, especially lead poisoning and chronic alcoholism.

Asking patients about their condition before the onset, often driving for a long time with a window open, catching a cold, extreme neck and shoulder tension, fatigue from overworking, and stress are common causes. There seems to be some hereditary factor, and some patients have many others among their family and relatives who have had facial paralysis. Be careful with patients who also complain of ear problems. Their prognosis is not good. As I said earlier, current medical opinion holds that the majority of facial paralysis is caused by viral infections.

7.3 Types of facial paralysis

Clinically, the majority of cases of facial paralysis involve the peripheral nerves. It is rare but there are cases with lesions in the central nervous system. It can occur along with strokes and brain tumors. The characteristic of facial paralysis associated with the central nervous system is that the forehead is not affected. The paralysis is limited to the lower aspect of the face, which is to say the cheeks and the lips. The reason the forehead isn't affected is because the muscles of the forehead are controlled by both hemispheres of the brain. If the facial paralysis comes from the central nervous system, it is important to consult a neurologist to determine the root cause.

7.4 Symptoms of facial paralysis

1. Paralysis in the facial muscles
2. Sweating-related dysfunctions (dyshidrosis) of lack of sweating (anhidrosis) or excessive sweating (hyperhidrosis)
3. Dysfunctions in taste and saliva excretion (drooling)
4. Dysfunctions in tear excretion and abnormal hearing (loss of hearing, hearing abnormal sounds, and/or extreme sensitivity to sounds)

The latter symptoms indicate that the facial paralysis is associated with the central nervous system, and the prognosis is therefore not good. You can be pretty certain that the patient will recover when the only symptom is paralysis in the facial muscles. Be sure to ask the following questions at the intake:

"Do you sweat more than usual?"

"Is there any change in your sense of taste?"

"Is there anything different about your hearing?"

"Did you have any pain or ringing in the ears, or sensitivity to sounds?"

"Did your tear glands dry up?"

In addition to the above symptoms, occasionally there is facial pain. Also, if the paralysis continues for a long time, there can be spasms and contracture in the affected facial muscles.

7.5 Functional examination of face and eye movements

The muscles innervated by the facial nerve are called the mimetic muscles. These are 23 facial muscles including the frontalis. The primary examinations consist of the following three:

1. Movement of the eyelids: Have the patient close their eyes (orbicularis oculi muscle). Position yourself above their head and pull up on both eyelids. The normal side will not open much, but the affected side will open easily. Remember the strength of the weak eyelid. When the eyelid is really weak, the eye cannot be closed fully and they exhibit what is called "hare's eye." When attempting to close the eye forcefully, the eyeball rotates upward and laterally so that the lower and medial sclera or the whites of the eyes are exposed. This is called Bell's phenomenon.

❷ Movement of the mouth: Have the patient close their mouth. The orbicularis oris muscle must relax and allow ten different muscles that radiate outward from the mouth to contract. Make sure to have them also pucker their lips.

❸ Movement of the forehead: The horizontal wrinkles in the forehead are caused by the frontalis muscle. Have them raise their eyebrows and make horizontal wrinkles.

Perform the above movement examinations every time before starting treatment to track the patient's progress. These are simple exams that don't take much time. It is common to mistake the normal side for the affected side before one becomes used to seeing patients with facial paralysis. It is good to perform these exams for this reason as well. There are other exams that you can do such as having them whistle, blow out a candle, or puff their cheeks out.

7.6 Treatment of facial paralysis

Ancient texts such as *Tracing the Symptoms of the Illnesses to their Origins (Zhū bìng yuán hòu lùn)* and *Restoration of Health from the Myriad Diseases (Wàn bìng huí chūn)* state that recovery from paralysis is better when the pulse is slow or floating. According to a commentary by Okamoto Ippo,[6] "The penetration of the wind-cold pathogen is shallow in those with slow or floating pulses. This is why it is considered good. Those with rapid and excess pulses have a deficiency of qi and blood, which allows the pathogen to penetrate deeply. This is why it is considered bad." Regardless of the validity of this viewpoint, it seems to me that patients with pulses that are tight or wiry don't recover well. A soft or moderate pulse is best. As far as the diagnosis, Liver and Lung deficiency are common, but the pattern can be anything. The most important meridians in the treatment of facial paralysis are the *yáng míng* meridians (Large Intestine and Stomach) and I often use LI-11 or ST-36 for this problem.

❶ The points I use most often on the face are GB-14, BL-2, ST-4, and TB-17. In cases of paralysis, you can assume that there will be no tenderness or indurations at treatment points. Position yourself above the patient's head and palpate the same points on both sides at once. Stroke with your fingertips and feel the condition of the skin surface. If it is slightly swollen, look to see if it is reddened or there are vascular spiders. Sometimes a drop or two of blood comes out after removing the needles retained at these points. I take this as a good sign. I mostly use acupuncture on the facial points, but when the paralysis is serious or recovery is slow, I sometimes apply very small cones of string-like moxa on points like GB-1 and ST-5.

❷ Give treatment to relieve tension in the neck, shoulder, and upper back. My favorite points are GB-20, GB-21, BL-13, and BL-43. Apply direct moxa on the most reactive points.

❸ Acupuncture and moxibustion on abnormal points on the abdomen. Treat points that are excessive with tenderness, induration, or sensitivity to pinching.

---

6. Okamoto Ippo 岡本一抱 (1654-1716): A prolific Japanese writer and commentator on medical classics in the early Edo Period.

❹ For patients who are anxious or depressed, it is important to convince them that acupuncture will make them better. Check for tenderness in the upper Governor Vessel points like GV-9, GV-19, GV-11, and apply direct moxa. Also apply moxa on M-LE-5 *(shitsumin/shī mián)* to help them sleep.

❺ Direct moxibustion facilitates recovery so points like TB-17, GB-21, BL-43, LI-11, and ST-36 can be marked for home treatment. Those who live far away and can't come for frequent treatments can achieve good results if they are willing to receive amateur moxibustion treatments at home.

7.7 Other aspects of treating facial paralysis

❶ The sooner treatment is started, the better the outcome. All varieties of paralysis show strong natural recovery within one month. Take full advantage of this and maximize the results.

The chances for recovery diminish with the passage of time. After one year it is very difficult to achieve any improvement. Cases more than one month after onset, however, can recover slowly even if not completely if acupuncture treatments are continued regularly, so the results are worth the effort. Don't let the patient give up too soon.

You must explain to first-time facial paralysis patients that timing is everything. Peripheral nerve paralysis, unlike other types of disease, will not respond to treatment after a certain period of time. Tell them, "The first month is your window for treatment." Even if they want to wait until they have more time and money, once the window closes, no amount of treatment will make a difference.

❷ If a patient happens to come on the day of onset, it is necessary to forewarn that the symptoms often become the worst on the third day. Also, cases that have or have had pain in the ear tend to recover poorly, so this must be explained also.

❸ Treatment frequency should be every day for the first week, every other day for the second week, and depending on the outcome, about twice a week after that. From my experience, it is better initially not to have too much time between treatments. Home moxibustion is very helpful in the early phase.

❹ Advise your patient to avoid those things that cause neck and shoulder tension, like sewing and knitting, office work, and computer work. Anything that chills the body, like air conditioning and fans, must be avoided as well.

❺ In cases of nuclear palsy and supranuclear palsy, that is, when there is central nervous system involvement, the patient must be referred to a specialist. Even in cases of peripheral nerve involvement, the patient needs to be referred if there are enigmatic symptoms.

❻ Acupuncture treatments can be effective even when the facial paralysis originates from the central nervous system. Treatments can be undertaken after consulting with the doctor and getting the patient's agreement.

7 For those patients who cannot close their eyes completely, it is important to advise them to wear dark sunglasses to avoid conjunctivitis and keratitis.

8 "Skin needling" of the face on the affected side is also effective (Fig. 1-9).

Summary

- To treat facial paralysis, give a root treatment, retain needles superficially in facial points, and release neck and shoulder tension.
- Begin treatments as soon after onset as possible, give frequent treatments, and aim for recovery within one month.

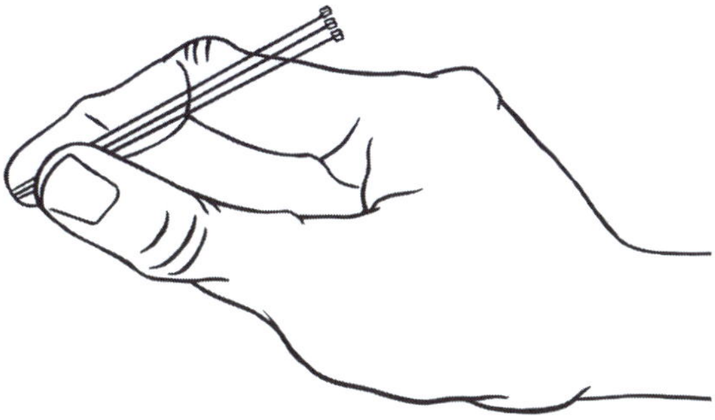

Fig. 1-9 Skin Needling. Hold three Chinese needles together between the thumb and index finger. Tap the skin quickly and lightly over the area. Be careful because it can be painful if the needle points protrude too much. This method can also be used for pediatric acupuncture.

Case Study 22

Patient: Male, 27 years old

FOC: October 17, 1969

Symptoms and Condition: Facial paralysis on right side, Bell's Palsy, lacrimation, altered taste, heaviness in head on right, stiffness in neck and shoulders, dizziness, and halitosis

Tongue Diagnosis: Thick yellow coating

Pulse Diagnosis: Spleen deficiency

Treatment: Root treatment and standard treatment on facial points and neck and shoulders (see discussion above)

Direct moxibustion on SI-19, TB-17, TB-15, BL-43, LI-11, and right GB-21. In some treatments, right BL-13 and ST-24 as well as both TB-22 were added to the above.

Progress:

(5th) Starting to recover around mouth.

(7th) Halitosis and tongue coating gone.

(8th) After treatment he is able to close his eyes.

(12th) Dizziness is gone.

(18th) Effects of facial paralysis no longer visible. He can wink.

Treatments concluded after 24 sessions.

Case Study 23

Patient: Female, 44 years old

FOC: June 29, c. 1971

Symptoms and Condition: Facial paralysis on left side that began three days ago. She has Bell's Palsy as well as stiffness in her neck and shoulders. Blood pressure is 160/90.

Pulse Diagnosis: Liver deficiency

Treatment: Root treatment and standard treatment on facial points and neck and shoulders (see above)

Direct moxibustion on TB-15, BL-43, LI-11, left GB-21, left BL-13, CV-12, TB-17 and TB-21

Progress:

(2nd) Blood pressure 125/75.

(3rd) Pain in front and behind ear on affected side.

(6th) Blood pressure 120/70.

(8th) Starting to show signs of recovery in forehead and mouth.

Treatments concluded after 13 sessions over 19 days.

Comments: This patient terminated treatments just shy of being completely recovered. Today, fourteen years later, you can't tell that she still has a problem unless you look closely. Her face tends to distort when she becomes fatigued. Some patients stop treatments before we are completely satisfied with the results.

Case Study 24

Patient: Male, 37 years old

FOC: July 5, 1979

Symptoms and Condition: Facial paralysis on right side that began five days ago. He is on medication for high blood pressure.

Pulse Diagnosis: Lung deficiency

Treatment: Direct moxibustion on BL-43 on both sides as well as GB-21, SI-9, and TB-17 on the right side

Root treatment – Superficial non-retained needle (simple insertion) in LU-9, SP-3, LI-10, and ST-36

Branch treatment – Retained needles in GB-14, ST-2, ST-4, ST-5, ST-7, and GB-3. Simple insertion in CV-12, right ST-24, left ST-21, Upper BL-10, GB-20, GB-21, BL-43, and M-BW-25 *(jōsen / shí qī zhuī xià)* (see Fig. 1-10), TB-15, LI-11.

Progress: This patient also came on the two following days for three treatments over three days. He recovered completely even though he could not continue with the treatments due to his schedule.

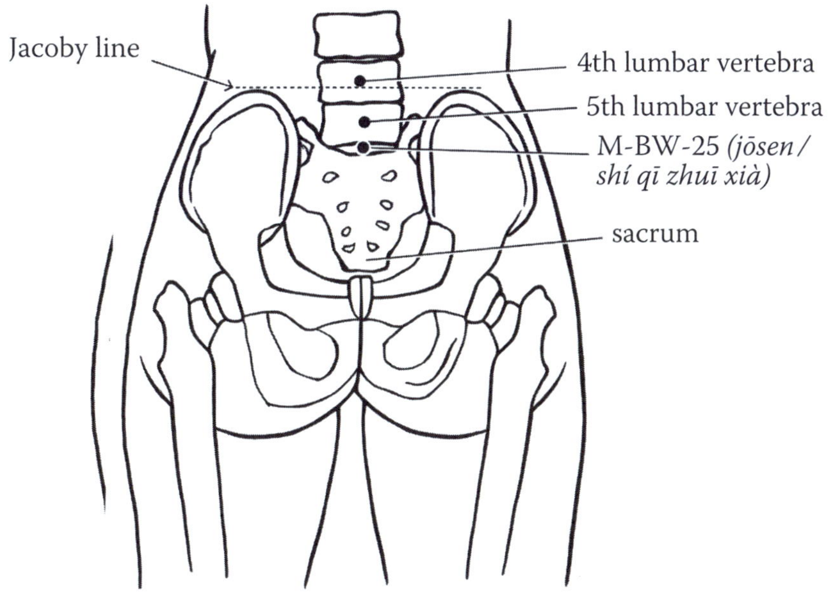

Fig. 1-10 The Jacoby line connects the top of the iliac crests. In adults this line intersects the spinous process of the 4th lumbar vertebra. M-BW-25 is between the 5th lumbar vertebra and the sacrum, in a depression a little below the Jacoby line.

Case Study 25

Patient: Female, 32 years old

FOC: April 26, 1982

Main Complaint: Facial paralysis on right side that began five days ago. She has altered taste and increased sensitivity to noise.

Situation: She received some medication and acupuncture at a hospital and now can move her forehead a little.

Pulse Diagnosis: Lung deficiency

Treatment: Direct moxibustion on TB-15 on both sides as well as TB-17, BL-43, and LI-11 on the right side

Root treatment – Superficial non-retained needle (simple insertion) in LU-9, SP-6, and left SP-9

Branch treatment – Retained needles in GB-14, BL-2, GB-1, ST-2, and ST-4

Simple insertion in Upper BL-10, GB-20, BL-43, TB-15, and right LI-4

Progress: This patient came for three treatments on April 26, 27, and 30. Both this and the previous case recovered in just three treatments. Was it the result of acupuncture or natural healing? It is hard to say.

Case Study 26

Patient: Female, 29 years old

FOC: September 19, 1981

Symptoms and Condition: Facial paralysis on right side that began three days ago. She presented with extreme neck and shoulder tension as well as Bell's Palsy, otitis externa with hearing problems in the right ear, and altered taste.

History: She suffered facial paralysis after an automobile accident. She is overweight. Blood pressure 110/70.

Pulse Diagnosis: Liver deficiency

Treatment: Direct moxibustion on GB-21 and right TB-17

Root treatment – Superficial non-retained needle (simple insertion) in LR-8 and KI-10

Branch treatment – Retained needles in GB-14, BL-2, ST-2, ST-4, ST-7, GB-20, and GB-21

Simple insertion on the right in LI-10, LI-4, and BL-43

Progress: She complained of swelling in her right upper arm when she came for treatment on September 29. Her grip strength was 20 on the right, 25 on the left. I referred her to a doctor for an exam which showed nothing abnormal. She received nine treatments until October 2 and recovered completely. No problems at all four years later.

Case Study 27

Patient: Female, 45 years old

FOC: October 25, 1982

Symptoms and Condition: Facial paralysis on left side. She had a fever of 37.5°C five days ago. She can close her eyes even though eyelids are weak. She can move her forehead muscles a little.

Pulse Diagnosis: Changed from Lung deficiency/Liver excess to Spleen deficiency/Liver excess to just Liver deficiency.

Treatment:

Root treatment – Superficial non-retained needle (simple insertion) in LU-9 (tonification) and right LR-3 (dispersion)

Branch treatment – Retained needles in GB-14, ST-2, ST-4, ST-7, and auricular vertigo point. Simple insertion in GB-21 and left LI-11.

Progress:

(2nd) Oct 28 – Felt nauseous and unsteady the day after treatment and could not come for treatment. The pattern was Spleen/Lung deficiency, Liver excess, but I treated her for a Liver deficiency pattern. I retained needles superficially in LR-8 and KI-10.

(4th) Nov 11 – Pulse quality was tight on the left and soft on the right. I treated her for the Liver deficiency pattern. She has not had any nausea. Superficial simple insertion used at LR-8 and KI-10.

The final treatment was on December 23, and this patient recovered completely with a total of 14 treatments.

Case Study 28

Patient: Female, 44 years old

FOC: December 26, c. 1978

Main Complaint: Facial paralysis on right side from three days ago. She exhibits Bell's phenomenon.

Pulse Diagnosis: Liver deficiency

Treatment:

Root treatment – Superficial non-retained needle (simple insertion) at LR-8 and KI-10

Branch treatment – Simple insertion in BL-43, GB-20, GB-21, and Upper BL-10. Retained needles in BL-2, GB-1, GB-14, ST-2, ST-4, and auricular vertigo point. ST-2 bled a little when the needle was removed.

Progress: (5th) Dec 30 – Able to close eyes a bit.

She was unable to come over the New Year's holidays and recovered without further treatment.

Case Study 29

Patient: Female, 18 years old

FOC: September 19, 1979

Symptoms and Condition: Facial paralysis on right side from 8 months ago. Ten days after starting medications, her face broke out in eczema all over. The facial paralysis has not completely resolved. Being a young woman, she is particularly concerned about facial distortion and eczema.

Pulse Diagnosis: Lung deficiency, Gallbladder excess

Treatment: Direct moxibustion on GB-21. Retained needles in BL-2, GB-14, ST-4,

TB-17, CV-12, ST-25, and right ST-19. Simple insertion in LU-9, SP-3, GB-20, GB-21, BL-13, BL-19, LI-11, ST-36, and GB-38.

Progress: During the long course of treatments, I encouraged this patient not to give up. After 29 treatments over 110 days, both her facial paralysis and eczema cleared up completely.

Case Study 30

Patient: Female, 75 years old

FOC: September 25, 1971

Symptoms and Condition: Facial paralysis on right side. She collided with a cow that she raises and hit her head hard. She has a headache and Bell's phenomenon. Tendon reflexes slightly exaggerated on the right. Blood pressure 180/80. She leans to the right sometimes when she stands up or walks.

Pulse Diagnosis: Changed from Liver deficiency to Lung deficiency to Kidney deficiency

Treatment: Direct moxibustion on LI-10, TB-15, and BL-43. Patient also instructed to apply moxibustion at home. The points were GB-21, BL-43, as well as TB-17 and GB-2 on the right.

Progress:

(4th) She can close her eyes and wrinkle her forehead.

(5th) Blood pressure 160/75. She can move some facial muscles.

(6th) Oct 6 – 80% recovered.

(12th) Oct 22 – 90% recovered.

This patient recovered in about one month with the help of home moxibustion.

Case Study 31

Patient: Female, about 40 years old

This was a patient I saw just a few years after starting my practice and I have no record.

She walked over to her elder sister's place where I had gone for a house call.

Symptoms and Condition: Right-sided hemiplegia and facial paralysis. She has speech impediment and a history of high blood pressure.

Comments: As I continued treating this patient, first she recovered from her facial paralysis, and then her hemiplegia symptoms, and finally her speech impediment. She died many years later from a stroke. In any case, from the first day of onset, I began giving this patient my stroke treatment detailed in a previous section along with some treatment of local facial points. This seems to have contributed to the good outcome. This shows that even facial paralysis from the central nervous system associated with a cerebrovascular accident can be treated successfully.

Case Study 32

Patient: Male, about 45 years old

This is another patient I saw in the early years of my practice and my records about it are incomplete.

Symptoms and Condition: Right-sided facial paralysis with Bell's phenomenon. He felt unsteady, tinnitus in the left ear, and pain behind his ears. He had received acupuncture and massage at a hospital.

Treatment & Progress: His pulse at the first treatment was flooding and Liver deficiency. He stopped coming for treatments before he recovered completely. Two years and five months later he came again for treatment because he had a recurrence. His pulse pattern was Lung deficiency. This time it was mild and he recovered with a few treatments. But then a year and a half later he contracted right-sided facial paralysis again. This time his pulse pattern was Liver deficiency.

Comments: This is a difficult case of a patient who stopped coming for treatment as soon as there was some sign of improvement, and he didn't like the idea of having moxibustion done at home either. Can recurrence be prevented by hanging in there until completely better, or by coming in occasionally for prevention? Or perhaps his case was recurring facial paralysis that couldn't be prevented. It is hard to say.

Case Study 33

Patient: Female, 62 years old

FOC: June 17, 1983

Symptoms and Condition: She had pain below her right ear, and then three days later she developed facial paralysis on the right side. She had extreme tension around GV-14 and was having people press on it, but the tension disappeared after she got facial paralysis. She has no other symptoms. Blood pressure 160/85.

Palpation: She has an enlarged thyroid and large masses of an unknown type in her lower abdomen (perhaps uterine fibroids). She said she had an operation to remove the lumps but that they just grew back. These masses made her lower abdomen protrude as if she were pregnant, and they were also hard. It didn't seem like she could lie comfortably on her stomach so I did not treat her back.

Pulse Diagnosis: Rapid and tight; Lung deficiency/Liver excess

Treatment: Retained needles in LU-9, SP-3, and GB-21. Intradermal needle retained in right auricular vertigo point. Direct moxibustion applied as follows: 10 cones on right GB-21 and 5 cones on LI-11, ST-36, and TB-17.

Progress:

(2nd) Blood pressure 140/80. Pulse is no longer rapid.

(5th) Liver deficiency. Eyes and mouth seem to have recovered a little. No change in forehead.

(7TH) She can wrinkle her forehead a little.

(9TH) July 1 – LI-10 and BL-43 added as moxibustion points on the right side. Needles retained in the face on the left side also.

(11TH) July 7 – She can wrinkle her forehead, but her eyelid closure is weak.

After the above treatment her husband was hospitalized and she could no longer come for treatments. I was concerned about her stopping with incomplete recovery, but when I met her sometime later her face was back to normal, so she must have recovered without further treatment.

Case Study 34

Patient: Male, 23 years old

FOC: August 20, 1983

Situation and Symptoms: He contracted facial paralysis on right side on July 25 and was hospitalized right away. He had stellate-ganglion block and intravenous infusions every day but showed no signs of recovery. On August 19 he met a neighbor who happened to come down with the same condition on the same day as him. She had fully recovered and told him that she had been treated in my clinic, so he left the hospital and came to me for treatment. He presented with altered taste, hearing problems, sensitivity to sounds, and lacrimation. Upon examination I found his forehead was severely affected, his eyelids were significantly affected, and his mouth was moderately affected.

Pulse Diagnosis: Lung deficiency

Treatment: Direct moxibustion applied on right GB-21, BL-13, LI-11, and ST-36. Retained needles in BL-2, GB-14, ST-4, and TB-17. Intradermal needle retained in right TB-17.

Progress: He received 14 similar treatments until September 28, but there was no change in his appearance and he stopped coming for treatment. I was pessimistic, believing that we couldn't expect much recovery when starting treatment one month after onset, but some time later he referred another patient with facial paralysis. I asked after him and found out that he had completely recovered. It's hard to say if the effect of the treatment appeared some time after a course of treatments or if natural healing kicked in.

Case Study 35

Patient: Female, 57 years old

FOC: August 9, 1984

Situation and Symptoms: Facial paralysis on left side that began 50 days ago. She went to a hospital and received acupuncture and injections in her throat (stellate ganglion block) every other day, as well as medications, but recovery was unsatisfactory. She knew about my clinic, but she didn't come because my location was inconvenient.

From the very beginning she also had tinnitus, altered taste, neck and shoulder stiffness, and strong pain in her external ear. Exposure to sunlight sometimes caused eczema and itching over her entire body. Blood pressure was 135/80.

Abdominal Palpation: She had fullness in the chest and hypochondrium, and pain on percussion in her right subcostal region.

Pulse Diagnosis: Rapid and hard; Liver deficiency

Treatment and Progress: She pinned her hopes on me and continued to come for regular treatments. Typical treatment consisted of retained needles in BL-2, GB-14, ST-4, and TB-17 as well as simple insertion in points such as LR-8, KI-10, LI-11, ST-36, CV-12, CV-6, right ST-19, GB-20, GB-21, BL-43, BL-18, BL-23, and BL-58. Over the course of the treatments she complained of symptoms like nasal discharge on the affected side, itching all over. Once she looked mystified when itchiness went away right after needling LU-9. She also had a sensation of heavy eyelids, fullness and distention in her costal region, and extreme fatigue. As we continued treatments, however, first the fullness and distention in her costal region disappeared. The distortion in her face did not change much, but she continued to come for treatments 2-3 times a month because her fatigue went away after treatment, and gradually her face started to improve. After 16 months of treatment the improvement was such that it became barely noticeable.

Comments: It is ideal when patients can receive treatment immediately after the onset of paralysis, but there are times when this is just not possible. I learned from this case that acu-moxa can also be effective in cases where some time has elapsed.

Case Study 36

Patient: Male, 19 years old

FOC: October 28, 1985

Situation and Symptoms: He worked at a pharmaceutical company manufacturing various drugs. Two days ago he contracted facial paralysis on the left side. He has pain behind that ear and outer canthus, tearing of the left eye, and no sensation in the left side of his tongue.

Pulse Diagnosis: Floating and wiry; Liver deficiency

Treatment and Progress: The typical treatment (as in the last case) with retained needles in BL-2, GB-14, ST-4, and TB-17 as well as simple insertion in points such as LR-8, KI-10, LI-11, ST-36, CV-12, CV-6, right ST-19, GB-20, GB-21, BL-43, BL-18, BL-23, and BL-58. Treatment was continued intensively for two months and his mouth recovered, but there was inadequate improvement in his ability to close his eyes and make wrinkles in his forehead. I tried various things like retaining needles on the normal side of the face and placing intradermal needles in the affected side of the face, but the outcome was disappointing.

Comments: I had counted on his youth and natural healing power, but I had to eat my words after having told him that I would help him get better within one month. This was the first time the response to regular treatment was so lackluster and it makes you hesitate to make any bold statements. This young man did eventually recover, but it took many treatments over the period of a year and two months.

Case Study 37

Patient: Male, 12 years old (1st year of middle school)

FOC: April 7, 2007

Symptoms and Condition: He contracted facial paralysis on right side 2-3 days previously. He has been on steroids for two weeks and he is still on them. He had severe paralysis in the frontalis muscle and medium level paralysis in the orbicularis oculi and orbicularis oris muscles.

Pulse Diagnosis: Liver deficiency

Treatment and Progress: SRT applied on BL-2, GB-14, ST-4, TB-17, LR-8, KI-10, ST-36, LI-11, CV-12, CV-6, right ST-19, GB-20, GB-21, BL-43, BL-18, BL-23, BL-58. Intradermal needle retained in right TB-17. Direct moxibustion on the right side only to TB-17, GB-21, ST-36, and LI-11.

Progress:

(4th) Forehead improved a little.

(10th) Recovery about 80% in forehead, 80% in eyelids, and 100% in mouth.

(13th) Recovery about 90% in forehead, and mouth went back to 90%.

Comments: It took a total of 40 days for complete recovery for a boy in middle school.

A slight backtracking in recovery occurred in this case. Ideally, recovery would be a steady progression, but often there are ups and downs, especially in cases of paralysis. Considering that my sister, who got facial paralysis at about the same age, never recovered at all and suffered her entire life, it was a great relief to see this young person recover completely.

7.8 Concluding remarks on facial paralysis

In order to present a variety of cases, I included those from early in my career, but I think this gives you a good idea of the development of my approach. According to the statistics on 500 cases of idiopathic facial paralysis by Park and Watkins, 66% recovered naturally, 21% recovered substantially, 9% recovered partially and 4% showed very poor recovery.[7] In other words, facial paralysis has a large rate of natural recovery. Usually the

7. Park HW, Watkins AL. Facial paralysis; analysis of 500 cases. *Arch Phys Med Rehabil.* 1949 Dec; 30 (12):749–762.

medical opinion about acupuncture is that it is hard to say whether there is an effect or it is just spontaneous recovery. From my experience, I can say acu-moxa is a wonderful therapy that facilitates spontaneous recovery.

Considering the cases with poor recovery, those with pain in and around the ear, abnormalities in the tongue and taste, and wiry, tight, or hard pulses do not fare so well. The former symptoms indicate a viral infection close to the central nervous system, and the latter pulse qualities indicate a lack of Stomach qi or vitality. I believe knowledge about this will help you with the prognosis.

8. Facial spasms (myokymia)

I just discussed facial paralysis in the section above and it happens to be one of the top conditions indicated for acu-moxa. What then about facial spasms, which are also a pathology of the facial nerves? From my experience, the outcomes are not as good. If it's a mild case, the symptoms will resolve and recurrence is unlikely. When it is severe, however, and patients cannot even see straight, it's out of our league. I can say it's not possible to treat this condition at my level of technique.

There didn't used to be a medical treatment for facial spasms, but a cure has been found with advances in neurosurgery. Why do facial spasms happen anyway? The current medical explanation is that they are caused by contact between a facial nerve and a blood vessel. So they can insert an insulator between the nerve and vessel to prevent contact. The pain stops just like that, so the above explanation has to be valid. Many people are happy with the surgery, so if the patient at first impression is in severe facial pain, I refer them to a neurosurgeon for surgery.

But then there are those patients who dislike surgery. It is rather disturbing to have someone cut into your head when you think about it. They say there must be some way to help them with acupuncture. When a patient pleads with me, I generally agree to give it a try for a few treatments. It is, however, also important to know when to refuse cases that are beyond your scope. I recently treated two cases of severe facial spasms, and I think they may be instructive.

Case Study 38

Patient: Female, 86 years old

FOC: June 1, 2010

Symptoms and Condition: Facial spasms on the left side. Facial muscles spasm continuously. The movement is visible down to the neck (platysma muscle). She has also experienced low back pain (spinal curvature due to aging) for the last six months.

Pulse Diagnosis: Liver deficiency. On the surface, pulses on the left are stronger than on the right.

Treatment and Progress: SRT applied on LR-8, KI-10, ST-36, LI-11, BL-18, BL-23, BL-58, GB-20, BL-2, ST-2, ST-4, and TB-16 on the left

Direct moxibustion on LI-11, ST-36 and BL-23 as well as GB-5 and GB-21 on the left side

Progress: After nine treatments and three months, there was no effect so I asked her if she wanted to give the treatments a rest, but she said she just didn't want to go through surgery so she wanted to continue with acupuncture.

(11th) Sept 17 – In addition to the above treatment I inserted needles in both LI-4 and ST-36 and added minute lifting and thrusting.

(13th) The spasms are a bit better.

(15th) Much better, but trimming trees in her yard brought the spasms back.

(17th) No spasms are visible during treatment.

(18th) No spasms during treatment, but she says there are mild spasms several times a day.

(19th) Spasms are down to about three times a day.

Case Study 39

Patient: Female, 75 years old

FOC: August 25, 2010

Symptoms and Condition: Facial spasms on the left side for the last six months, which have gradually become more and more intense. Pain of the spinous process of L1.

History: Hyperthyroidism and hypertension

Pulse Diagnosis: Liver deficiency

Treatment and Progress: SRT applied on LR-8, KI-10, ST-36, LI-11, BL-18, BL-23, BL-58, GB-20, BL-2, ST-2, ST-4, and TB-16 on the left

Direct moxibustion on LI-11, ST-36, and BL-23 as well as GB-5 and GB-21 on the left side

Intradermal needle retained in tender point over spinous process of L1

Progress: She received one treatment in August and nine in September.

(4th) Feels a little better. Added retained needle and direct moxibustion afterward to right LI-4.

(11th) Oct 1 – Needles inserted in both LI-4 and ST-36 and minute lifting and thrusting added.

(14th) Facial spasms are smaller.

(19th) Hard to see any spasms.

Comments: In both case 38 and 39 the effect clearly came from the lifting and thrusting technique applied on LI-4 and ST-36 and not SRT. It is not hard to understand the effect because the face is the domain of the *yáng míng* meridians, but why did these particular points work? One could say it's the function of these points, but why do they require lifting and thrusting?

Case Study 40

Patient: Female, 81 years old

FOC: March 29, c. 2011

Symptoms and Condition: Facial spasms on the right side. She had surgery for this five years previously, and while the spasms stopped, bitter fluids dribbled out from the right side of her mouth. Furthermore, she still had discomfort from the right side of her face down to her neck. Recently the facial spasms returned. Her appetite, sleep, and bowel movements are normal.

History: Last year, on Dec. 25, she fell backward onto her hips and had a compression fracture in T12. She has had back pain ever since. She's also had knee pain.

Pulse Diagnosis: Liver deficiency

Treatment and Progress: SRT on LR-8, KI-10, LI-11, BL-18, and BL-23.

Minute lifting and thrusting on left LI-4 and both ST-36, followed by direct moxibustion.

Needle inserted 5mm in right TB-16 and retained, followed by direct moxibustion.

Progress:

(3rd) Still has occasional spasms.

(4th) Still having slight spasms.

(5th) No more spasms.

Comments: This patient still complains of pain in various parts of her body, but her facial spasms went away completely. At first I thought she would be a difficult case since a problem that resolved with surgery had recurred, but not only did the spasms cease completely, the discomfort in her face from the surgery also went away. This is the power of acu-moxa.

I believe the sparrow pecking technique on left LI-4 was especially effective. The flow of the Large Intestine meridian crosses over to the other side on the face. That is why I treat distal points on the side opposite from the affected side on the face. LI-4 is effective for facial spasms, and my experience bears out that needle insertion on the opposite side works better. In the case of the Stomach meridian, the flow doesn't cross over so the same side can be treated, but treating one side still affects the other so I tend to treat both sides.

Summary

- To treat facial spasms do minute lifting and thrusting on LI-4 on the opposite side, and ST-36 on the affected side.
- Insert the needle 5mm and go in and out just 5 times.

9. Glossopharyngeal neuralgia

I tend to stick with what I like. With my personality it's an effort to try new things. I have been going to a certain bar for almost 40 years. It is owned by one of my patients. One night a woman sitting next to me at the counter was complaining loudly. Her mother had been suffering greatly with pain in her mouth. The pain was so bad she couldn't eat or speak. At the university hospital she was told there was no disease, and there was nothing to do but wait for the pain to subside. The woman at the bar was casting about for anything that her mother might do to get relief. The matron behind the counter said, "Ask Shudo Sensei. He might be able to help." So the ball was in my court.

So I told this woman that there might be a way. There are 12 cranial nerves, and one of them is the glossopharyngeal nerve. Probably her mother had neuralgia of this nerve. While I don't have much experience treating this particular nerve, I've cured many cases of trigeminal neuralgia, which is another one of the cranial nerves. I thought I might be able to treat it with the same method, but that was only a guess, so we would have to see.

You can't be definitive about a condition you have never treated, but you can make a guess from past experience, and with my experience, often my guesses turn out to be correct. In any case, she may have been grasping at straws, but the lady I met in the bar came to my clinic with her mother a day or two later. I presented this case at the symposium of the Japan Traditional Acupuncture Society several years ago, so the details are fresh in my memory. I will present an abridged version here.

Case Study 41

Patient: Female, 64 years old

FOC: January 11, 2002

Main Complaint: Pain in the mouth that makes it difficult to eat or speak

Symptoms and Condition: Pain in the throat and mouth on the left side for the last two months, which causes spasm and extreme discomfort on the left side of the face when swallowing water or food. She had a thorough exam at a university hospital including CT scan and MRI, but no abnormality was found. She was told, "Just wait for it to resolve naturally. Be careful not to catch a cold." She had the same symptoms 11 months ago, but they were mild and resolved by themselves.

She does have an appetite, but eating is painful so she takes a limited amount of liquid foods. Her sleep is good. Her urination is normal and she has four bowel movements a day. Speaking is painful so her daughter explained all of this to me.

Examination: Her face has luster, but perhaps because of the constant pain she looks depressed. Her eyes are narrowed. Tongue has light yellow coating. She told me sometime later that it felt like her mouth was inflamed. Blood pressure was 125/78; pulse rate was 45.

Pulse Diagnosis: Sunken, slow, deficient, and rough pulse. Liver deficiency, and also Triple Burner and Large Intestine deficient.

Palpation: The left cervical region was tense and hard posterior to GB-12 and around TB-16. Left protrusion and tenderness at BL-14, BL-15, and BL-17.

Treatment: SRT on LR-8, KI-10, CV-12, CV-6, LI-11, BL-18, BL-23, TB-17, Upper BL-10, GB-21, and BL-58. On the left side only: BL-14, BL-52, LI-1, and TB-1.

Direct moxibustion on GB-21, GV-10. On the left side only: LI-11, TB-9, BL-14, TB-17, and TB-16.

Progress:

(3rd) Pulse is no longer rough; Liver deficiency. She can speak a little, but cannot swallow solid foods.

(4th) She can speak a lot more. Eating liquid foods is fine, but there is pain when chewing solid foods.

(5th) She can eat some solid foods. Tongue coating is normal.

(8th) She can eat without pain. She eats rice and solid foods.

(9th) Enunciation of "p" sound is clearer. Able to eat normally. Hot foods are fine. She is gaining some weight and her face has more color.

(14th) Symptoms are all gone.

Comments: This is an unusual case, but I found a reference text, and I decided that it had to be a case of glossopharyngeal neuralgia. The physician did not make this diagnosis, however, so it's not definitive.

Case Study 42

Patient: Male, 84 years old

FOC: September 25, 2002

Main Complaint: Pain in the mouth and inability to chew solid foods

Symptoms and Condition: He had pain in the mouth a year before between October and December. He was told it was trigeminal neuralgia at the public hospital. For a month and a half he has had pain on the right side of his mouth and inside of his cheek during meals. When it's really bad it hurts even to brush his teeth, so he has to hold his cheek away from his teeth to brush them. He is on pain medication. His sleep is poor. His appetite and elimination are good. Blood pressure is 155/65; pulse rate 78.

Pulse Diagnosis: Sunken and deficient; Liver deficiency, Gallbladder excess

Tongue Diagnosis: Yellow coating

Treatment: SRT on LR-8, KI-10, CV-12, CV-6, LI-11, BL-18, BL-23, GB-21

On the affected right side: ST-36, GB-38, BL-58, TB-16, and TB-17 (marked induration)

Direct moxibustion on the affected right side: GB-38, LI-11, GB-21, TB-16, TB-17, and BL-43

Progress:

(**3rd**) Oct. 7 – He had excruciating pain three days ago while washing his face. Pulse diagnosis shows Spleen deficiency, Liver excess with Triple Burner deficiency. I added SRT on LR-1, and direct moxibustion on ST-36 and Sawada's TB-9 (see Fig. 1-11).

(**4th**) Not much pain even when eating solid foods. Pulse diagnosis shows Spleen, Pericardium, and Triple Burner deficiency with Liver excess.

(**6th**) Pulse diagnosis shows Spleen, Pericardium, and Triple Burner deficiency. He can eat solid foods. Pain is 80% better.

(**8th**) No severe pain.

(**10th**) No more pain.

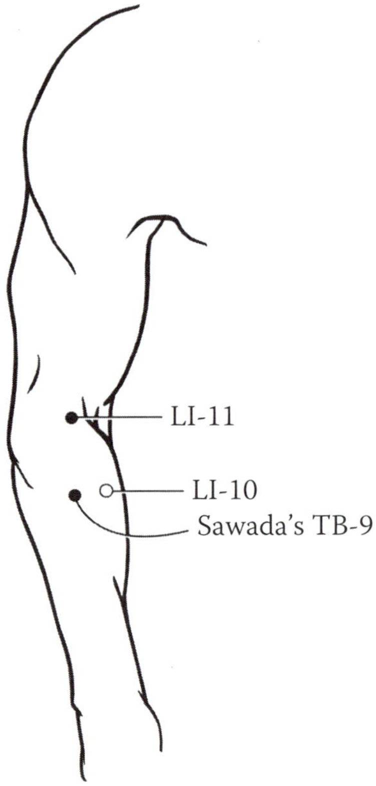

Fig. 1-11 Sawada's TB-9

Case Study 43

Patient: Female, 64 years old

FOC: April 2, 2003

Main Complaint: Pain in the gums

Situation: This patient started having pain in the left lower molars three years ago. Now she has a stinging pain and numbness in her mouth and spasms in the left corner of her mouth. Two years ago her wisdom teeth were removed to see if that would help, but the symptoms only got worse. She has received the stellate-ganglion block procedure 10 times at a pain clinic. She is on pain killers and tranquilizers.

Symptoms and Condition: In addition to the above she experiences heaviness in the head, sores in mouth, flushing, coughing, stiffness in the neck and shoulders, neck pain, numbness in her right arm, cold arm and leg on the left, right knee pain, pain in the upper back, fullness in the abdomen, constipation, is easily fatigued, insufficient saliva on left side, unable to have long phone conversations, food doesn't taste good, sleep is disturbed by pain. Blood pressure is 155/65; pulse rate 78.

Pulse Diagnosis: Sunken, slow, and wiry; Kidney deficiency

Tongue Diagnosis: Red tongue with yellow coating

Abdominal Diagnosis: Surgical scar in lower abdomen. Upper and lower abdomen as well as thoracic area are all deficient.

Treatment: SRT on KI-10, KI-7, LU-5, LU-1, CV-12, CV-6, BL-13, BL-23, LI-10, LI-4, BL-58, ST-36, GB-21, and TB-15, and on the left side only TB-1 and TB-16

Direct moxibustion on TB-15, and on the left side TB-16 and Sawada's TB-9

Progress:

(2nd) Apr. 7 – The stinging pain in the mouth is about 70% better. It has never been this good since it first began. There is pain around the molars. Left ear feels blocked. Liver deficiency, Large Intestine deficient. LI-11 tonified in addition.

(4th) Pain all around the inside of the mouth has disappeared to be replaced by one painful spot. There are moments when there is no pain. It feels like the bite is not right. She finds it hard to speak. Liver deficiency.

(5th) There are times when she forgets she has pain. She had no pain after the last treatment all through the following morning. Tongue appears normal.

(6th) May 2 – She has good days and bad days. Liver deficiency. Instructed her to do moxibustion at home on LI-11, TB-15, and TB-16 only on the left. She could close her mouth completely after this treatment, and there was little pain.

(7th) The pain is much better. She can chew and taste her food better, especially rice.

(8th) Pain is even better. There is no more feeling of having peppers in her mouth. There is still some discomfort inside her cheeks. There is pain and numbness in the rear-most molars. The quality of pain has changed.

(9th) She feels more like eating.

(10th) She is doing well, and less self-conscious when going out. No more numbness in fingers.

(11th) June 3 – She has stopped thinking she wants to die. Liver deficiency. Induration and tenderness at TB-17, and acu-moxa applied to this point.

(12th) No pain in the root of the tongue, but there is still pain and numbness on the tip of the tongue and on the inside of the cheeks.

(15TH) About 70% better. Some numbness just inside the lips.

Comments: Pain in the mouth for three months was resolved with three months of treatment. This patient was unable to continue treatments due to her schedule, but I advised her to continue moxibustion at home. The following two points can be raised concerning her slower recovery compared to the first two cases:

- It had been three years since the onset of her condition.
- I did not suggest moxibustion at home in the first half of the treatment period.

9.1 Concluding remarks on glossopharyngeal neuralgia

As detailed above, I have performed acu-moxa on three cases presenting with pain in the mouth and also deep in the ear. The first case had no diagnosis, and the other two cases had received the diagnosis of trigeminal neuralgia. These three cases can be surmised to be glossopharyngeal neuralgia based on the medical literature and all showed good results with acu-moxa. Unlike neuralgias such as sciatica, the glossopharyngeal nerve doesn't travel close to the body surface, so local treatment is difficult. I was able to get good results by performing the root treatment of Meridian Therapy and treating the stiffness in the neck and shoulders. Among the points that I used on all three cases, TB-16 stands out as being particularly tender and indurated. It is presumed that this point had an effect as a local treatment.

The cause of glossopharyngeal neuralgia is attributed to blood vessels pressing on the nerve. It is hard to imagine that the impingement of blood vessels can be removed by acu-moxa, so there must also be other causes. In terms of the yin and yang organs and meridians of East Asian medicine, from these three cases the cause can be attributed to an imbalance in the Liver and the Liver meridian as well as the Triple Burner meridian. So let us consider the pathway of the Triple Burner meridian for a moment.

A branch of the Triple Burner meridian ascends from CV-17 up to ST-12 and continues up to the occipital region. It continues straight up to go around the posterior ear to the top of the ear and then descends to the cheek down toward the mandible. Another branch of this meridian enters the ear from the posterior end and emerges anterior to the ear. It then goes past GB-3 to reach the outer canthus.

As stated in chapter 10 of the *Divine Pivot,* when the Triple Burner meridian is affected by a pathogen the ears pound and hearing is impaired. Also the throat swells and becomes sore. When the disease originates in the Triple Burner meridian there is sweating, pain in the corner of the eyes, cheeks, behind the ear, and the posterior aspects of the shoulder, arm, and elbow. Therefore the Triple Burner meridian flows from the ear to the cheek and toward the jaw and connects with the leg *shào yáng* Gallbladder meridian which flows in the same area. The above cases experienced pain in this area, which was the symptom common to all three of these cases. Chapter 10 of the *Divine Pivot* doesn't mention the course of the Triple Burner meridian inside of the cranium, but if we surmise that it also flows around the glossopharyngeal nerve, it would make sense that treatment of this meridian would serve to alleviate glossopharyngeal neuralgia.

Summary

- Pain in the mouth could be glossopharyngeal neuralgia.
- Liver deficiency is common.
- The key is to relieve stiffness in the neck and shoulders and also to treat TB-16.

10. Occipital neuralgia

This type of headache is quite different from tension headaches that come from neck and shoulder stiffness. I have experienced occipital neuralgia on occasion and the pain is sharp and cutting. In my case, every time it strikes, I can't help but cry out, "Ouch!" This must be characteristic of neuralgic pain. It depends on where in the head the pain appears, but sometimes it is occipital neuralgia and at others it is trigeminal neuralgia. There is spontaneous pain (unrelated to movement) and they say it hurts even to touch their hair. I have quite a few patients who come in with this complaint. Examining them, I find that they have muscular tension in the shoulders and upper back. When a person does manual labor or is under stress, symptoms tend to appear above the shoulders and neck. Sometimes it appears as neuralgia, or a neurological deficit like paralysis. It can even go inward to cause an embolism or a stroke. So we shouldn't take it lightly because it's just muscular tension in the neck and shoulders. It is really too bad that neck and shoulder stiffness doesn't receive that much attention in Western medicine or even in East Asian medicine.

The key to treating neck and shoulder stiffness, and the conditions it can precipitate like occipital neuralgia, is to regulate the condition of the entire body with the root treatment of Meridian Therapy. In addition, we must find at least one *Ahshi* point in the local area and apply direct moxibustion if possible. In the case of occipital neuralgia, the point could be covered with hair, so it takes special care, but it is worth the trouble.

Case Study 44

Patient: Female, 57 years old

FOC: July 9, 2008

Symptoms and Condition: Spontaneous pain in the left occipital and temporal regions since July 5. There is throbbing pain around the clock, and she can't sleep. She was told she had neck and shoulder stiffness in the hospital, and no CT scans or X-rays were taken. She has poor vision, neck and shoulder tension, shortness of breath, stomach pain, and a heavy sensation all over her body.

Her appetite, urination, and bowel movements are fine. Blood pressure 145/80.

Pulse Diagnosis: Liver deficiency

Treatment: Root treatment for Liver deficiency – SRT on LR-8, KI-10, ST-36, and LI-11

Local treatment – SRT on Yanagiya's GB-20 and Upper BL-10 on the left side; also SRT on GB-21, BL-15, and GV-11

Direct moxibustion on Yanagiya's GB-20 and Upper BL-10 on the left side; also applied on GB-21, BL-15, and GV-11

Progress:

(2nd) Liver deficiency. There is occasional mild pain.

(3rd) Liver deficiency. The pain is gone. Treatment terminated.

Comments: Patients become upset when there is sudden pain in the head, especially when it's never happened before. They think it's a stroke or something serious and run to a neurologist. Usually they are told there is nothing wrong. The doctors who say that you have excessive neck and shoulder tension are the better ones. In the above case, the doctor identified the cause of the pain as neck and shoulder stiffness and gave the patient some medication, but it took acu-moxa to bring true relief.

CHAPTER 2

Diseases of the Eyes, Ears, and Teeth

1. Eye diseases

There is a saying in Japan, "First eyes, second legs." The most difficult thing is not being able to see, and the second most difficult thing is having trouble walking. This is a saying that probably emerged from the suffering of people over centuries. When a person with normal vision loses sight, it is said that they are sure to contemplate suicide at least once.

In Ohita where I live, there is a colloquialism, "flushing eyes." Just like "flushed face," when heat and tension builds in the neck and head, it can cause eye problems. Many ophthalmologists used to advise their patients, "This eye problem is caused by excess tension in the neck and shoulders. You need to get some acupuncture" or "Get a massage." These days few consider tension in the neck and shoulders to be the cause of eye problems. The majority of doctors now think there is no connection.

1.1 Indications for acupuncture

It has been all but forgotten, but there used to be a folk remedy in Japan in which points on the shoulder and upper back areas were burned using a lamp wick. This remedy left small burns all over the back, but it was held to be effective for eye diseases. The aim must have been to reduce neck and shoulder tension, but it does make some sense. There is a deep connection between eye diseases and neck and shoulder tension.

When we think of organs related to the eyes, the Liver is the first one that comes to mind. This association is clinically correct. When it comes to the ocular fundus, however, the Kidney becomes involved. In general, diseases on the surface of the eyes, even if they are rather serious, tend to heal well. This is most appropriate for acupuncture treatment. It becomes more difficult as the disease goes deeper into the eyeball or the fundus. Cataracts, for example, respond slowly to acupuncture, but fortunately modern medicine has achieved startling advances in this area. It used to take couple of days in the hospital, but now treatment doesn't even require hospitalization, and vision recovers immediately.

Where modern medicine still has trouble is glaucoma. They have some eye-drops for it, but it doesn't always bring full recovery. Acu-moxa, on the other hand, can yield surprising results. Often intraocular pressure returns to normal right away. The goal is to get it down to 15 mmHg, and try to keep it from going over 20 mmHg. When patients are examined after my acupuncture treatments, their intraocular pressure is normal so their ophthalmologists are mystified. Even when my patients say they received an acupuncture treatment, many ophthalmologists don't believe it. "That's impossible," they say. Then my patients become annoyed and say things like, "If you won't believe me, I won't tell you about it anymore." Ophthalmologists rarely give thought to how intraocular pressure can go down so quickly. It is too bad they are so narrow-minded.

In terms of disease of the ocular fundus, one that has become common these days is fundal hemorrhage due to diabetes. Ocular specialists attempt to cause coagulation with a laser and stop the bleeding. I get pretty good results in cases of fundal hemorrhage these days, but it's better to leave it to specialists when the bleeding is extensive. There was one case, however, in which a patient being told that it was beyond treatment at a university hospital came to me for regular treatments, and his vision, which had become basically nonexistent, became clear again. Even I was surprised by this. It is true for all diseases, nevertheless, that the sooner patients are treated after onset, the better the results. When it comes to disease of the ocular fundus, we are really in the dark so it's important to consult a specialist and get some guidance. It is ideal if an ophthalmologist is aware of the efficacy of acu-moxa for eye diseases and is willing to collaborate with us. This I believe brings the best results for patients.

1.2 Treatment of eye diseases

Pulse diagnosis: Liver deficiency is common, but also consider Kidney deficiency.

Meridians to treat: Liver, Kidney, Large Intestine, Bladder, and Gallbladder

Points to consider: Yanagiya's GB-20: Often this point is indurated. The needle can be inserted right into the highest point of the induration, but first press it from all sides. It is also good to insert the needle into the hardest place. Insert the needle if the patient has normal physical strength. The needle is angled medially and superiorly. When you slowly advance the needle as you rotate it, you will reach the hard spot. This is the arrival of qi. I retain the needle briefly, from 30 seconds to a minute. Longer is fine too. When you get the point just right, the patient is very satisfied. When you miss the point, the patient won't feel anything, and this point only has a good effect when there is some sensation. When you don't get the expected sensation, you can reinsert the needle. For patients who are deficient, I recommend SRT followed by direct moxibustion.

GB-20: When there is an induration this point is effective.

GB-21: Eye problems indicate neck and shoulder tension. The condition will not improve unless the neck and shoulder tension is released with points like GB-21. This is why balancing the whole body with the root treatment is also important for eye diseases.

LI-14: This point is effective when there is an induration. The point is located over a large area and often is found proximal or distal to the standard location, so you need to search for it skillfully. It is usually 2-3 finger widths below LI-15. This is a Fukaya moxibustion point for eye diseases. Have the patient apply moxibustion at home when the symptoms are severe.

LI-15: Both acupuncture and moxibustion are effective on this point.

BL-43: Look broadly for an induration on the medial margin of the scapula. The induration can sometimes be found on the first or second bladder line.

GB-38: This point is effective when there is Gallbladder excess.

Points around the eyes: BL-2, GB-5, GB-14, M-HN-9 *(tài yáng)*

Associated and Alarm points: BL-18, BL-23, LR-14

1.3 My standard treatment for eye diseases

Supine: SRT on LR-8, KI-10, and LI-11. Retained needle in BL-2 and GB-14.

Direct moxibustion on LI-11.

Sidelying: Retain needle briefly in Yanagiya's GB-20.

Prone: Retained needle in BL-18 and BL-23. Simple insertion (non-retained) in BL-43 and BL-59.

Sitting: Direct moxibustion on GB-21 and LI-14.

1.4 Other considerations in treating eye diseases

Advise patients to avoid work that causes neck and shoulder tension. This includes sewing and knitting and other work requiring manual dexterity. These days many people get neck and shoulder tension from computers. Some people work at computers for more than six hours a day. They often have indurations around SI-9. They must take some measures to reduce this tension.

Does the patient have diabetes? Diabetes influences all conditions. We must add treatment for diabetes when the blood sugar is borderline, or clearly indicative of diabetes. Have the patient keep a record of blood sugar levels as they undergo treatment. They tend to have a ravenous appetite and everything tastes good so it's quite difficult to control their diet, but wise counsel is necessary. Acu-moxa on CV-12, CV-6 and both ST-21 and BL-20 on the left is the best treatment for diabetes.

High blood pressure: Those who have hypertension and arteriosclerosis tend to get sclerosis of the fundal artery, and consequently hemorrhage or occlusion. We must advise and treat these patients to control their blood pressure. The main points for hypertension are LR-8, KI-10 (or KI-7), ST-36, and LI-10 along with CV-6, CV-12, GB-20 and 21 (or TB-15), BL-18, BL-23, and GB-38.

Tuberculosis: It is rare these days, but there were a lot of eye diseases due to tuberculosis in Japan before the war. These patients tended to have fundal hemorrhaging.

Ocular pressure: The eyes become hard when ocular pressure rises with glaucoma. One simple test is to gently press the closed eyes of patients. (Be sure to use a light touch and refer to an ophthalmologist if the patient has had eye diseases or surgeries.) Use the index, middle, and ring fingers to press both eyes. With normal ocular pressure the eyes feel soft. When they are hard like pressing on a board or a glass ball, chances are the ocular pressure is high. These days many people wear contact lenses so ask the patient first before pressing. Hard contacts can make the eyes feel hard. When patients with hard eyes have not seen an ophthalmologist recently, suggest that they do so. If test results show the ocular pressure is in the normal range, there is no worry, but we must stay on top of hardening of the eyes. Advise treatment for prevention of abnormal ocular pressure. When patients present with hard eyes, they always have subjective symptoms such as headaches, neck and shoulder stiffness, and eye strain.

Summary

- Eye diseases are often associated with Liver deficiency; use LR-8 and Yanagiya's GB-20.
- With eye diseases ask about diabetes, check hardness of the eyes, and palpate neck and shoulder for stiffness.

1.5 Varieties of eye disease

Cataracts: My teacher used to treat cataracts with acu-moxa, but I recommend surgery. I highly recommend acu-moxa when there is some problem after eye surgery or when surgery is not possible. The occurrence of cataracts is a sign of aging and patients will be elderly. The whole body is aging so we must pay attention to the body as a whole and give a whole-body treatment. In other words, we must focus not on the eye problem but the meridians. For best results we need to regulate the meridians.

Glaucoma: Always inquire about the ocular pressure number. 15 mmHg is the ideal, and strive to keep it under 20 mmHg. Tonifying LR-8 for Liver deficiency and inserting needles in Yanagiya's GB-20 is everything. Especially concentrate and put everything into the insertion in Yanagiya's GB-20. When there is good focus, the ocular pressure tends to go down. It takes skill. Also find and treat the induration at LI-14.

Retinal disease: These days most cases of retinal disease are due to diabetes. There are other issues such as neovascularity and fundal hemorrhaging. So in cases of diabetes, the problem is not limited to the eyes but extends to the all blood vessels and affects the kidneys, lower limbs, heart, and brain. We must pay attention to all these issues even as we seek to resolve the eye problems. As mentioned above, I had a patient who was told at a university hospital ophthalmology department that the hemorrhaging was too extensive to do anything about it. His vision was 0, but he was able to see again after a course of acu-moxa. Of course, such miraculous results cannot always be expected, but acupuncture can sometimes yield unexpectedly good results. Also there are cases that ophthalmologists don't want to deal with. Patients are grateful even if there is a few percentage points of improvement. I would like to see acupuncturists have more courage to take on difficult cases like this.

Conjunctivitis: The eyes become very red, painful and sensitive to light. It is a very difficult condition to bear. It is often related to tension in the neck and shoulders. Treat this excess condition of tension in the upper body. In times past eye doctors would say, "get a massage" or "acupuncture is good for this." This is correct. I discussed this in my previous text, *Finding Effective Acupuncture Points,* under the topic Yanagiya's GB-20, but I once treated a farmer who was injured by getting poked in the eye by a leaf of a rice plant. Treatment by the ophthalmologist did not help, and she came to me in hopes that acupuncture might. There was inflammation on the surface of the eye and pain. The pain subsided on the way home from treatment. When this patient came for treatment the next day, all the symptoms had resolved and the conjunctiva was clear. Problems on the surface of the eyes heal relatively easily.

Subconjunctival hemorrhage: You look in the mirror while washing your face in the morning and you are stunned. One of your eyes has turned completely red. There is no pain or other symptoms. You rush to the ophthalmologist and are told that there's nothing to worry about, it will be reabsorbed after a while. You are relieved and disbelieving at the same time. Even if they say it's no big deal, it can't be right, something is not normal. With the right acupuncture treatment, the eye will go back to normal the next day. Doctors will say it's due to stress or excessive neck and shoulder tension, but in traditional acupuncture we attribute it to imbalances in the five yin organs, in other words, deficiency and excess in the meridians. Tonifying and dispersing points appropriately will restore the eyes to normal. But here again, one must be aware that it's not just a problem of the eyes.

Dry eyes: The well-known condition with dry eyes is Sjōgren's syndrome. This is an autoimmune disorder in which the eyes, nose, and mouth dry up. Even when eye drops are used for the dry eyes, it is pretty difficult. Acupuncture and moxibustion are highly recommended since currently there is no other treatment than eye drops.

Computer screen overexposure: In Japan this is called video display terminal disorder or VDT disorder. In an age where the use of computers is commonplace, symptoms and disorders related to overexposure to computer screens have become widespread. People stare for hours at glaring computer screens. They use the mouse with their right hand and keep moving their fingers. It is fine when you use the computer for a couple of hours a day for the fun of it (like me), but when it's for work, people are on the computer for 5 to 8 hours a day. When this goes on year after year, it is only to be expected that the shoulders, upper back, and arms become tense and stiff. And this affects the rest of the body from the shoulders to the head and eyes, and eventually the entire body. Along with periodic exercise for the whole body as well as eye and neck exercises, proactive prevention with acu-moxa is recommended. In addition to points around the eyes, treat points like GB-21, ST-12, SI-9, SI-11, BL-43, LI-11, and ST-36.

Phlyctenular keratoconjunctivitis: In this condition white specks appear on the conjunctiva. Acu-moxa to treat neck and shoulder stiffness is sufficient to cure it. When it is associated with tuberculosis, a constitutional improvement is required. For inflammation of the conjunctiva, steroidal eye drops are most effective.

Sty (Herdeolum): This is not an eye disease, but an infection in the eyelid. The eyelids are governed by the Spleen meridian. The pulse of patients with sties is usually Spleen or Liver deficiency. In the Sawada style, direct moxibustion is applied on LI-2 (see Fig. 2-1).

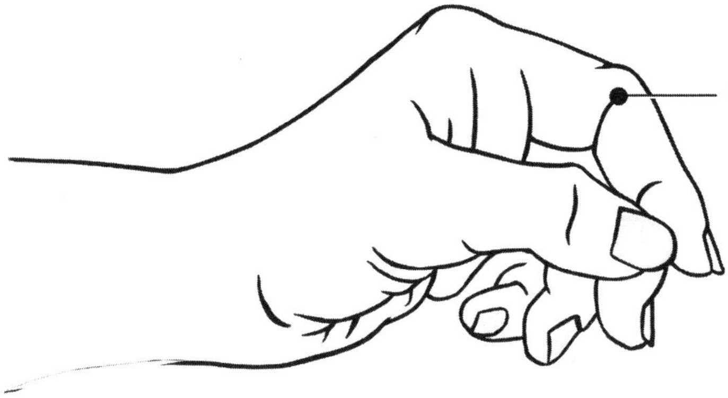

Fig. 2-1 In the Sawada style, LI-2 is located on the radial side of the index finger at the end of the crease on the distal end of the proximal phalanx when the finger is flexed.

Declining vision: As we age our vision and hearing decline. Some seniors are unable to renew their driver's license because they fail the eye exam. I've helped people like this by helping them successfully passing the eye exam the day after acupuncture treatment. Yet we must be very careful because some elders have weakened physically to a point where there is danger of an accident. We can't just be happy that they have managed to keep their driver's licenses. We must encourage them to be careful and continue to come in for acupuncture treatments.

Eye pain: Sometimes there is pain or discomfort in the eyes even where there is nothing specifically wrong with the eyes. This kind of pain often appears along with trigeminal neuralgia. The pain can be alleviated with SRT in the domain of the affected trigeminal nerve and points, especially BL-2 and GB-5.

Diplopia (double-vision): This condition is not related to the optical nerve. It is caused by paralysis in the extra-ocular muscle that moves the eyeball. It is often associated with diabetes. I also see many cases related to trauma such as auto accidents. Acupuncture and moxibustion are indicated. There is no specific treatment in modern medicine, so acupuncture is strongly recommended.

Upper eyelid ptosis (blepharoptosis): This condition is also not really an eye disease, but a dysfunction of the levator palpebrae superioris muscle which raises the upper eye lid. Many cases aren't paralysis or complete ptosis, but quite often the upper eyelid becomes difficult to open. Perform a root treatment and add local points like GB-14, GB-20, and Yanagiya's GB-20.

Case Study 45

Patient: Female, 48 years old

FOC: September 25, 2006

Main Complaints: She has normal-tension glaucoma.[1] There is narrowing in her field of vision. She also has asthma and knee pain due to a sports injury.

Pulse Diagnosis: Lung deficiency, which changed to Liver deficiency in later treatments

Treatment: Needles were retained every time in points around the eye including BL-2, GB-14, *Taiyang*, and GB-5 along with insertion in Yanagiya's GB-20. She has received treatments for six years, once a month on average.

Progress: The asthma and knee pain subsided and her physical condition has been good. In recent years her glaucoma has improved to a point where the ophthalmologist said it no longer needs to be treated. I have forgotten about treating her glaucoma recently, and writing this book reminded me of it.

Case Study 46

Patient: Male, 54 years old

FOC: September 18, 2010

Main Complaints: He has double vision from two weeks ago. He has had glaucoma in the left eye for three years. Ocular pressure is 14 mmHg on both sides. He has had diabetes for five years. He has stiffness in the neck and shoulders.

Pulse Diagnosis: Liver deficiency

Treatment: SRT was applied on LR-8, KI-10, ST-36, LI-11, GB-20, GB-21, BL-18, BL-23, BL-58. Needles were retained in BL-2, GB-14, CV-12, and right ST-21. Needle inserted but not retained in Yanagiya's GB-20. Direct moxibustion on LI-11 and GB-21.

Progress:

(3rd) No more double vision.

(6th) Ocular pressure up to 30 mmHg on both sides. No double vision.

(8th) Ocular pressure normal in right eye.

(13th) Dec 25 – Ocular pressure 35 mmHg on left, right remains normal. Needled Yanagiya's GB-20. Teishin used on all points except those around the eyes.

(15th) No double vision.

---

1. Normal ocular pressure glaucoma: Even though glaucoma is usually associated with high ocular pressure, for unknown reasons normal-tension glaucoma is not uncommon in Japanese people.

(16TH) Ocular pressure down to 15mmHg on left. Field of vision has narrowed.

(19TH) Ocular pressure 18mmHg on left, 11 mmHg on right.

(22ND) May 2011 – Ocular pressure 25 mmHg on left, 15 mmHg on right. Blood sugar in the 200s.

(27TH) Ocular pressure 18 mmHg on left, 10 mmHg on right. Blood sugar up to 388.

(29TH) Blood sugar 280.

(30TH) Ocular pressure 10 mmHg on left, 11 mmHg on right. Blood sugar 180.

(33RD) Blood sugar 189. Ocular pressure remains low along with the lowered blood sugar.

Comments: The main complaint of diplopia was resolved in the first few treatments, and has not recurred. It must have been paralysis in the abducens nerve from diabetes. I deduced this from the position of his eyes when he looked left. His ocular pressure was unstable, starting off close to normal and going up to 35 and then back down. He continues to receive weekly treatments.

Case Study 47

Patient: Female, 41 years old

FOC: March 14, 2001

Main Complaints: Iritis in left eye, high ocular pressure

History: Grave's disease and hay fever

Temperature: 37.6°C (normal = 37°C). Note that I often take the temperature of patients with a floating, rapid pulse.

Pulse Diagnosis: Floating, rapid, deficient; Lung deficiency, Liver excess

Treatment: Patient is new to acupuncture. Only SRT used, no retaining of needles.

Root treatment – LU-9, SP-3, LR-4, LI-11, BL-13, BL-18.

Branch treatment – points around the eye (BL-2, GB-14, *Taiyang*), CV-12, CV-6, Yanagiya's GB-20, and Upper BL-10, BL-58, LI-4, and LI-1 on the left. These treatments will be given weekly until her ocular pressure normalizes.

Progress:

(2ND) Liver deficiency. 37.1°C.

(3RD) Liver deficiency. 37.2°C. The hospital she had been going to twice a week cut back her visits to once every two weeks.

(4TH) 37.0°C

(5TH) 36.7°C. She is using medicated eye drops to dilate her pupils, and her ocular pressure went up as a result.

(6TH) Liver deficiency. Inflammation has subsided according to her ophthalmologist.

She continues to be Liver deficient in subsequent treatments.

(9TH) Her eye still has lesions inside, but the surface is fine according to her doctor.

(12TH) Medication reduced by one tablet. She is making good progress according to her doctor.

(14TH) Her use of medicated eye drops reduced from four to three times a day.

(16TH) Her visits to her ophthalmologist reduced to once in two months.

JUNE 2002: She had an operation to remove uterine fibroid tumors.

EARLY 2003: She had an operation on her ovaries.

AUGUST 2003: She experienced some blurriness in her vision and began to use strong medicated eye drops. Ocular pressure in the left eye rises.

DECEMBER 2003: Ocular pressure goes back to normal.

APRIL 2004: Ocular pressure rises without the eye drops so she resumes their use.

SEPTEMBER 2004: Ocular pressure 17 mmHg on the left, 15 mmHg on the right. Vision in left eye is 0.5 with glasses.

NOVEMBER 2004: Ocular pressure 21 mmHg on the left.

APRIL 2005: With three different eye drops, ocular pressure kept down to 15 mmHg on the left.

FEBRUARY 2006: Ocular pressure 15 mmHg on the left without medication.

2007: Ocular pressure 16 mmHg on the left, 17 mmHg on the right. Duodenal ulcer and polyps.

2008: Ocular pressure 16 mmHg on the left, 16 mmHg on the right.

2009: Ocular pressure 15 mmHg on the left, 15 mmHg on the right.

Subsequently her ocular pressure stabilized at 15 mmHg.

COMMENTS: Perhaps the treatment for her iritis caused glaucoma in this case. The relatively quick resolution of iritis can be attributed to regular acupuncture treatments. Later her ocular pressure started to rise and her vision began to decline. Her ophthalmologist told her there wasn't much hope and that she would probably go blind. This immediately made her distraught, and she probably wasn't exaggerating about what the doctor told her because her mother told me the same story. This patient dislikes moxibustion, so the treatments primarily consisted of acupuncture. It's been 11 years since I started seeing her, but now her ophthalmologist says she doesn't have to go in for exams and she doesn't need to use eye drops. So this positive outcome had to come from regular acupuncture treatments.

Incidentally, the mother of this patient makes an appearance in the section for kidney diseases. She was scheduled to have kidney dialysis the next day, but her condition resolved with acu-moxa alone. Today, 23 years later, she still comes to me once a month for treatment. So the outcomes for this mother and daughter seem like a script from some drama, and they could be actors in a play. The almost miraculous effect of acu-moxa is amazing indeed.

2. Ear diseases (especially hearing impairment)

Visual impairment is very inconvenient, but difficulty in hearing must be a big problem for those who experience it. Complete loss of hearing, a world of silence, can be endured once a person becomes used to it, but the symptoms of headache, tinnitus, heaviness in the head, and dizziness seem to be harder to endure. Since there are cases of people suffering from such symptoms who take their own lives, it must be difficult indeed. I know of an elderly woman over 80 years of age who couldn't bear the incessant ringing in her ears and opted for surgery with a specialist. Unfortunately, she didn't make it out of the operating room alive. Since she didn't have any other symptoms, I do wonder about her choice of treatment. Of all the patients who come to my clinic for ear problems, tinnitus is the most common problem. There is a wide range from those who only notice it at night when it gets quiet to a ringing in the ears that is heard all the time and is quite loud. I get nervous when, instead of being just one of the symptoms, tinnitus is the main complaint that a patient wants treated, as it is hard to resolve.

2.1 Questions pertaining to tinnitus

When did it start? The longer one has had tinnitus, the more difficult it is to cure. It's difficult when someone has had tinnitus for over 10 years, but it doesn't mean their tinnitus will not improve at all. I recommend attempting treatment. Continue for three months, and stop if there is no improvement at all. Nevertheless, a person's general condition such as neck and shoulder tension and balance improve, and one may feel more energy and enthusiasm, so in many cases tinnitus patients will continue to come in for regular treatments anyway.

What does it sound like? Is it a buzzing, ringing, or popping sound? Is the sound always the same (continuous) or does it come and go (intermittent)? Is it a high-pitched sound or a low sound? Conductive tinnitus, which is a low sound that is intermittent, is relatively easy to cure. High-pitched tinnitus that is continuous is difficult to cure.

How is hearing? Check the patient's hearing. Position yourself opposite to the head of a patient lying supine. Rub both your thumbs and index fingers back and forth together right in front of both ears simultaneously. When the patient can hear this sound in both ears equally, to me their hearing is basically normal. Sometimes patients will say they hear it when they don't. If you have a doubt, do this test in a way that they can't see where your hands are. When the finger rubbing is not heard, rub the nails of the thumb and index finger together in front of the ears. When even this is inaudible, the loss of hearing is quite advanced.

Are there other symptoms? Symptoms that accompany tinnitus include dizziness, neck and shoulder tension, and general fatigue. This can be treated the same as "vertigo syndrome." (See Chapter 14.)

Is there a medical diagnosis? Ear and nose specialists are the experts when it comes to ear diseases. If the patient has seen a specialist, it is important to take the diagnosis into account. Antibiotics are very effective, especially in cases of acute inflammations like otitis media. Acupuncture can be effective against acute symptoms, but modern medical treatments also have wonderful effects. There is no reason to discount this.

2.2 Treatment of ear diseases

How do we approach the treatment of ear problems? When it comes to the pattern, the classics say, "The ear is associated with the Kidneys." It is true that the ear and Kidneys have a deep relationship. See if the pulse is Kidney or Liver deficient, and ask the patient if there are any Kidney meridian symptoms like cold feet, tension in the lower abdomen, soreness or heaviness in the low back, fatigue, loss of motivation, loss of hearing and tinnitus. If you decide it is Kidney deficiency, start with the root treatment, carefully tonifying points like KI-7 or KI-10. Also tonify LU-5, or LU-8 can be used instead. The lower abdomen is the domain of the Kidneys, so palpate the Conception Vessel between CV-6 and CV-4 and needle the most depressed point, or otherwise the tightest point. On the back, tonify BL-13 and BL-23. This takes care of the root treatment.

Now, how to approach the local (branch) treatment on points around the ears? In my experience, symptoms of the ears can get worse if too much treatment is done on points around the ears. This is especially true in cases of tinnitus. Therefore it is better to keep the treatment around the ears short and put your effort into distal points. This is difficult, and presents an additional problem of dosage. I recommend SRT on all points including the root treatment, but if there is an induration at TB-17, the needle can be inserted a little. In the occipital region GB-20 often has an induration, or otherwise there is one just anterior at TB-16. If there is an induration, insert the needle a little and retain.

GB-2 just in front of the ear, TB-20 just above the ear, GB-11 just behind the ear, and GB-12 just under the ear are good treatment points if you can find a reaction. I also use ST-5, which was Yanagiya's favorite point for ear problems. When needled right, a sensation can be felt in the ear. Yet it is safer to use SRT on these points than to insert.

Among auricular points, I find the auricular vertigo point to be quite effective. I either retain a needle or intradermal needle in this point. In the shoulders I use TB-15 or GB-21, ST-12. As for distal points, TB-1, TB-2, TB-5, and GB-38 or GB-41.

Direct moxibustion is also very useful. Moxibustion at home tends to create large marks (with overenthusiastic application) so instruct patients to treat distal points. For home moxibustion prescribe KI-3 or KI-7, and KI-2 if there is inflammation in the ear. Also prescribe TB-5 (or LI-11) and GB-21 (or TB-15). Treat patients once a week for three months.

Blocked feeling in the ears. This usually happens when climbing a high mountain or when the airplane is landing. The ears feel blocked, and there is pain in extreme cases. It usually resolves by itself, but it's very uncomfortable when it goes on for days. If it just goes on like that, sometimes it can cause loss of hearing. In my experience, retaining an intradermal needle in the auricular vertigo point is most effective. This, coupled with a treatment for whole body regulation, should resolve this problem.

Summary

- Root treatment for Kidney deficiency – KI-7, LU-5 & BL23
- Branch treatment – TB-17, TB-16, GB-21, TB-1 (or 2)
- Moxibustion – KI-1, BL-23 & GB-21

Case Study 48

Patient: Female, 60 years old

FOC: January 7, 2008

Main Complaints: Sudden hearing loss that started two years ago. Left ear feels blocked and tinnitus in right ear. Discomfort deep in both ears. She cannot hear rubbing of fingers next to ears. She can hear scraping of nails on the right but not on the left.

History: Intestinal volvulus, Ménière's disease, and otitis media

Other Symptoms: Anxiety, constriction in throat, neck stiffness, shoulder joint pain, numbness in arms, left knee pain

Pulse Diagnosis: Liver deficiency

Treatment: Root treatment – SRT at LR-8, KI-10, KI-3, ST-36, LI-11, BL-18, BL-23, BL-58

Branch treatment – Needles inserted in TB-17, GB-20, auricular vertigo point, and GB-21. SRT on BL-2, CV-12, CV-6, and M-LE-16 (the inner 'eye' of the knee).

Direct moxibustion – TB-17, GB-21, BL-23, M-LE-16

Progress:

(2nd) Jan 21 – Liver deficiency. She can hear scraping of nails next to both ears. Intradermal needle retained in auricular vertigo point.

(7th) Kidney deficiency. No feeling of ears being blocked.

(8th) She can hear rubbing of fingers next to ears. She notices that the tinnitus is no longer constant.

(9th) Kidney deficiency. She no longer has to take medications.

(11th) Lung deficiency. Throat pain and hoarseness.

(12th) Doing well. Treatments discontinued.

Comments: I mentioned the saying "First eyes, second legs" at the start of this chapter, but losing your hearing is also difficult. It seems that sudden hearing loss is on the rise recently. It is true for all diseases, but the sooner treatment is started, the better the prognosis. The longer it goes on, the worse the prognosis. Treatment was started two years after onset in this case, but fortunately it proved to be an exception to this rule.

Case Study 49

Patient: Male, 59 years old

FOC: August 12, 2006

Main Complaints: He has had hearing issues for six months, but on July 20 he noticed sudden hearing loss of the right ear. He also developed dizziness and tinnitus. The dizziness went away in one day, but the tinnitus remains and he still feels off balance and unsteady.

History: Operation for herniated lumbar disk in 1998

Pulse Diagnosis: Liver deficiency

Treatment: Root treatment – Needle inserted and retained in LR-1 only. SRT at LR-8, KI-10, LI-11, BL-18, BL-23, BL-58.

Branch treatment – right TB-17, TB-16, TB-1, GB-20, and GB-21

Direct moxibustion – TB-17, TB-16, and GB-21 all on the right side only

Progress:

(9th) Oct. 10 – Tinnitus better.

(10th) Oct. 17 – He has diarrhea that doesn't stop. Applied 20 cones of direct moxa on BL-52.

(16th) Liver deficiency. No back pain.

(20th) Kidney deficiency.

(23rd) Aug 11, 2007 – Lung deficiency, Liver excess. Ringing in right ear. Intradermal needle retained in right auricular vertigo point.

(38th) Ringing in right ear a few days ago.

(43rd) 2008 – Lung deficiency; sore throat.

(45th) Kidney deficiency, almost symptom free.

(48th) Kidney deficiency, decided to continue treatments once a month for prevention.

Comments: Unlike the previous case, treatment was started within one month of onset. Despite this his recovery was slow for some reason.

Case Study 50

Patient: Male, 73 years old

FOC: January 23, 2010

Main Complaints: Tinnitus and loss of hearing in the right ear

History: Pneumonia 13 years ago

Situation and Symptoms: About a month ago when he was directing traffic, his right ear suddenly felt blocked, his ear started ringing, and he had difficulty hearing. The left ear has had hearing loss for 30 years. He has been told that the eardrum was torn.

Examination: Rubbing of fingers next to ears not heard. Scraping of nails next to ears not heard. Metal sound is audible (hitting metal tube against stainless steel needle tray).

Pulse Diagnosis: Lung deficiency, Liver excess

Treatment: SRT at LU-9, ST-36, BL-13, BL-18, BL-20, LI-11, TB-5, GB-20, GB-21, right TB-15, TB-17, right TB-16, BL-58

Direct moxibustion – TB-17, GB-21, right TB-15. Intradermal needle retained in right auricular vertigo point.

Progress:

(2nd) Jan 30 – On the way home from the first treatment his hearing suddenly returned. Rubbing of fingers next to ears is not audible but scraping of nails is.

(6th) Liver deficiency

(7th) He is doing well. Treatments concluded.

Comments: He is an elderly man who is busy as a volunteer, but his recovery was quick because the onset was just one month before. Even when patients are elderly, we can get unexpectedly good results by beginning treatment early. This applies to all conditions.

Case Study 51

Patient: Male, 76 years old

FOC: December 22, 2001

Main Complaint: Tinnitus

Situation and Symptoms: He was hospitalized for treatment of his liver and he had tinnitus after being discharged (right > left). He also has neck and shoulder stiffness.

Rubbing of fingers next to ears not heard. Scraping of nails next to ears is audible.

Pulse Diagnosis: Liver deficiency

Treatment: Root treatment – SRT at LR-8 (retained), KI-10, ST-36, BL-18, BL-23, CV-12, CV-6

Branch treatment – SRT at GB-38, LI-11, GB-21, Upper BL-10, BL-2, CV-22, right ST-19 (retained), right GB-20 (induration), right TB-17, left auricular vertigo point

Direct moxibustion – CV-22, GB-21, LI-11, BL-23

Progress:

(2nd) Dec 25 – Liver deficiency. Tinnitus was better the day of treatment but resumed the next day. Triple Burner was deficient, so I did SRT at TB-1 and the tinnitus stopped.

(3rd) Dec 29 – Spleen deficiency. No tinnitus at all for two days, but sleep is not good since the last treatment.

(4th) Jan 4 – Spleen deficiency. Both sleep and tinnitus are much improved.

(8th) No more tinnitus.

Comments: This case is from nine years ago. He still comes in for treatment for hotness in head, shoulder tension, back pain, and ear symptoms. Tinnitus and hearing loss rears its head when his neck stiffness centered around GB-20 gets bad. His pattern constantly changes from Liver to Kidney to Lung to Spleen deficiency, but recently he is mostly Kidney deficient. When tinnitus is viewed as a symptom of aging, slight tinnitus may be considered natural. The treatments are working when there is no headache, neck and shoulder tension, and he is in good spirits. He tells me that he gets a little worried when there is no tinnitus at all, and he feels better with just a little tinnitus. Go figure!

2.3 Other ear diseases

I recently treated a case of otitis media. The patient is a 60-year-old male and complained of difficulty getting to sleep, but he sleeps fine once he falls asleep. He has been taking sleeping pills to get to sleep. So he's an insomnia patient with Liver deficiency, but he wrote down on the intake form that he contracted otitis media on the right side four months ago.

Palpating TB-17, I found an induration on the right, so I did both acu-moxa on this point for prevention. As for the rest of the treatment I used SRT on KI-7, LU-5, CV-6, and BL-23 for Kidney deficiency. For the branch treatment I needled KI-2, TB-17, TB-16, GB-21 and retained an intradermal needle in the auricular vertigo point.

So it was a standard treatment with standard results. This patient didn't come back for treatment of otitis media, but he told me that it cleared up with just one treatment when he came in four months later with sleep issues. Before coming to me he had gone to an ear, nose, and throat specialist for two months without any relief, but after the acupuncture treatment some pus came out of his ear and the otitis media cleared up.

Case Study 52

Patient: Female, 51 years old

FOC: November 16, 2010

Main Complaint: Tinnitus since a week ago. When she goes to bed at night, she hears a ringing in the back of her head that disturbs her sleep. She doesn't have much of an appetite. She has shoulder tension.

Examination: Blood pressure: 135/90. Rubbing of fingers next to ears audible.

Pulse Diagnosis: Lung deficiency, Liver excess

Treatment: SRT at LU-9, SP-3, LI-11, BL-2, TB-16, GB-21, BL-13, BL-20, BL-23. SRT with dispersion only at LR-2. Needle inserted and retained at auricular vertigo point. Direct moxibustion on TB-17.

Progress:

(2nd) Liver deficiency.

(3rd) Lung deficiency. Ringing in crown of head. Appetite insufficient. White tongue coating.

(4TH) Dec. 14 – Lung deficiency. She has insomnia and feels depressed. She also has eye fatigue and heaviness in the occipital region. I used teishin instead of needles.

(5TH) Dec 18 – She feels nauseous. She also feels tension between her left temporal region down to her ear and neck. I added acu-moxa on GB-20.

(6TH) Dec 25 – Tinnitus is a bit better and there is no more nausea. Appetite is normal, but sleep is poor.

(8TH) Slight tinnitus.

(13TH) No more tinnitus.

COMMENTS: This case seems a bit different from the usual tinnitus. Her hearing is normal and the ringing is not in the ear, but somewhere outside. I believe this is a psychological issue judging from the patient's symptoms and pulse.

3. Dental problems

3.1 Dental cavities (caries)

Even when one has a cavity there are times when it hurts and times when it doesn't. It tends to hurt more when one is in poor physical condition, when there is a lot of neck and shoulder tension for example. Where I come from this is called "upset teeth." Often dentists do not treat as the pain will calm down by itself. It is one approach to wait for the pain to subside, but it is good to use acu-moxa. The teeth pain often disappears when neck and shoulder tension is alleviated. Then the patient can go to the dentist right away for the dental work. This is a benefit for both parties. Just like with eye diseases, however, there are few dentists who recommend acupuncture treatment for neck and shoulder tension. They just don't view the teeth pain as being part of the whole picture.

More recently it is being said, however, that dental problems are not only about the teeth. One issue is periodontal or gum disease. Germs from gum disease can dispose a person to diabetes or arteriosclerosis. One cannot be careless about dental care. Along with treatment of the periodontal disease, one has to be diligent about oral hygiene. The second issue is not about the teeth per se, but there are temporomandibular joint (TMJ) problems. TMJ problems can impact the brain as well as the health of the whole body. So Western medicine is coming around to this understanding. East Asian medicine has always treated the whole body, so even for dental problems the whole body is treated to resolve dental issues. The whole-body treatment in Meridian Therapy is, of course, the root treatment. When it comes to local treatment, more than the teeth, the treatment of the neck and shoulders is better. When there are other problems besides neck and shoulder tension, treatment of these is also a priority. Again, the root treatment is helpful in resolving a variety of problems.

3.2 Treatment of dental problems

Among the meridians related to the teeth, there is the famous "Tooth Meridian" in *Moxibustion Classic of the Eleven Yin and Yang Meridians*, which was found among the Mawangdui manuscripts buried in 168 BCE and unearthed in 1973. This meridian generally corresponds to the Large Intestine meridian. Furthermore, the upper teeth are on the pathways of the Large Intestine meridian and the lower teeth are on the pathways of the Stomach meridian, so the *yáng míng* meridians are connected to the teeth. In *Divine Pivot* it says, "The teeth are where the bones terminate." The bones are associated with the Kidneys, so the teeth are also related to the Kidney meridian. The gums are flesh and therefore associated more with the Spleen. So periodontal disease is related to the Spleen meridian. I therefore perform the root treatment for Lung, Kidney, or Spleen deficiency according to the pulse.

As for the branch or symptomatic treatment, measures to alleviate neck and shoulder tension need to be used. Points like GB-20, GB-21, and TB-16 have a direct result for this. My favorite points on the Large Intestine meridian are LI-4, LI-10, and LI-11. On the Stomach meridian, ST-36 is good.

What about direct treatment of the painful places? This is not a smart approach. Painful places are usually swollen and have heat. Avoid inserting needles in such places, but contact needling and SRT are fine. I also like to do moxibustion on points like LI-4, LI-10, and GB-21. Multiple cone moxibustion on GB-21 on the painful side is also very effective. You must apply over 20 cones.

For teeth pain that persists despite a dental exam showing no abnormalities, refer to the sections on trigeminal neuralgia or glossopharyngeal neuralgia in the previous chapter.

■ *Example of treatment* (Lung deficiency)

- SRT on LU-9, SP-3, and LI-11.
- Insert needle 5mm and retain at TB-16 and GB-21.
- Direct moxibustion at LI-10 or 11, GB-21, and BL-43.

Progress: The pain resolves quickly. Have the patient keep track of the amount of pain and swelling and then decide on further treatment.

■ *Point for periodontal disease*

In Fukaya-style moxibustion there is a special effect point for periodontal disease called *Jyoshitsu* (Fig. 2-2). It is at the center of the posterior heel, between the red and white flesh. It can be painful, but direct moxibustion is most effective if the patient is willing to bear it. Apply five cones; remove the cone before it burns all the way down if it's too strong.

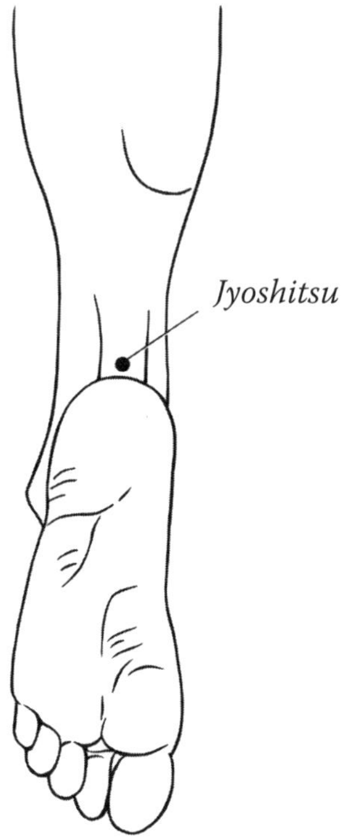

Fig. 2-2 *Jyoshitsu*: Fukaya's moxibustion point for gum disease

Q&A

QUESTION AND ANSWER NO. 1

(Featured in *North American Journal of Oriental Medicine*, issue #38, Nov. 2006)

Whether to treat one side or both sides

Q. When treating points with SRT (other than Five-Phase points), is it enough to treat the reactive point on one side, or should points be treated bilaterally?

A. First, let us think about root treatment. Take a case of Liver deficiency, for example. We stroke both LR-8 points with a fingertip. This is done to locate the point, and one's most sensitive finger can be used. Comparing the points on the right and left, one is more depressed. The more depressed LR-8 is selected and SRT is applied. The needle is removed after the arrival of qi is felt. Now the pulse must be checked. If the pulse has come up and has become normal, the root treatment is concluded. When the pulse is not so good, the other LR-8, or both KI-10, are needled in an attempt to normalize the pulse.

Among non-root treatment points, let's consider the back associated points and front alarm points. I often use back associated points, so in cases of Liver deficiency, I palpate BL-18 and BL-23 to see how they are. It is possible to needle all four points on both sides, but when only the points on the left side are depressed, I needle only those associated points. If all four are depressed, you can needle all four. Why do I do this? It comes from many years of experience, but if I were to explain it in a rational American way, I would say the depressed points are the reactive ones, and that there isn't much of an effect when we needle points that show no reaction. In other words, the manifestation of reactive points on a living body varies. It is interesting precisely because it varies. It is our job as professionals to find these reactions.

From classical principles and experience, in cases of Liver deficiency, the pulse balances when LR-8 and KI-10 are needled. Therefore, it is a smart approach with no hit or miss to needle all four (tonification) points when you are not confident about pulse diagnosis or the pulse is not clear. In my own practice I sometimes needle one point, and sometimes all four. The issue is whether the pulses are balanced as a result. In branch or local treatment, it is enough to needle just the side with the reactive point. There is no need to needle places that are normal.

CHAPTER 3

Diseases of the Shoulders and Arms

1. Neck and shoulder tension *(katakori)*

While *katakori* is not a medical term, it is a word every Japanese person knows. It refers to a commonly experienced sensation of stiffness in the neck and shoulder muscles associated with stress. It has become even more widespread with the prevalence of computer work and viewing video monitors.

1.1 Muscles and points associated with *katakori*

I have a long relationship with *katakori*, or neck and shoulder stiffness. My mother also suffered from *katakori* and I remember she used to call an acupuncturist several times a month to receive acupuncture and massage. Her tension was such that, if she didn't receive acupuncture and massage regularly, she would start to feel sick and take to bed.

My first experience with strong neck and shoulder tension was when I had a pleural effusion (tuberculous pleurisy) in my youth. I recall the unbelievable amount of tension on my affected side. My next episode of *katakori* came after I reached middle age when I was extremely stiff in my shoulders for almost a year. The place that felt stiff was around GB-21, but putting a needle there didn't seem to hit the center of the stiffness. I finally found a point that worked, and it was closer to ST-12. It was a tight area in the anterior scalene muscle. It was as hard as a stick. The moment the needle tip hit the center of this tension, I knew that would do it. I was sure that would alleviate the stiffness. And sure enough, the tension dissipated like fog.

After that, even when the stiffness returned, I would find tight and tender points in the scalenes and needle them for relief. And I started to check the scalenes on my patients, and a large percentage of them had tight points. I would treat those points on the spot, and of course my treatment results improved. Even among those who do massage rather than acupuncture, there is a big difference between those who palpate and treat the scalene muscles and those who don't. I think it marks the difference between those who are good and those who are not.

Once an acupuncturist who had attended one of my lectures came to my clinic for a treatment. He complained of neck and shoulder tension and the area around ST-12 was very hard on the left so I inserted a needle there. I advanced the needle to the center of the hardness and he said it felt good and that the sensation reached his left interscapular area. I explained to him that this was the arrival of qi, and that was fine but he was sweating quite a bit. It was a good experience, but I don't think the treatment was a success. With a good treatment, sweating stops. He might have been tense.

ST-12 (Scalene Point): The scalenes cover a much larger area than ST-12. We have to find the hardest point in the thoracic outlet area in the supraclavicular fossa. If you are not used to palpating this point, stand behind the patient who is seated on the treatment table and grasp their shoulders from behind with both hands. The thumbs are placed on the backside and the four fingers on the front. Palpate especially with the middle finger, and compare the tightness on the right and left sides. Once you are used to palpating this area, you can find the tight spot right away in the supine or side-lying position. Use contact needling or SRT on those patients who are new to acupuncture. Insert the needle when the patient is used to acupuncture. It works when the needle tip reaches the hard spot. When the patient is an old goat like me, you can advance the needle into the center of the hardness. There is an indescribably good sensation when the needle reaches the right place. The stiffness will go away for a while. Acupuncture is enough, but pain at rest, which is rare, requires extra stimulation, as in direct moxibustion.

Another group of muscles that gets stiff at the same rate as the scalenes is the trapezius. With respect to acupuncture points, it corresponds to GB-21 and BL-43. These two points are widely known as *katakori* points, and in Japan it is common knowledge to "go to an acupuncture clinic for *katakori.*" I will start by explaining how to find and treat GB-21.

GB-21: As I have explained in my point location text, *Finding Effective Acupuncture Points*, the reactive area for this point can appear over a wide area. The point moves right and left, forward and backward. It can be palpated in the seated position, prone position, or the side-lying position. When I palpate the point in the latter two positions, I tend to insert the needle. Usually the shoulder tension will go away with one or two treatments, but it is safer not to insert the needle when the patient is new or deficient. It's better not to try too hard in the beginning. When the needle is inserted 5 to 10mm in the side-lying position there is a radiating sensation in many places. It can be felt in the occipital region, temporal region, or the interscapular area. A pleasing sensation is elicited wherever the patient is feeling the tension. Sometimes there is twitching in the muscle, which is fine for those who are used to acupuncture and can handle the stimulation. Patients will be happy when the twitching feels pleasant, but some will be put off if it feels too uncomfortable.

BL-43: This point can be palpated with the patient in three positions.

First is the seated position. Get the interscapular area to open up as much as possible. Some patients sit up straight and assume a posture that closes the interscapular area. This usually happens when they don't realize they are better off relaxed. In such cases, have the patients cross their arms or grasp opposite shoulders to open up the space. Press the point with your most sensitive finger, up and down, right and left to find a reactive point. It will be indurated or depressed. It's good when you find a point that feels right to the patient. Practice finding the most reactive point with feedback from your patient. But you have to be careful because patients tend to want to get as many needles as possible. This is just their desire and it makes psychological sense. Yet our objective is not the same. We want to find which point is the most reactive. So we must focus our inquiry and limit our questioning. Even if you want to needle many points in this area, it's better to treat only about two. If possible, keep it to just one.

Next is palpating BL-43 in the side-lying position. Some patients cannot be treated in any other position than side-lying. Have the patient bend the elbow of the arm on top furthest away from the table and bring the forearm close to the face to open up the interscapular area. In this position, palpate the point on the topside. The needle insertion technique is the same as in the seated position, but it tends to be a bit awkward.

Last is palpation in the prone position. I explained this in detail in *Finding Effective Acupuncture Points*, so please refer to that text also. It is good to have the patient hug the pillow. The neck must be straight (in a face cradle). The head can be turned to one side but then you have to locate each side separately with the head turned in different directions. You can position yourself to the right or left of the patient. I find it easiest to position myself to the right of the patient, but just find the side that is easier for you. Aim the needle under the scapula, and in my case it points left, superior and diagonally. It can be an awkward position to needle but I am used to it and usually can hit the point right on. Be careful with patients who are thin, or those who have asthma and tend to cough easily. We must pay close attention to avoid a pneumothorax.

Let me explain how to insert needles here. It is best to avoid starting the needle by tapping it in. Set the needle as if you were doing SRT by just touching the top of the needle and side of the tube at the same time. Slowly advance the needle diagonally in a lateral and superior direction. Keep rotating the needle and move the needle in and out. Of course, the needle doesn't go in very much. When the needle tip reaches the right place you will feel it. The patient will feel as if you have gotten the needle into the epicenter of their tension. If you hit it just right, the tension should dissipate like fog in the sun. At least that's the way it's supposed to work. When you have reached this sweet spot, it feels like a shame to remove the needle right away. It is fine to keep manipulating the needle for a while. I move the needle in and out very slightly as I rotate it rapidly. It is a very minute, sparrow-pecking motion. It's not easy to add a slight in and out motion at a superficial depth. In any case, if you manipulate the needle too vigorously or too long, it can cause pain or discomfort in the upper back. So it's better not to overdo it. As they say, "Too much is good for nothing." There is no risk if you use a teishin or stick with SRT.

BL-13 & BL-15: The point BL-43 discussed above is on the second Bladder meridian line on the back, but stiffness can also occur at associated points on the first Bladder meridian line. The most common are BL-13, BL-15, and BL-16. These points become stiff mainly in response to visceral diseases, but indurations can also form here with rheumatic joint diseases in the upper limbs. When a needle is inserted in the reactive point, sometimes the patient feels a sensation reach the very center of their stiffness. When this happens, a direct connection is made between the feeling of stiffness and the muscle holding the tension.

BL-11: Sometimes the cause of stiffness in the neck and shoulders comes from tension next to GV-14. This tension is difficult to pinpoint. In my experience, patients feel extreme tension and pain in the base of the neck at the back when there is misalignment or abnormalities in the cervical vertebrae. This is the place where the neck transitions to the shoulder. The patient feels a pleasurable sensation when a needle is inserted here and reaches just the right place. The problem is that this point is difficult to palpate. In terms of the position, I prefer to have the patient side-lying. I press the intervertebral spaces from below the 7th cervical vertebra down to the 3rd thoracic vertebra. I also press the side of the spinous processes toward the vertebral body to rotate it toward the side I am pressing. Often an induration can be palpated in this area when there is cervical syndrome. In cases of cervical syndrome, TB-14 and TB-15 also show up as tight or tender points.

1.2 Causes of *katakori*

1. Overuse of arm and hand: Moderation is the rule for everything. Even in the classics, "overuse" is mentioned as the cause of disease. When it comes to the hand, however, especially since movements of the fingers stimulate activity of the brain and activate brain cells, it's more a matter of degree, approach, and how one feels about the activity. Overuse is not such a big problem if it involves muscles that are used on a regular basis. When we use muscles that we don't normally use, that is, when we move in ways we aren't used to, we fatigue quickly and tension accumulates. When the tension comes from such strain, it becomes important to question the patient in detail about the movement and the focal point of the tension.

2. Influence of computers: The more we use computers, the more we come to depend on them. Is this good for our body? Actually, it is harmful in some ways. It can cause *katakori*, tension in the arms, tension in the upper back, eyestrain, loss of appetite, and general fatigue. The fatigue especially multiplies when the computer is used for work. It's not so bad if you are using computers for the fun of it, but even then one must not overdo it. The negative effects can be prevented with regular stretching or exercise breaks as well as acupuncture treatments. We are moving more and more into an age when computers are indispensable, so this is a big opportunity for us acupuncturists.

3. **Eye diseases:** There is terrible *katakori* with eye diseases like glaucoma. The eyes become better when the neck and shoulder tension is relieved.

4. **Nose diseases:** Many patients with nose problems like sinus infections have tension in the occipital area. BL-10 is a very important point in such cases.

5. **Ear diseases:** There is terrible *katakori* with inner ear diseases like Meniere's disease, but treating the shoulder does not relieve the tension. The dizziness treatment[1] will make it go away like a miracle. In the case of otitis media or elderly patients with fluid accumulation in their ear, there tends to be strong neck and shoulder tension. It is good to have the fluid removed by a doctor, but acu-moxa for the ear is also good. It will stop the fluid from accumulating in the ear.

6. **Dental problems:** There is a deep relationship between toothaches and *katakori* because any dental problem is exacerbated by neck and shoulder tension. Many dentists even avoid dental work until the pain has subsided. When we relieve the *katakori*, then it is possible for patients to get dental work. Sometimes there is a toothache even when there is nothing wrong with the teeth. In such cases, treat the patient for neuralgia. SRT is the best approach. Usually it is related to the periodontal nerves, trigeminal nerves, or the glossopharyngeal nerve.

7. **Abnormalities around cervical spine:** Problems in the cervical vertebrae and cervical nerves and surrounding structures usually cause *katakori*. Orthopedic doctors don't seem to pay any attention to complaints of neck and shoulder tension. There seems to be an attitude that you can't win any awards by studying something as mundane as *katakori*. Nevertheless, there are a few rare doctors who study the treatment of *katakori*. They say there is nothing that corresponds to *katakori* in other countries. That *katakori* is just one type of pain. But that's not what it feels like. The feeling of tension or stiffness is not the same as pain.

8. **Heart and other visceral diseases:** Many patients with heart disease complain of *katakori* on the left side. It is interesting that patients with liver disease rarely complain of *katakori* on the right side. In any case, problems with an internal organ can cause pain to be referred to the neck and shoulders. The reactive points in the case of heart disease are most often at BL-15 and ST-12 (scalene point) on the left.

9. **Lung disease:** There was a lot of tuberculosis in Japan before the war, and much was said about the connection between *katakori* and pulmonary tuberculosis. In recent years the connection with lung cancer is more likely. I suspect lung cancer when the patient has a chronic cough, but I can miss it when there is no cough. It could happen that you see a patient for a long time for *katakori* and come to find out he has lung cancer. This is a serious issue because acupuncturists treat a lot of *katakori*. We must be very careful.

---

1. For the treatment of dizziness, see section on dizziness in Chapter 14.

1.3 Meridians and treatment of *katakori*

I began this section by discussing palpation of points and needle technique for treating *katakori*, but this is the branch or symptomatic treatment. What about the root treatment? *Katakori* is so common in my practice that I have never given much thought to this, but I will now consider the relationship to the meridians. It seems that potentially all meridians could be involved, but the main ones are as follows:

Lung meridian: In chapter 10 of the *Vital Axis* it lists "pain in the supraclavicular fossa" under diseases of the Lung. This makes one think of thoracic outlet syndrome. *Katakori* is up there with respiratory symptoms and colon problems.

Large Intestine meridian: In the Mawangdui manuscripts, this meridian is called the "tooth meridian." So this meridian is also deeply connected to *katakori*.

Small Intestine meridian: In the Mawangdui manuscripts, this meridian is called the "shoulder meridian," so obviously it too is connected with *katakori*.

Bladder meridian: This meridian flows from the inner canthus at BL-1 over the top of the head into the occiput and down the back, so it is related to tension in the upper back.

Triple Burner meridian: In the Mawangdui manuscripts, this meridian is called the "ear meridian," so it indicates a relationship between ear diseases and *katakori*.

Gallbladder meridian: This meridian has the deepest connection to the shoulders, but the cause of the imbalance often lies in the Liver. That is to say, the cold or heat that is generated by the Liver imbalance often spreads to the Gallbladder meridian.

Liver meridian: *Katakori* with Liver deficiency is usually accompanied by irritability and migraines.

1.4 Assessment of *katakori* and basic patterns

Through the history (and intake form) we must find out if there are visceral diseases or other conditions that patients are currently being treated for. Next determine if the *katakori* is chronic or a recent occurrence. If the onset is recent, is there any cause that comes to mind? When we mention a list including overuse of arms or hands, computer work, intensive reading, and stress, usually patients recognize a cause. Sometimes orthopedic tests identify a cause (e.g., thoracic outlet syndrome).

- In abdominal diagnosis pay particular attention to findings around the subcostal region and CV-12, especially indurations. When there is a reactive point in the right subcostal region, I suspect liver or gallbladder disease. With a reactive point in the epigastric region, I suspect heart disease. With a reactive point at CV-12, I suspect stomach disease. With a reactive point between the left subcostal region and ST-21, I suspect heart, stomach, or pancreatic disease.
- In pulse diagnosis I pay attention to the pulse quality in addition to the relative pulse strengths. When the pulse is rapid, qi moves quickly so be careful not to over treat.

When the pulse is slow, sunken, and thin, it is also better to treat them gently.

- For Liver deficiency cases, ask about dizziness and vertigo, and especially pay attention to the pulses at the Gallbladder and Bladder positions.
- For Lung deficiency cases, ask about respiratory problems including asthma and tonsillitis as well as about any loss of motivation. Check for indurations in the supraclavicular fossa (scalenes).
- For Spleen deficiency cases, ask about sleep, appetite, stomach issues, and depression. Look for tongue coating.
- For Kidney deficiency cases, ask about fatigue and heaviness or soreness in the low back. Palpate Upper BL-10, BL-12, and Bladder meridian points in the upper back for tension.

1.5 Hypothetical *katakori* treatment

We have a 70-year-old man with *katakori* that has persisted for many months. Orthopedic exams show there is pain with internal and external rotation of the shoulders bilaterally. Palpation reveals tenderness or indurations at M-UE-48 (*mae kengū/jiān qián)*, SI-9, SI-11, BL-13, and LI-11. It appears to be shoulder tension and stiffness from shoulder joint pathology, or pain that is being experienced as stiffness. He has no findings on the abdomen. His pulse is Liver deficiency.

We apply simple (non-retained) insertion at LR-8, KI-10, GB-38, and LI-11. We then retain needles at the auricular vertigo point, M-UE-48 (*mae kengū/jiān qián*), and SI-9. Then we perform a 5mm horizontal insertion in LI-15 and gently lift and thrust a few times. This is followed by simple insertion at GB-20 and GB-21. We finish up with five small cones of direct moxibustion on LI-11, M-UE-48 (*mae kengū/jiān qián*) and SI-9.

The actual focus of the treatment, after getting a good idea of the pulses and performing the root treatment, is to figure out if there are any reactive points in the abdomen which can treat the stress associated with *katakori,* and also which local point to treat. It only has to be one point. What must happen is for the needle tip to reach the center of the key point.

Case Study 53

Patient: Female, 30 years old

FOC: January 14, 2012

Main Complaint: *Katakori*

Palpation: No abnormalities found in orthopedic tests. Tension in the scalenes is not extreme with the left side being just a little tighter. GB-21, however, is tense with R < L. Her eyes are hard. She doesn't wear contact lenses. She says the ocular pressure is high since having surgery to correct her myopia. Yanagiya's GB-20 is also hard with R < L. She also has indurations at BL-13 and BL-52, and tenderness at SP-6.

Pulse Diagnosis: Liver deficiency

Treatment: Root treatment – SRT on LR-8, KI-10, LI-11, CV-12, CV-6, BL-18

Branch treatment – SRT on GB-21, BL-2, BL-13, GB-14

Simple insertion at ST-12 (Scalene point) and Yanagiya's GB-20

Direct moxibustion on SP-6, LI-11, BL-13, left GB-21. One cone each of stick-on moxa at BL-52.

Comments: This patient was a third-year student at an acupuncture college who wanted to experience one of my treatments. The thing that stood out in her examination was her high ocular pressure. I thought she might have glaucoma, but she said it was due to eye surgery. She told me her eyesight became normal, but still her high ocular pressure is a concern. It would be ideal if we could bring the pressure down with acupuncture treatment. The hardness at Yanagiya's GB-20 also points to an eye problem. When I inserted a needle it was very hard, and almost made me break out in a sweat. The indurations BL-52 and tenderness at SP-6 seem to indicate dysmenorrhea. Rather than inquiring about this, I just treated her with the aim of improving hormonal balance. Her scalene muscles were hard, especially the left side, so I inserted the needle up to the hardness and rotated it there for a short while, and called it good. She probably was stressed out working and going to school. I showed her points she could treat herself on a regular basis. The treatment of *katakori* is like this—very individualized.

2. De Quervain's tenosynovitis (stenosing tenosynovitis)

In this condition flexing the wrist toward the ulna causes pain, as in Finkelstein's test.[2] The radial wrist is also extremely tender, so it must be examined gently. This condition is said to be the most painful among all the varieties of tendonitis. It is important to locate the most tender point. For example, imagine pressing with the head of a match to pinpoint the tender point within a millimeter. Instruct the patient to apply moxibustion at home. Just retaining an intradermal needle at the point will not be enough to cure it completely. It takes time, but this condition responds to acu-moxa.

Case Study 54

Patient: Female, 70 years old

FOC: January 8, 2010

Main Complaints: Severe pain on the radial aspect of the left wrist for about a month. She also has neck *katakori*.

Palpation: Radial side of wrist swollen and extremely tender. Finkelstein's test positive.

2. Patient makes a fist with the thumb across the palm and flexes the wrist toward the ulna. Pain distal to the styloid process of the radius indicates de Quervain's disease.

Pulse Diagnosis: Liver deficiency

Treatment: Root treatment – SRT on LR-8, KI-10 and LI-11

Branch treatment – tender point on wrist, LI-10, GB-21, SI-11, BL-43, BL-17

Direct moxibustion applied on left on last four points, and patient instructed to apply moxibustion at home on left arm at the tender point on wrist, LI-10, and LI-11.

Progress:

(2nd) Less swelling. Tenderness and pain in wrist diminished.

(3rd) About 70% better.

(4th) Occasional pain when moving the wrist.

(5th) Feb. 26 – Tender point moves more toward the Lung meridian. Direct moxibustion applied on new point. Had patient continue with home moxibustion even though tenderness in the local area has diminished.

(6th) Tenderness mild, but Finkelstein's test is still positive.

(7th) Tenderness mild, and Finkelstein's test is only moderately positive. Not experiencing much pain.

Comments: This case, as expected, took three months to recover, but the recovery was complete. Doing moxibustion every day at home is a challenge, but not nearly as much as trying surgery, so it's an ideal form of treatment.

Summary

- Locate the most tender point on the wrist to within one millimeter.
- Moxibustion at home for three months.

3. Carpal tunnel syndrome

When patients complain of numbness in their fingers I think of the possibility of cerebral infarction, cervical syndrome, thoracic outlet syndrome, and carpal tunnel syndrome. I see quite a bit of the last. The carpal tunnel is a passageway of bones and connective tissue on the palmar side of the wrist. Narrowing of this tunnel can cause median nerve entrapment neuropathy. This condition is especially common in middle aged and older women. The orthopedic doctors perform surgery and this brings quick relief, but acu-moxa can cure this condition as long as it's not severe. Striking the affected wrist at PC-7 or PC-6 with a reflex hammer will cause a strong sensation to radiate to the fingers (Tinel's Sign). There are sensory abnormalities in all the fingers except the little one. Pushing the back of the hands together to hold the wrists in flexion increases the paresthesia (Phalen's test).

Looking for reactive points, you find that there is an induration around PC-6 and the point is tender with light pressure, which can cause numbness in the fingers. It is good to do the examinations and orthopedic tests for cervical syndrome (Jackson and Spurling tests, check neck range of motion) and thoracic outlet syndrome (Wright's test and look for indurations and radiating pain by pressing the scalenes) because other pathology can also be present.

For treatment, insert a needle in the tightest point, PC-6. A radiating sensation is felt in the fingers when the needle is inserted just a few millimeters. It is better not to create too strong of a sensation. Going too deep tends to miss the point. The same effect can be obtained by superficial insertion in PC-7 or a point just distal (about 2mm) to it. Moxibustion treatment at home is also good. Treat once a week for three months. If the results are unsatisfactory, it is best to refer the patient to an orthopedic surgeon.

Case Study 55

Patient: Female, 82 years old

FOC: c. 2010

Main Complaints: Right hip pain and numbness in fingers R > L

Symptoms and Condition: The patient points out the location of the hip pain, around BL-53. She has difficulty walking. The numbness in her fingers is such that it interferes with their movement, and there is also some pain.

Treatment & Progress: Weekly treatments alleviated her hip pain so that she could walk and move about quickly. I initially forgot about her fingers in my attempt to cure her hip pain, but she kept reminding me to treat it so I performed the superficial insertion at right PC-6. The numbness in her fingers was greatly improved in about three months.

Comments: This patient had gone to an orthopedic doctor who had recommended surgery for the numbness in her fingers, but she had refused.

Summary

- Check for Tinel's Sign. Insert needle up to 5mm in PC-6.

4. Arm pain

In this discussion of arm pain I will exclude joint pathology such as arthritis, which is discussed in Chapter 6. The most common cause of arm pain is neuralgia, especially that of the radial nerve. The root cause is often an abnormality in the cervical vertebrae. At one time it used to be popular in the acupuncture and massage professions to study chiropractic and osteopathic techniques. I'm sure that the massage practitioners, especially, wanted to incorporate new techniques. I once was a model in one of these practice sessions. This may be the cause, or otherwise it could be the frequent neck spasms I would get in bed, but I once got neuralgia in my right arm. The pain was in the lateral aspect of my upper arm, and occasionally I have some numbness in my thumb. It must have been radial neuralgia.

Another common cause of arm pain is thoracic outlet syndrome (see next section), which is often missed by orthopedic doctors. This syndrome responds well to acu-moxa and it presents an opportunity for us. Chickenpox and herpes zoster can also be the cause of arm pain (see Chapter 14). Finally, there are cases where the cause cannot be pin-pointed in which the abnormality is the whole area. This is called "cervical-omo-brachial syndrome." This condition also responds to acu-moxa treatment.

Orthopedic tests are indispensable for understanding the causes of arm pain. Once when I gave a presentation at the Japan Traditional Acupuncture and Moxibustion Society, someone commented that orthopedic tests were not appropriate for traditional acupuncturists. But we don't give treatments to be true to the classics. We study and utilize the classics to treat disease. So we need to understand disease from a Western medical perspective as well. At least this is what I believe. When the arm is in pain, it is not enough to understand which yin or yang organ or which meridian is out of balance. We can treat a patient when we figure out that the pain is associated with an abnormality in the Lung and Large Intestine meridians. Yet we must subtly change our treatment according to whether it is from cervical syndrome, thoracic outlet syndrome, shoulder joint pathology, or frozen shoulders (adhesive capsulitis). At times we need the help of Western medicine like MRI imaging to fully understand what is going on. So please refer to other texts[3] and learn simple tests like neck flexion/extension, Wright's test, Jackson Compression test, and the Apley Scratch test. Another test that is very useful is that for grip strength.

Summary

- Use orthopedic tests to determine the cause of the arm pain.

4.1 Cervical syndrome[4] and arm pain

The neuralgia that I experience in the arm is not that bad, but it can be excruciating in some cases. I recall back when I used to retain a lot of needles in my practice. I had a patient with cervical syndrome resting on his side with retained needles. I noticed after a while that his face was beaded with sweat. I was so surprised. His whole face was drenched in sweat. It was almost amazing how much sweat there was, but I had no time to be amazed, I had to alleviate his pain somehow. I removed all the needles and gently

3. One very good source is Joseph J. Cipriano, *Photographic Manual of Regional Orthopaedic and Neurologic Tests.* Philadelphia: Lippincott Williams & Wilkins, 2010.

4. Cervical syndrome in Japan is defined by degeneration of the cervical spine or intervertebral discs that causes neuropathy and radicular pain.

moved the painful arm back and forth. This movement thankfully served to alleviate his pain. In cases of spontaneous pain, where there is pain without any movement, it is good to ask about the pain during treatment and make sure that it isn't getting worse. One more thing is that the range of motion and many orthopedic tests for neck pain can compress the cervical nerves, so we have to be careful when performing the physical exam that we don't aggravate the pain.

To treat this type of arm pain, it is best to have the patient lie on his side with the affected side up. Even the supine position can initiate pain in extreme cases. The prone position is the worst. It will aggravate the pain. One more thing is not to massage the neck. Even when a professional massage therapist does it, it is tricky. Alcohol, compresses, low frequency electro-stimulation, and hair work (getting shampoos in the recumbent position) are all to be avoided. When there is spontaneous pain, the pain can be alleviated or even eliminated by the right arm position in the side-lying position. This is probably due to the position of the cervical vertebra that impinges on the nerve.

In mild cases of cervical syndrome, the pain can be alleviated right on the spot, but there are severe cases where nothing seems to help. You wonder why on earth the pain doesn't ease. It makes you want to cry along with the patient. Once I asked the question at a symposium about what we can do as acupuncturists for intense spontaneous pain that doesn't respond to treatment. The responses were to send the patient to a medical clinic for detailed examination, and be sure that the case was indicated for acupuncture, but there was no instant answer about what kind of technique we could use to alleviate the pain. A long time ago I asked Okabe Sodo[5] the same question. He responded that no treatment worked well at the peak of any disease; you must wait until the peak has passed. This reminds me of something I read. In chapter 55 of the *Vital Axis* there is a passage listing situations in which acupuncture should not be done. Acupuncture is proscribed when a patient is drenched in sweat, running a high fever, the pulse is beating wildly, and when the pulse and the disease state do not match. I wonder about when the pain is extreme.

There is also a passage in Sunzi's *Art of War*, an ancient Chinese military treatise, which suggests that the authors of the *Vital Axis* were referencing Sunzi's work:

> Do not rise against that which is at the peak of vigor; do not attack a large and strong defensive position.

Be that as it may, we still want to ease the pain, if not stop it, with acupuncture. As a strategy, I suggest first starting with the root treatment. Use SRT and keep it short, as inserting and retaining needles is not a good idea. In some cases, applying SRT with a teishin is good. On the upper arm, use points like LI-11, Sawada's TB-9, and SI-11. On all these points, go slowly and gently. Ask the patient about the pain as you needle. Use a lot of direct moxibustion. I recommend multiple cone moxibustion (20-30 cones) on SI-11.

When the arm pain is moderate, you can insert a needle directly between the trans-

---

5. Okabe Sodo (1907-1984), one of the founders of Meridian Therapy.

verse processes of the affected cervical vertebrae, but there is risk of exacerbation when the arm pain is strong. Use a teishin instead. Other points to treat on the neck and back include BL-10, GB-20, and GB-21. Also have the patient bring the arms together in front of the chest to open up the interscapular area. Palpate tender or tight points and treat points like BL-13, BL-15, and BL-43 with a teishin or SRT. I finish up with the patient in a seated position and insert a needle in a reactive point next to the spinous process of C7 followed by a few cones of direct moxibustion.

Summary

- Perform orthopedic tests gently to avoid exacerbating pain.
- Perform treatment with patient lying on side.
- Be careful about retaining needles because it can make the pain worse.

Case Study 56

PATIENT: Male, 60 years old

FOC: November 28, 2009

MAIN COMPLAINTS: Pain and stiffness in the right neck shoulder and arm that started three years ago. Pain in lateral aspect of right elbow (lateral epicondylitis). Eye fatigue from use of computer.

PULSE DIAGNOSIS: Liver deficiency

TREATMENT: Root treatment – SRT on LR-8, KI-10 and LI-11

Branch treatment – SRT on GB-20, GB-21, reactive point on right of lateral epicondyle, BL-18, BL-23, BL-2. Needles inserted in tight point on the right SI-11 and tight point of the spinous process of C7.

Direct moxibustion applied on LI-11 and right lateral epicondyle, right SI-11, and right of spinous process of C7.

PROGRESS: Grip strength before and after the first treatment was 40 and 46 on the right, and 42 and 45 on the left. So the results were immediate, but the increase on the right could have been more.

COMMENTS: I continue to treat this patient 2-3 times a month. It has been over two years since he first came in, but he no longer experiences much pain. He still has symptoms, including stiffness, but with regular treatments he is able to work without problems.

Case Study 57

PATIENT: Male, 69 years old

FOC: December 6, 2010

Main Complaints: Pain and numbness in the right upper arm that started six months ago. The pain is such that he finds it difficult to sleep. He also has stiffness in his neck and shoulders.

History: Gastric ulcer

Orthopedic test: Jackson Compression test mildly positive

Pulse Diagnosis: Liver deficiency

Treatment: SRT on the following points with the patient lying on the left side – LR-8, KI-10, GB-38, LI-11, Yanagiya's GB-20, tender point between transverse process of C5 & C6, SI-11, BL-18, BL-23, and BL-58. SRT on GB-21 and tight point on the right of spinous process of C7 with the patient seated.

Direct moxibustion (all on right side only) SI-11 (10 cones), LI-10, LI-11, point lateral to space between spinous process of C5 and C6, and point lateral to spinous process of C7.

Progress:

(2nd) Arm pain is better.

(3rd) Lung deficiency. No arm pain.

(4th) No more arm pain. Treatments concluded.

Comments: In simple cases, just treatment of the arm is enough. When the cervical vertebrae are the cause, to get results in some cases you also have to treat the cervical region. On the other hand, treating the cervical region sometimes actually increases the pain. Arm pain doesn't always resolve in a prescribed way, so it is tricky.

Case Study 58

Patient: Male, 56 years old

FOC: April 21, 2012

Main Complaints: Fatigue and loss of strength in right arm, but there is no pain or numbness

Examinations: Grip strength 40 on the right and 45 on the left. Jackson compression test mildly positive. Spurling test mildly positive on right. Neck flexion to right mildly positive. Patient is right-handed.

Pulse Diagnosis: Liver deficiency

Treatment: Root treatment – SRT on LR-8, KI-10 and LI-11

Branch treatment – SRT on LI-11, SI-11, and tight points next to spinous process of C7

After treatment, grip strength increased to 50 on the right and remained 45 on the left.

Progress:

(3rd) Grip strength 52 on the right and 52 on the left. No more fatigue in the arm, but still feels off.

(5th) Grip strength 60 on the right and 50 on the left.

Comments: The grip strength returned to normal after the first treatment, but more treatment was required to resolve the symptom in the right arm.

5. Thoracic outlet syndrome (TOS)

This condition is one that acupuncturists should be especially interested in, but it is often overlooked by acupuncturists in Japan. For massage therapists also, the difference between excellent and terrible depends on their understanding of this condition. TOS is an entrapment neuropathy of the thoracic outlet that often occurs in conjunction with other problems in the region. An understanding of the anatomy of this region is essential, so please study texts for more detail on this syndrome.

The muscle group that crosses through the supraclavicular fossa, consisting primarily of the scalene muscles, tends to get hard for some reason. We can often find tender points and indurations in the supraclavicular fossae by palpating from behind. Pressing these points sometimes causes a radiating sensation in the interscapular region and down the arm. This sensation is caused by the induration compressing the nerves and blood vessels that go to the upper arm, forearm, and fingers. The key point that determines the outcome of treatment is how skillfully we palpate the indurations in this area.

5.1 Needling the scalene muscles

The easiest way is to palpate and treat the patient in the seated position, but it is safer to treat patients in the side-lying position when they are new to acupuncture, or the acupuncturist is inexperienced. Three levels of acupuncture—SRT, superficial insertion, and shallow insertion—can be distinguished. When you have experience, you can insert the needle and the needle tip hits a hard point in the muscle. There are cases (usually new or sensitive patients) where I rotate the needle at this depth and do not insert deeper. In other cases, I insert the needle a bit deeper, but when the induration is very hard, the needle is not easy to advance. I rotate the needle and advance the needle gradually and eventually the needle tip reaches the center of the induration. Rotation and very slight motion along the longitudinal axis of the needle produces a sensation that is hard to describe. The sensation reaches the spot that the patient feels the most tension. Sometimes it is around BL-43, and GB-21 at other times. It is an indescribably pleasant feeling, and it makes me salivate. Once you hit the center of the induration, the sensation of tension and stiffness dissipates. But as long as the induration is still there, the discomfort will return. Regular treatment is desirable.

In my experience, indurations in the scalene muscles don't go away so easily with acupuncture. You will have to skillfully explain to the patient that they need to be patient and come in for regular treatments. Remember that when the stiffness in these muscles becomes extreme, one begins to suffer from arm pain even when one is not using the arm. Orthopedic doctors have a hard time finding this problem. That is because it doesn't show up with imaging.

Once I had a patient whose doctor found TOS, and he said let's operate on it. I told this patient, "There are cases where acu-moxa cures such problems. Why not save surgery as the last option if it doesn't get better?" So this patient came in for regular treatments. I actually applied direct moxibustion on the induration in the supraclavicular fossa, and also asked her to do moxibustion on this point at home. The pain went away in about three months, and she was able to avoid surgery. I rarely apply moxibustion in the supraclavicular fossa (due to the sensitivity of the area and its visibility). In this case, however, the symptoms were severe and the patient was middle-aged and less concerned about her appearance.

These days I find this problem in younger women. They dislike moxibustion. It would be ideal if I could treat them while it is still mild. As for local points, in addition to the induration in the supraclavicular fossa, look for an induration at KI-27 and LU-1. SI-11 is also good (and better for direct moxibustion).

Case Study 59

Patient: Female, 68 years old

Date of Treatment: February 16, 2011

This is a patient who has been coming to me off and on for 40 years. This time was the first time in over a year.

Main Complaints: Neck and shoulder stiffness. She has discomfort all over.

Pulse Diagnosis: Liver deficiency

Treatment: I began with SRT on left LR-8, and that balanced her pulses. Then I palpated her neck and shoulders. She was extremely tight in her right infraclavicular fossa. The left was tight too, but not as much as the right. She also had indurations at GB-20, TB-16, and BL-43. I had the patient lie on her left side and inserted a needle in the right scalene point. I used a 30mm x 0.12mm needle, and I felt a lot of resistance. I removed the needle and tried again. After advancing the needle 1cm, I hit a hard wall. I couldn't get the needle in any further. I rotated the needle at that point and the needle advanced a little more. I worked the needle in an out at an amplitude of a couple of millimeters, and then felt the needle tip hit the core of the induration. This patient is always quiet during a treatment, no matter which points I treat, but this time she spoke up.

"That's it. I feel the sensation spread into the space between my shoulder blades."

Certainly, it was a pleasant sensation for both of us. I told her that now the tension would go away for a while. Even so, it is not good to allow your stiffness to progress to this point. I had her turn over and inserted a needle in the left scalene point, but the response was less in accordance with what I had palpated.

Comments: As I reviewed this patient's chart, I went back to years before. I had used a blue marker to mark in the figure of a body in patient charts and had covered the area between the occiput and the shoulders, lateral neck, and the anterior neck. In addition to pain in these areas, she used to complain of pain in her mouth and throat. I knew that hers was not the usual case of neck and shoulder stiffness. Later I surmised that she must have a case of glossopharyngeal neuralgia.

6. Fingertip sclerosis (localized scleroderma)

When you practice for as long as I have, you sometimes encounter rare diseases. If you've never treated the disease before, you experience some tension as well as curiosity as to whether acupuncture will work. If you get some result, chances are you can treat similar diseases and obtain similar results. Other acupuncturists can also use your approach. This case is about such a disease.

Fingertip sclerosis, also called localized scleroderma or sclerosis of the extremities, is a rare condition and is associated with the autoimmune connective tissue disease, progressive systemic sclerosis (PSS). One of the precursor symptoms is Raynaud's syndrome, a vasospastic disorder that causes discoloration of the fingers and toes due to localized ischemia. Typically, Raynaud's syndrome is aggravated in the winter and diminishes in the summer. The characteristic progression in scleroderma begins with the edema phase, goes through a sclerotic phase, and then ends in the atrophy phase. The sclerotic phase is the longest and lasts from several years up to several decades. Most cases begin in the distal ends of the four limbs and gradually spread proximally.

Case Study 60

Patient: Female, 63 years old

FOC: Feb 8, 2012

Main Complaint: Pain in the forearms and especially the fingertips for one month. Touching things causes unbearable pain. At the hospital she was told it was a collagen disease called localized scleroderma. She is being medicated for it, but the pain does not diminish at all.

Situation and Symptoms: This patient's mother contracted glossopharyngeal neuralgia, and after being told at the university hospital that the cause was unknown and there was no treatment, she came to me for acupuncture and was cured. Knowing about this, this patient decided that she would try acupuncture as a last straw since Western medicine didn't help.

She is taking time off work because she can't touch anything without pain. It seems to me that this is a case of type II progressive systemic sclerosis. She also has Raynaud's syndrome. In fact, during the treatment I could see some of her fingers and parts of her hand turning white, and pink, and light blue. The hands and fingers feel stiff in the morning.

Pulse Diagnosis: Liver deficiency

Treatment: Root treatment (see Case 56 above)

Branch treatment – SRT on LI-10, LI-11, SI-11 and GB-21

Direct moxibustion applied on LI-10, LI-11, BL-13 and SI-11

Progress:

(4th) Feb. 29 – Added direct moxibustion to the center of the nails of affected fingers.

(5th) March 6 – Pain is worse in the left hand. SRT on PC-4 and LU-5.

(6th) March 14 – Needle inserted in SP-6 followed by five cones of direct moxibustion.

(7th) Pain in fingertips when touching something has decreased.

(8th) Pain in fingertips when touching only in four fingers on left. No pain in thumbs and other fingers. Dark color of necrotic tissue on fingertips as follows: 2nd, 3rd, and 4th digits on the left, 1st, 2nd, 4th, and 5th digits on the right. Patient was able to return to work.

Comments: With difficult diseases like this there is always uncertainty. But you just don't know until you try. There was no change at all after three treatments. In addition to the above standard treatment, I palpated reactive points on the meridians proximal to the affected fingers and retained needles in TB-9 for the ring finger, for example. The patient was able to return to work after eight treatments, but judging from the nature of this disease, I am concerned that she needs to continue regular treatments to prevent recurrence.

Summary

- Perform the Wright's test to see if the radial pulse weakens.
- Assess the degree of tension in the scalene muscles.
- Try to get the needle tip to the center of the induration.
- There is intense pain when touching something with the fingers.
- Ask about Raynaud's syndrome. Acu-moxa has hidden potential.

7. Other diseases of the shoulders and upper extremities

7.1 Cervical-omo-brachial syndrome

This syndrome is characterized by a broad area of pain, stiffness and numbness affecting the neck, shoulders, upper back, and arm. This label is applied in Japan when no specific cause can be found in a medical examination. It is often seen in people in occupations like cashiers and computer operators who tend to have repetitive stress in their arms. Even when the cause is not discovered in Western clinics, I often find the cause by performing both the traditional examinations of acupuncture as well as orthopedic testing.

One of the advantages of acupuncture is that we don't need an exact diagnosis to undertake treatment. So we can employ all the techniques we can to treat as many conditions as possible.

7.2 Ganglion cyst

A ganglion cyst, also called synovial cyst, is a benign soft tissue tumor that can occur on any joint, but appears most often on the dorsal wrist joint around TB-4. These thin-walled, multi-chambered cysts are soft in the early stages when they contain mucous fluid. They harden after time with fibril formation. Usually there is no pain. Acupuncture and moxibustion are indicated. Ganglion cysts can be unsightly and this poses a problem, especially for young women. They can be surgically removed, but this can leave a large scar, which is even worse.

To treat a ganglion cyst, insert a thick needle into the hardest part of the cyst—usually the highest point. Be sure to carefully disinfect the point first. Lift and thrust the needle five times and remove it and then press down on the hole with the palmar surface of the distal thumb joint. Press gently at first and gradually increase the pressure. Don't press too hard. Moderate sustained pressure is best. Soft cysts will disappear on the spot but older, harder cysts will not go away with one treatment. The dissolving of the cyst can be facilitated by the patient applying five cones of direct moxibustion on the cyst every day.

Ganglion cysts also appear in other places, such as the dorsal foot or ankle. Direct moxibustion is the best treatment. Small cysts will disappear when moxibustion treatment is continued at home.

7.3 Heberden's node

Heberden's nodes begin with pain in the distal interphalangeal joints (close to the well points) that eventually develop into hard or bony swellings. The pain goes away as the nodes form. There is a strong genetic disposition. To treat Heberden's nodes, hold the end of a thick needle (about 0.2mm) and give the node a quick poke. Apply one cone of direct moxibustion right afterward.

Those who get Heberden's nodes also have a tendency to develop arthritis in the sternoclavicular joint. It is a good idea to prevent this progression with acu-moxa.

Q&A

QUESTION AND ANSWER NO. 2

(Featured in *North American Journal of Oriental Medicine*, issue #38, Nov. 2006)

Retaining needles after SRT

Q. When using SRT as the main treatment protocol, how does the practitioner decide whether to retain the needle?

A. Reasons for choosing SRT or retaining needles are a little complicated. When I first started practicing Meridian Therapy, I followed Sodo Okabe's method and retained many needles. This is convenient in many ways. First off, when we retain needles and allow patients to rest for a time, the body and the needles naturally harmonize. It also gives you time, and you can treat other patients in this time. Things work out okay even if you don't know how to feel the arrival of qi. Also the whole body feels lighter after needles are retained all over the body.

On the other hand, there are cases where the patient actually becomes fatigued or feels dizzy. Furthermore, you can't feel the arrival of qi if you retain a needle. I changed my approach once I became interested in the arrival of qi and began to seek it. I became curious about the effect of each and every needle in the root treatment, and it became harder to retain needles. In this way, SRT became the mainstay and I no longer need to retain needles. From my many years of experience, however, there are cases where retaining needles a little works even better (even though I haven't actually done clinical trials). I do retain needles for such cases.

Dizziness, for example, is usually a sign of Liver deficiency. It is more effective to retain needles at GV-22, the auricular vertigo point, and LR-1, than to apply SRT at LR-9 and KI-10. These days I don't retain needles very much except in cases of dizziness. Your treatments gradually change when you practice for many years. There is the term "the unchanging and the changeable." Some things are subject to change and some things remain unchanged.

Reflecting on the points where I retain needles in my practice, there are the following:

- Yanagiyas GB-20 for headaches and eye problems
- GB-21 for *katakori* (neck and shoulder stiffness)
- SP-3 for knee problems with heat and swelling
- Onoderas point for cramps in the leg

A question related to the above is when to insert needles instead of using SRT. In what situations is the needle actually inserted? I do insert needles occasionally. Often this is when there is marked induration or tenderness, when there is a strong feeling of stiffness, or when SRT is ineffective. Points that are very tender or indurated are therefore candidates for retaining needles. So SRT is not almighty. This means I am still working on my treatment strategy. This is something I will do until I die.

CHAPTER 4

Diseases of the Low Back and Legs

1. Overview of diseases of the low back

The common perception in Japan is that acupuncture is for someone with low back pain or neck and shoulder stiffness. But although there is a strong association between low back pain and acu-moxa, treating low back pain is not so easy. We have to think deeply and determine the location and extent of the pathology. If you are good at treating low back pain, you become busy. One can say there is a direct correlation. How can we give a treatment that suits each patient? I will outline the key to treating various types of low back pain.

1.1 Questioning

First of all, questioning the patient gives us important hints about the low back pain. If we skillfully question the patient, we quickly get an idea of the pathology, treatment approach, treatment points, and depth of insertion.

❶ When did the pain start?

If the pain is chronic we can treat it slowly and thoroughly. There is no hurry. If the pain started recently (acute), however, we have to be careful. We must ask what brought it on. Was there a sudden onset; was the back overworked or strained? If this is the case, myofascial back pain or a muscle strain is likely. It could also be a presage of lumbar disc herniation.

❷ When do you feel the worst pain?

When there is pain in moving the low back it is generally a back spasm or damage to the muscles and soft tissue. When there is pain at rest and difficulty lying supine, suspect acute neuropathy or lumbar disc herniation. When there is low back pain at night that has been getting progressively worse, suspect cancer. Back pain that comes on while getting out of bed in the morning and eases after more than an hour is an arthritic pain known as "morning back stiffness." Low back pain only while walking can be spinal stenosis, lumbar disc herniation, or arteriosclerosis obliterans.

3. Where does it hurt?

   The low back is a broad area so we need to know the location of the pain. Have the patient point to the place that hurts. The location of where the pain comes from and the place a patient points to is sometimes different, so remember that the pathology and the site of pain are not always the same.

4. What is the cause?

   Often patients respond that they don't know, but have them reflect a bit because sometimes they remember that they did some yard work they weren't used to, standing on a ladder trimming a tree. If we know the cause of the back pain, we can treat them without worry.

5. Have you had surgery recently?

   If a patient has had surgery for cancer in the last five years, we must rule out recurrence and metastases.

   Other important questions are whether they have been treated in a medical facility, and what the diagnosis was. This type of diagnosis is useful information.

1.2 Orthopedic tests

When patients have symptoms below the waist, I perform a few simple orthopedic tests. Some people are surprised that a classical acupuncturist like myself does such tests, but these tests are useful for gaining evidence as to the pathological condition from a Western medical perspective as well as deciding what kind of branch treatment to perform. They are also useful for explaining what is going on to the patient. The tests I perform most often are as follows:

1. Palpate the dorsal pedis artery (ST-42) and the posterior tibial artery (KI-3). Difficulty in feeling the pulse indicates arteriosclerosis obliterans.

2. Extension and flexion of big toes against resistance. Diminished strength on one side could be impingement of L4 or L5 spinal nerves.

3. Straight leg raising test: With patient supine, raise affected leg up to 90 degrees if possible. Severe pain in the back indicates disc lesion, while pain down the leg indicates sciatica.

4. Bonnet test: Flex the hip and knee joints of the affected leg and place the foot on the lateral side of the normal leg, then press the knee of the affected leg toward

the opposite side (medially rotate hip). This test is positive when this movement causes pain in the hip or posterior leg (along the course of the sciatic nerve) and lateral rotation diminishes it.

5. Patrick test: Abduct and laterally rotate the leg, bend the knee, and place the foot over the opposite knee. If there is pain when pressing down on the flexed knee, this indicates hip or sacroiliac pathology.

6. Deep tendon reflex: Strike patellar tendon with reflex hammer. Decreased reflex indicates a lesion in L2 to L4 spinal nerves. Exaggerated reflex indicates central nervous system involvement.

All of these tests give better information when one is proficient with them, so it is important to practice them. Once I inquire about the main complaint and perform a few orthopedic tests, I proceed to abdominal and pulse diagnosis.

Summary

- Question skillfully and perform orthopedic tests to determine the cause.

1.3 Abdominal palpation and pulse diagnosis

Abdominal palpation: Palpate to see if there are any tight or hard areas. I palpate lightly over the surface to see if there are any depressed or tense areas to help determine the pattern. This process is described in detail in my first text, *Japanese Classical Acupuncture: Introduction to Meridian Therapy.*

Pulse diagnosis: It is important to be able to discern at least the six basic pulse qualities of floating or submerged, rapid or slow, and excessive or deficient. Again, refer to my first text for more details on pulse diagnosis. Be careful with patients with a rapid pulse. Also, those with submerged or excessive pulses are hard to treat. In terms of pulse diagnosis and patterns for low back pain patients, I find that back sprains and pain with movement are often Liver deficiency. Dull and heavy pain in the back are often Kidney deficiency. I suspect Spleen deficiency in cases of "morning back stiffness," but it is hard to say until I check the pulses.

Prognosis: It is possible to guess if the back pain will resolve quickly or if it will be a long process. This is based on the orthopedic tests and whether there is neuropathy or arthritis, but in general the more recent the pain, the faster the recovery. Explain this to the patient.

1.4 Types of low back pain and basic approach

In my practice I make a quick assessment of the type of low back pain, and then I continue to carefully examine the patient to check my assessment. Here I will provide a quick summary of different types of low back pain—what I look for and how I treat them.

Back strain (myofascial low back pain): The key to treating back strains is to precisely locate the site of soft tissue injury (usually an Ahshi point around the Iliac point, BL-27 or BL-52). The trick is to get the needle tip right to the center of the problem area. If we can do this, the pain resolves with a few treatments. It will take a lot longer if it progresses to become a disc lesion. The pattern is often Liver deficiency. LR-8 is the principal point—use SRT to tonify this point.

Lumbar disc herniation & sciatica: Some cases resolve relatively quickly, while others take time. The pattern is often Liver deficiency. Apply SRT on LR-8 or LR-1. For branch treatment, apply SRT on BL-25, Ischial point, and BL-59 (see Fig. 4-1).

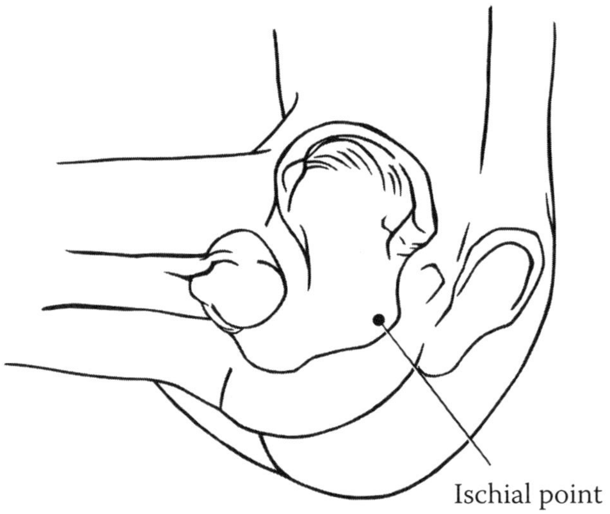

Fig. 4-1 Ischial point

Osteoporosis & spondylosis deformans: Do not press on the spine if the integrity of the vertebrae is compromised. Stroke over the back to locate and treat points. Recovery takes a long time. The pattern is usually Kidney or Spleen deficiency.

Morning back stiffness (osteoarthritis): The pattern is often Spleen deficiency. Perform SRT or superficial needling at SP-3.

Back pain in bed: The symptomatic treatment points are the Iliac point, BL-25 or BL-27, BL-52, and BL-23. Usually there are not many reactions like tenderness and induration, so instead perform SRT or superficial needling in depressed points.

Damage to interspinous ligaments: This problem can occur at any level of the spine. The tender points over the spine serve as treatment points. Use multiple-cone moxibustion (over 10 cones) on local points. Also retain intradermal needles.

Pain over spinous processes: Retain intradermal needles in tender points over affected spinous processes.

Urethral calculus (kidney stone): This type of low back pain is best treated using tonification points based on the pattern. For example, if it is associated with Spleen deficiency, retain needles superficially in points like SP-3 and SP-8 (cleft point).

Menstrual low back pain: Apply stick-on moxa to BL-52.

Occlusive arteriosclerosis: It is difficult to walk any distance. Can the pulse be palpated in arteries in the foot? (See section on occlusive arteriosclerosis in Chapter 5.)

Spinal stenosis: The pain makes it difficult to walk any distance, but resting in a bent forward posture brings quick recovery. Pulses can be felt on the foot. Do they have numbness in their legs? Insert needle in BL-25.

2. Back strain (myofascial low back pain)

One look and it is easy to tell a back strain patient. They walk bent forward or to one side. Most cases come on suddenly with a casual movement. When the pain is extreme, the patient cannot lie supine. Examine them in any position they can assume. When I tell them, "Please rest in a comfortable posture," most always they lie on their side. Usually they lie with the painful side up. If possible, have them bend the knee of the top leg and place it down in front on the treatment table. This posture tends to relax the back muscles and makes palpation easier. If the patient has difficulty with this posture, suspect an abnormality in the hip joint that is on top.

Confirm that they don't have spontaneous pain (pain at rest) and begin the examination of the spine and lumbar region. It is probably damage to interspinous ligaments if there are big spaces between the spinous processes or there is tenderness between them. This is best treated with multiple-cone moxibustion.

Next palpate the Iliac point. Use the middle finger and press toward the iliac crest as if to scoop under it. This is the area just lateral to the top of the sacro-iliac joint. If you can find an obvious induration you are in luck. Now slide your finger toward the spine from the Iliac point and look for a reaction at BL-27. If you can find a tight point that is clearly different from the others, this could be the center of the lesion. Next palpate BL-52, which is easier to find a reaction at in the side-lying position. Finally, examine the muscle tension around BL-23. Again, this is easier to do than in the prone position. Note any indurations, tender points, depressions, and abnormally warm points. (Leave these local points alone in treatment; instead, see if you can get them to change with the root treatment.)

So these are the key points: M-BW-25 *(josen/shí qī zhuī xià),* the Iliac point, BL-25, BL-27, or BL-52 are the places most likely to be at the center of the lesion. BL-23 is the next most likely point. Mark all the reactive points. Ask the patient as you palpate to find the most painful point. Usually it is just one point, but occasionally there are several lesion sites.

When the patients aren't able to lie supine, I take their pulses in the side-lying position. If I find that they are Liver deficient, for example, I palpate the five-phase points of the Liver and Kidney meridians of the leg on the bottom. I tonify the points that are the most depressed. Then I find and treat indurated points on the yang meridian of the leg on top—the Bladder and Gallbladder meridians in the case of Liver deficiency.

There are the following associations of patterns and meridians with different types of low back pain:

1. Pain with movement, Liver deficiency: Bladder and Gallbladder meridians
2. Deep pain, Kidney deficiency: Bladder and Large Intestine meridians
3. Spontaneous pain (pain at rest), Spleen deficiency: Stomach and Triple Burner meridians

2.1 Order of treatment

I begin the treatment with distal points—usually the root treatment. It is not necessarily wrong to treat the local area first, but the more severe and complicated a pain case is, the more careful you need to be with the local area and leave it for later. So in the case of Liver deficiency, I would tonify LR-8, KI-10, and perhaps LR-1. Then I would also do SRT on indurations at points like BL-59, BL-39, and GB-38. After this I have patients move and see how their back pain is. If it is any better, their prospects are good. When the damage in the muscles is extensive or they have symptoms like mild fever, rapid pulse, feeling chilled and dark urine, the pain does not improve at all.

I then move to the local treatment. I apply SRT on the tender points that I have marked on the back. I use quite a bit of focus and give it my best. This is followed with direct moxibustion. The top candidate for direct moxibustion on the leg is BL-59. I have five cones applied on two or three points on the low back or hips. It is also helpful to find a point that is tender with deep pressure close to the source of the pain, often in the quadratus lumborum or the glutes. Once this point is found, I apply 10 cones on it.

Then I have the patient move again. Sometimes the pain is better, and at other times there is no change at all. When there is no change, I consider slightly inserting the needle in the point closest to the problem. I begin with SRT, and then carefully advance the needle. I am in luck if the qi arrives near the surface. Then the pain will ease.

If the pain improves without extra treatment on the local area, I have the patient lie supine and recheck the pulse and do a few orthopedic tests. I have the patient get up from the treatment table and move their waist to assess the extent of relief. In cases of severe pain, it is rare for the pain to go away in one treatment. It takes repeated treatments, if possible every day, so that it can be resolved quickly. Sometimes I retain an intradermal in the local reactive point. Moxibustion at home is also good. Prohibit immersive bathing and the use of alcohol. They can toast after the back pain is cured.

In cases of mild low back pain, I have the patient lie supine, check the pulse, do some orthopedic tests, determine the pattern, select points, and start a distal treatment. SRT is sufficient. I then have the patient lie prone and palpate for reactive points in the problem area. I insert needles in these points. The needles inserted in the Iliac point hits right on the damaged spot in 5 to 10mm if things go right. I feel the arrival of qi. It is an indescribably good feeling. The patient also says that the needle reaches the most painful spot. When the patient feels nothing, either the point location is off, or the patient is insensitive. If the former is the case, we have to repalpate the point and try again. If the latter is the case, the patient may say after a while, "Oh, I feel it!" So if we are sure we feel the arrival of qi, we don't have to ask the patient. Have them move their waist while still on the table and inquire about the pain and continue needling. Sometimes I will insert two needles in the same point. But it's better stop at twice. More stimulation can make the pain worse. This is what makes local treatment so difficult.

In mild cases one treatment is all it takes. With younger patients, even if the pain doesn't go away completely, it will resolve by itself without treatment. That is because their natural healing powers are robust. Some people have financial constraints, so it's better to conclude treatments as soon as possible.

There are cases where a back sprain resolves, but then pain develops in the hips or a leg. This means the back sprain was actually a precursor symptom to herniation of a lumbar disc. In such cases, we need to give treatment for disc herniation (refer to the next section). When patients have repeated back sprains, there is a high probability that they will develop sciatica. Moxibustion at home in the early stage can serve as a preventative.

3. Cases of damage to interspinous ligaments

Low back pain caused by damage to interspinous ligaments is actually quite common, but recovery is delayed when we fail to find this problem. Rather than developing gradually, the damage tends to manifest all of a sudden. The German term for acute low back pain, *hexenschuss* (literally, a shot unleashed by a witch), describes it perfectly. Sometimes there is a snap when the interspinous ligament tears. In severe cases, the interspinous ligament tears apart completely. There is a snapping sound and a person is instantly immobilized. Be that as it may, this condition does not require surgery, and acu-moxa can cure it.

Treatment outcomes are good when direct moxibustion is used. The key to treatment is to locate the lesion precisely. To find the lesion, palpate over the lumbar spine, pressing gently with a fingertip. You will find a space between the spinous process that is soft, one might even call it boggy. This is clear when you compare it with the spaces one spinous process above and one below. Sometimes the lesion is chronic. In any case, precise location is the key to successful treatment.

Looking out from my clinic at an approaching patient it is clear how a patient is doing. The following patient arrived bent forward and leaning to one side. He appeared to be in a lot of pain. Thus the looking exam begins even before the patient enters the clinic.

Case Study 61

Patient: Male, 32 years old

FOC: Year unknown: February 18

Questioning: He thinks that lifting a washing machine on the evening of February 14 was the cause. His low back was in so much pain the next morning that he couldn't walk without bending forward. He forced himself to go to work, but it only got worse.

Q. "Is the pain only in the low back, or does it extend into the hips and legs?"

A. "It's only in the low back."

Q. "Is there pain without movement?"

A. "The pain is intense when I move."

He couldn't lie on his back, let alone face down, so I asked him to lie on his side. He elected to lie with his right side up. I had him extend his left leg and flex his right leg and place the knee down on the treatment table. He says this movement was painful, so I asked him to get in a more comfortable position. He moved his upper body and waist and seemed to settle down.

Q. "Where does it hurt the most?"

A. "It hurts all over the low back, and it's hard to say where in particular."

Pulse Diagnosis: Wiry and slightly rapid. It is hard to tell which position is weakest in the side-lying position, so I just call it Liver deficiency.

Examinations: The dorsiflexion of his big toes are normal. I lightly strike his ischial tuberosity on the leg on top, but this does not exacerbate the pain. It appears that the sciatic nerve is not affected.

Treatment: I palpated reactive points especially carefully – BL-52, BL-23, BL-27, and the Iliac point, but there is no clear reaction. BL-59 on the leg is the only reactive point. I went ahead and applied SRT on all the above points. Then direct moxibustion was applied on BL-23, the Iliac point, and right BL-59.

Probably due to assuming strange postures to avoid pain, his neck and shoulders are stiff. I also applied SRT on GB-20 and GB-21. Then I had him turn over to lie on his right side. With this movement, it was clear that his pain was no better. Palpating reactive points in this position, I found the same thing as the other side. When I was palpating the Governing vessel with my middle finger, however, he said, "Ouch!" Palpating more carefully I found a tender point between the spinous process of the 5th lumbar vertebra and the sacrum. This is the point called M-BW-25 *(josen/shí qī zhuī xià)*. Depending on how much pressure I applied with my middle finger, it was extremely tender. After doing the same acupuncture as the other side, I applied 30 cones of direct moxibustion on M-BW-25 *(josen/shí qī zhuī xià)*.

I had the patient lie supine after this, and he said it felt much better. So I told him

"It's easier when you bend your knees, so you can bend them." But he replied, "It's alright, they can be straight." So I checked his pulse again, and found it showed Liver deficiency after all. I applied SRT on LR-8, KI-10, LR-4, LU-8, and ST-36. Then I asked the patient to get up. His movements looked better. I had him sit up on the table. He had no pain. I asked him to stand up. He could stand straighter. He still couldn't stand completely straight. He was bent slightly forward because there was still some residual pain. But he appeared almost normal walking away.

Point Selection: LR-4 and LU-8 were needled to disperse the Lung meridian, which is in a five-phases controlling relationship with the Liver. BL-59 is especially effective for pain in the low back and legs. It is just as important as BL-58. BL-59 is effective for the low back and legs. BL-58 is effective for the head, occipital region, and upper back. In simple cases of back sprain, one root treatment point and one branch treatment point is enough to give dramatic results. The patient is mystified and can't understand where the pain went, but this is the work of a professional. We can provide an explanation, but it's hard to believe.

Comments: In this case, I did not palpate the tenderness over the spine right away because the patient was lying on his side and his back was in flexion. If I had missed this, quick relief would have been unlikely, and he would have had to suffer for several more days. This case highlights the importance of careful palpation and the need to hone the skill of finding the one point related to the lesion. This takes a lifetime of practice.

Case Study 62

Patient: Female, 61 years old

FOC: November 20, 2007

Situation and Symptoms: This morning she had a back spasm when she carried her mother. There is pain over the entire low back with movement, but no pain without movement.

Pulse Diagnosis: Liver deficiency

Treatment: SRT applied on LR-8, KI-10, BL-52, Iliac point, BL-40, BL-58, and BL-59. Then direct moxibustion was applied on BL-52 and the Iliac point.

I had the patient get up off the treatment table. She still had pain, but it was focused on the midline—on the Governing vessel. I had her sit down on the table and bend forward and palpated her spine from behind. It seemed like M-BW-25 *(josen/shí qī zhuī xià)* was slightly depressed, so I applied SRT with the patient seated. After I applied just a little rotation the patient exclaimed, "Oh, I really feel that!" It seems that she felt the needle sensation reach the center of her pain. I concluded the treatment with 20 cones of direct moxibustion on M-BW-25 *(josen/shí qī zhuī xià)*. I instructed the patient to come back one more time if her pain hadn't completely resolved.

Progress: This is another case where I didn't detect the damage to the interspinous ligament right away. The patient went to bed after returning home, and the pain was gone when she woke up. Treatment was concluded with her second visit.

Case Study 63

Patient: Male, 13 years old

FOC: March 26, 2011

Symptoms and Condition: Pain on the left side of the low back. He felt a spasm two weeks ago when he twisted his back. The pain has continued unchanged. He was told at a hospital that he had spondylolysis and a stress fracture, and he would have to wear a brace for six months for complete recovery.

Examination: Marked tenderness at M-BW-25 *(josen/shí qī zhuī xià)*

Pulse Diagnosis: Liver deficiency

Treatment: SRT applied on LR-8 and KI-10. Needles were inserted at BL-59 and only on the left side at BL-52 and the Iliac point. This was followed by 20 cones of direct moxibustion on M-BW-25 *(josen/shí qī zhuī xià)*. Finally, an intradermal needle was retained in this point.

Progress:

(2nd) March 30 – Lung deficiency. Pain is a little better.

(4th) April 13 – Liver deficiency. The pain is gone.

Comments: Based on the finding of marked tenderness at M-BW-25 *(josen/shí qī zhuī xià)*, it seems that this was a case of damage to interspinous ligaments. It would really be something if spondylolysis and a stress fracture could be cured in just three treatments.

Summary

- Apply multiple-cone moxibustion on M-BW-25 *(josen/shí qī zhuī xià)* when there is tenderness.

4. Lumbar disc herniation and sciatica

Leg pain that develops after myofascial low back pain, or that just happens by itself, is often caused by lumbar disc herniation. There are acute and chronic cases.

4.1 Acute cases

In acute cases there is often spontaneous pain (pain at rest). Many patients cannot lie supine because of the pain. Lying prone is even worse, but there are exceptions where lying prone relieves the pain. The position that relieves the pain most often, however, is side-lying. Lying on the good side with the bottom leg extended, and flexing the hip and knee of the top leg, puts the least stretch on the sciatic nerve. Lying prone puts the greatest stretch on the sciatic nerve. That is what causes the pain. As descriptions of the pain, there is a whole range from excruciating pain to dull pain. It can interrupt sleep and sometimes the pain even affects appetite.

> *"Do not treat when the symptoms are severe and the force of the disease is robust. This was the basic policy of ancient physicians."*
>
> —TRANSLATION BY Iemoto Sei-ichi of Chapter 55 of the *Vital Axis*

This approach was adapted from ancient military strategy. I once asked about treatment for extreme pain. Okabe Sodo (one of the founders of Meridian Therapy) referred to the above passage and said that one should "wait until the pain settles down." The other teachers in the symposium gave similar answers. They said patients had to be referred to a specialist, or that it was out of the scope of acu-moxa. Does that mean that we can't treat spontaneous pain or extreme pain with acupuncture? Is there no other option than hospitalization even when the patient has already received a medical exam and diagnosis? There had to be cases in classical times when treatments were occasionally given, even going against standard practices. There is a passage in the *Systematic Classic of Acupuncture and Moxibustion* (*Zhen jiu jia yi jing*) that says something to the effect that prohibiting treatment is because one doesn't yet have the skill. The reason it cannot be treated is because your skill is still underdeveloped. I believe it is possible if you have developed the skill.

4.2 Acute cases with strong spontaneous pain (pain at rest)

The patient who has severe spontaneous pain can only lie on their side. So I do the root treatment in this position with the leg closest to the table extended and the top leg flexed. Often they have Liver deficiency, so I do SRT on points on the bottom leg. Usually the pain increases the more I insert the needle, so I avoid insertion. I use points on the top leg like GB-38 and 41 on the Gallbladder meridian, and points like BL-59, BL-58, and BL-39 on the Bladder meridian. Next I start the branch treatment. I treat points like BL-25, BL-27, and the Ischial point. When I apply SRT on these points for a long time, the pain diminishes or even goes away. I ask about the pain time and again as I apply the SRT and stop once it has significantly decreased. The pain will return, however, in acute cases with severe pain. The pain relief will last for about an hour at best. When the above treatment is repeated every day, the pain relief extends to two hours, then six hours, then half a day, and eventually an entire day.

Of course, I use direct moxibustion as well. On important points, which for disc disease or disc herniation are BL-25, BL-59, and the Ischial point, I apply multiple cones. I start with 10 cones, and applying these, I will ask the patient if the pain has diminished. If it hasn't, I will do 10 more and ask again and continue until there is some change. The patient is exhausted from the pain, and the brain is over-excited, so SRT on points on the shoulders and upper back is also helpful. Inquire about the pain relief and reduce frequency of treatment to once every two days, then once every three days, and so on.

When the pain becomes bearable, reduce the frequency to once a week and see how they do. Usually, the pain goes away in one to three months, but some cases take longer.

I treated five cases of acute lumbar disc herniation in the same year that I treated the case described below. The pain didn't go away for one 80-year-old woman and she had to have surgery, but the other four patients achieved complete pain relief with acu-moxa and were able to return to normal activities. They had all been recommended for surgery, but they wanted to avoid that if at all possible. Even though it's true that surgery these days is much less invasive and quite effective, it is preferable not to come under the knife. I think it is worth giving acupuncture a try.

Be that as it may, surgery should be recommended when there is paralysis in motor nerves, bowel/bladder dysfunctions, or exaggeration of tendon reflexes. It would be best to recommend the patient to a good orthopedic surgeon. What I tell patients is this: "Some of my patients have recovered from this with acu-moxa. Why don't you consider surgery if this doesn't work out?" But then there are those who question back, "Are you sure that just a needle can cure this? Who is this patient you speak of?" I do understand their reservations. We could also say the Japanese public does not have that high of an opinion of acupuncture.

4.3 Chronic cases (orthopedic tests and palpation)

The treatment sequence is the same as for acute cases. You can also perform some orthopedic tests. If the pulse at the dorsal pedal artery is diminished or absent, this indicates occlusive arteriosclerosis and requires medical evaluation. When the Patrick test is positive, there is a hip joint problem. When straight leg raising test is positive or there is lack of strength in either flexion or extension of the big toe against resistance, the spinal nerves are involved and it will take time. The pain won't resolve in a few treatments. Palpate around BL-25 to find indurations. Usually, patients find this point tender.

Case Study 64

Patient: Male, 60 years old

FOC: April 5, 2010

Main Complaint: Low back pain on the left side. It began two weeks ago when he twisted his back. There is pain when moving.

Examination: All orthopedic tests negative

Pulse Diagnosis: Liver deficiency

Treatment: Root treatment – SRT on LR-8, KI-10, and LI-11

Branch treatment – SRT on left BL-23, left BL-25, and BL-59. 5mm insertion at left Iliac point. Direct moxibustion on LR-4, left Iliac point, and left BL-59

Progress: (2nd) April 6 – The back pain is gone, but there is hip pain on the left side since this morning. I added SRT to the Ischial point, BL-36, and BL-58.

Comments: It is actually quite common that as soon as the myofascial low back pain resolves, the patient feels spontaneous pain in the hips or legs. So this indicates the back strain was a precursor to neuralgia, or disc herniation. If we can explain this to the patient before we treat them, this would be what these days is called informed consent. Most cases do not get much worse, and the pain goes away with a few treatments.

4.4 A few interesting cases

A. Two-tiered pain and its treatment

A 57-year-old office worker had pain in his left calf muscle and numbness in the sole for two months. The pain kicked in when he walked 30 meters. He received some pain medications and a nerve block injection in the side of his left hip from an orthopedic doctor, but there was no effect. He was unable to walk anymore due to pain in his left hip, and the pain was keeping him awake. His pulse was slightly rapid and showed Liver deficiency. His body temperature was 36.7°C. His pain decreased to about half with a treatment consisting mainly of SRT. The pain resolved in five treatments, but it wasn't completely gone because he still felt mild pain from time to time.

Ten months later, and very suddenly, he experienced severe pain from his left low back to the lower leg. It was in the same places as before: the low back, hip, and posterior aspect of the lower leg on the left side. He couldn't walk, so he took two pain pills and barely got himself to my clinic. He couldn't lie supine, so he lay on his side. His pulse showed Liver deficiency. Palpation revealed an induration at BL-27 and tenderness at the Ischial point. I treated LR-8 and KI-10 on the unaffected side, and BL-27, the Ischial point, BL-58, and BL-59 on the affected side. I inserted 10mm at BL-27 and 5mm at the Ischial point, and all other points received SRT. I then applied 30 cones of direct moxibustion on the Ischial point.

I asked him to get up after this treatment, but he couldn't move due to the pain. I used a teishin and stimulated points on his neck, shoulders and head, and some on the low back. He was then able to move a little, but it still hurt more than when he had come in. Perhaps inserting the needles was too much. He told me the many cones of direct moxibustion on the hip point caused a stinging pain, so maybe I over stimulated it. I treated him rather casually as if it was a case of a back sprain, and this could have been a mistake. Looking at his chart for the last treatment, I realized that this was a case of neuralgia where inserting needles is best avoided. In this instance, I was under the gun because he called me at the last minute saying he really needed a treatment because of severe pain, and I squeezed him in at the end of my day. Of course, this is still no excuse...

He didn't have an appointment the next day either, but I squeezed him in for another treatment. He walked in using a cane, but he didn't appear to be in as much pain as the day before. Since he was able to sleep the night before, this meant that his spontaneous pain wasn't that bad. He was able to lie supine without great discomfort, so I did a few orthopedic tests. He had pain at 20 degrees flexion with the straight leg raising test. His pulse was floating and rapid with Liver deficiency. I gave him a treatment strictly adhering to SRT and applied just five small cones of direct moxa on the Ischial point. He was much better after this treatment. Carelessness leads to mistakes. One has to be careful about inserting needles. SRT is safer.

He came in for his third treatment the next day. The pain with the straight leg raising test was at 45 degrees flexion. He felt some pain lying on his stomach, so I treated him on his side. He felt numbness in his leg when he sat. Two days later he came for his fourth treatment. The pain with the straight leg raising test was at 65 degrees flexion. His pulse was still Liver deficient but it was no longer rapid and felt good. He had no trouble lying on his stomach. He had a bit of numbness in his leg when sitting. Two days after that he walked in without a cane for his fifth treatment. Eight days later he came in for his sixth treatment. He woke up in the morning with low back pain, but he didn't have any pain during the night. The straight leg raising test was negative. He could lie on his stomach without discomfort.

B. Root treatment corrects loss of strength in extension of big toe

A 37-year-old man had low back pain that began without incident, and examination by an orthopedic doctor showed no abnormalities. He felt pain when standing or extending his back. My orthopedic exam revealed diminished strength in extending the left toe. His subjective symptom, however, was pain on both sides of his low back. His pulse showed Liver deficiency. I palpated LR-8 on the right side and applied SRT. I rechecked his pulse and it had become balanced. I rechecked extension of his toes, but there was no change. So I applied SRT on LR-8 and KI-10 on the left side, and rechecked toe extension. This time the strength of extension was about the same on the left and right.

I was surprised, but the patient was also surprised. We had no idea how this was affecting his back pain, but he was amazed by this effect. Actually, there was little change in the low back, but palpating BL-25, I found the left side deficient and the right side somewhat hard. I inserted needles on both sides and felt the arrival of qi at about 5mm, but the feeling was different from what I expected from the palpation. I felt tightening around the needle on the deficient left side, and not that much on the right side. I applied SRT on BL-59, and then checked extension of the toes again. Both sides were equally strong. I had the patient get up and extend his back, and the pain was also gone.

C. Quick results for a chronic case

It stands to reason that acute cases resolve quickly and chronic cases resolve gradually, but there are exceptions. A 57-year-old man came to me with left-sided low back pain and posterior leg pain that had bothered him for a month, which intensified when walking. His diagnosis, received from an orthopedic doctor, was sciatica. The straight leg raising test on the left was positive (painful) at 40 degrees. His pulse showed Liver deficiency. I gave him a standard treatment with SRT. I followed this with direct moxibustion on both BL-25 and on the left side only, the Ischial point, BL-58, BL-59, and ST-36. The pain did not go away that day or the next, but the second day after the treatment it disappeared like magic. When he came for treatment 43 days later, the straight leg raising test was negative. There was no pain when striking the ischial tuberosity (possible sign of sciatica). All that remained was slight tension and heaviness in the back.

D. When it takes a very long time for an effect

In general, chronic cases and neuralgia take a long time to treat, but in some cases it can take so long as to become exasperating. I treated a 38-year-old woman who is a manager at a supermarket, who worked long hours. She had an outbreak of pain and numbness in her left low back and leg around New Years. She had spontaneous pain and standing was difficult. Three months later, in April, she had no change in her pain so she decided to try acupuncture. The hospital where she had been getting treatment gave her the diagnosis of lumbar disc herniation, but apparently it wasn't bad enough to operate on.

I first treated her on April 25. The straight leg raising (SLR) test on the left was positive at 10 degrees. This became the main indicator of progress, but it took four months before this test became negative. Otherwise, the pulsation of her anterior tibial artery (around ST-40) was hard to feel. Her pulse showed Liver deficiency and was deficient, sunken, and slow. Her progress was slow as follows:

(3rd) May 10 – SLR test positive at 35 degrees.

(4th) May 14 – The low back and leg pain is intense. Treatment done in side-lying position. Thirty cones of direct moxibustion on left BL-59.

(6th) May 17 – Sometimes there is no pain. Treatment in supine position is possible.

(7th) May 19 – Treatment in prone position is possible.

(8th) May 21 – Involved in MVA (rear ended). Treatment also done for MVA injury.

About a month after starting treatment, SLR test is still positive at 35 degrees. Sometimes the pain becomes intense and she uses prescription pain medication.

(23rd) July 7 – SLR test positive at 45 degrees. She takes pain medication once a day.

(25th) July14 – The induration at BL-25 on the affected left side and tenderness with pressure continues unchanged. I inserted a needle 5 to 10mm in this point. This reactive point remains even today when her symptoms have mostly resolved. It will be called a complete cure when this reaction finally goes away.

In early September (40th), four months since starting treatments, the SLR test has finally become negative. In October, MRIs showed no abnormalities. We continued weekly treatments until the end of the year. From January of the next year on, since the symptoms were mild even when they recurred, treatments were reduced to once or twice a month.

For this patient, the point selection was fairly standard, with root treatment on LR-8 and typical symptomatic points. The most reactive points were BL-25, Ischial point, and BL-59 on the left side. I used pretty much the same points in every treatment, and it felt a bit like it might have been a worn-out routine, but in this case we stayed on course and the symptoms naturally resolved.

Case Study 65

A case in which SRT wasn't effective

Patient: Male, 66 years old

FOC: May 31, 2010

Main Complaint: Spontaneous pain (without movement) in the right leg. He was told after an exam at a hospital that it was nothing serious. It hurts for 24 hours continuously.

Pulse Diagnosis: Liver deficiency

Treatment: I applied SRT on the points that were most painful and indurated. The tender points were BL-25 and the Ischial point on the right; LR-8, KI-10, ST-36, BL-37, BL-58, and BL-59 on both sides. Direct moxibustion was applied on ST-36, BL-37, BL-58, BL-59, BL-25, and the Ischial point (the last two points on the right side only).

Progress:

(6th) July 6 – The pain has not stopped.

(7th) July 12 – I used a teishin instead of needle and treated the same points.

(8th) Pain is much better.

(11th) No pain.

Comments: This patient was a taxi driver. He's been retired for a year and now gives rides to children to and from kindergarten. Perhaps I was fooled by his good physique, and his pulse was not that weak. In fact, it was strong and closer to a flooding pulse. I treated him six times over a 37-day period, but the spontaneous pain at rest continued unchanged. I used mostly SRT and inserted the needle a bit in points like BL-25 and the Ischial point. Since it wasn't having any effect, I switched to a teishin. I used a Yagi style gold teishin,[1] and rotated it. A teishin can't be rotated as rapidly as a normal needle, but I rotated it as much as I could. As soon as I switched to a teishin, his pain

1. Yagi style teishin: A large 24k gold teishin 90mm long and 4mm in diameter.

started to diminish and eventually disappeared. Two years since then, he has been getting treatments once a month, but the pain has not returned.

Case Study 66

A case in which SRT was effective

Patient: Male, 64 years old

FOC: May 8, 2012

Main Complaint: Spontaneous pain in the right low back and leg. Diminished strength in dorsiflexion of right big toe. He cannot lie on his back.

Pulse Diagnosis: Liver deficiency

Treatment: I applied SRT on LR-8, KI-10, ST-36, LI-11, CV-6, CV-12, BL-18, BL-23, GB-20, and GB-21 and only on the right side on the following points: BL-25, BL-37, BL-58, and BL-59. Direct moxibustion was applied on the right side to ST-36, Ischial point, BL-25, BL-58, and BL-59.

Progress:

(4th) The pain has diminished. He can lie on his back for short periods.

(5th) His pain is much better. No trouble lying on his back.

(6th) No more pain. Dorsiflexion of right big toe normal. Treatments concluded.

Comments: He had spontaneous pain so I played it safe and did not insert the needle even at BL-25.

Case Study 67

A case of pain in the lumbosacral area

Patient: Female, 66 years old

Main Complaint: Chronic low back pain

Observation: Her back was quite bent and she was stooped over.

Examination: Tender points found over sacrum. There were four points on each side. She said, "Right there!" when I press. The tender points were around BL-28 and about 2cm below bilaterally.

Pulse Diagnosis: Usually Liver deficiency, but sometimes Kidney or Lung deficiency

Treatment: For local treatment I inserted needles in 4-6 of the above mentioned tender points. I needled to a depth of about 1cm and then applied minute lifting and thrusting 4-5 times and then removed the needle. After that I placed intradermal needles in these points.

Comments: It's been about 40 years since I first started seeing this patient. I used to treat her parents, and she resembles her mother. She comes a few times a month for treatment. There is no cure for her deformed back, but acu-moxa serves to reduce her discomfort. When I speak of low back pain, it's usually above BL-25. Pain around the sacrum is not that common among people suffering with low back pain, but it is worth knowing about.

5. Femoral neuritis with paresthesia

This condition manifests as pain on the anterior aspect of the thigh along the pathway of the Stomach meridian. The femoral nerve runs quite superficially, so the quality of pain is different from other types of neuritis. Patients describe it as a stinging, burning, or numb sensation. The pain is exacerbated by standing or walking for a long time, or when the hip is extended. The pain diminishes when the hip is flexed. In hospitals in Japan, they say it's not as serious as sciatica, and don't pay much attention to it. In the practice of acupuncture, however, quite a few patients come in for treatment of this condition. It is caused by entrapment neuropathy in which the nerve is pinched, much the same as in carpal tunnel syndrome.

Reactive points appear between the inguinal crease and two-thirds down the course of the Stomach meridian on the upper leg. Palpate in the neighborhood of ST-32. Look for tender points, indurations, and points sensitive to pinching. Regular treatments for one month should be enough. Also GB-29 and GB-30[2] are good points to treat. The femoral nerve exits between the middle lumbar vertebrae, so also look for reactions around BL-22 and -23. You're in luck if you can find an induration there. If the patient has normal strength or better, you can insert the needle about 5mm and add minute lifting and thrusting. Usually there are no indurations on the healthy side.

Summary

- Femoral neuritis is a common cause of leg pain.
- Treat leg points around ST-32, and back points around BL-22.

For the sake of reference, below are the nerves in the legs that are related to common types of neuralgia. They are worth memorizing (see Fig. 4-2).

Sciatic nerve: 4th lumbar nerve to 3rd sacral nerve

Femoral nerve: 2nd to 4th lumbar nerve

Lateral cutaneous femoral nerve: 2nd to 3rd lumbar nerve

Obturator nerve: 2nd to 4th lumbar nerve

---

2. For the location of these points, refer to my locations in *Finding Effective Acupuncture Points.*

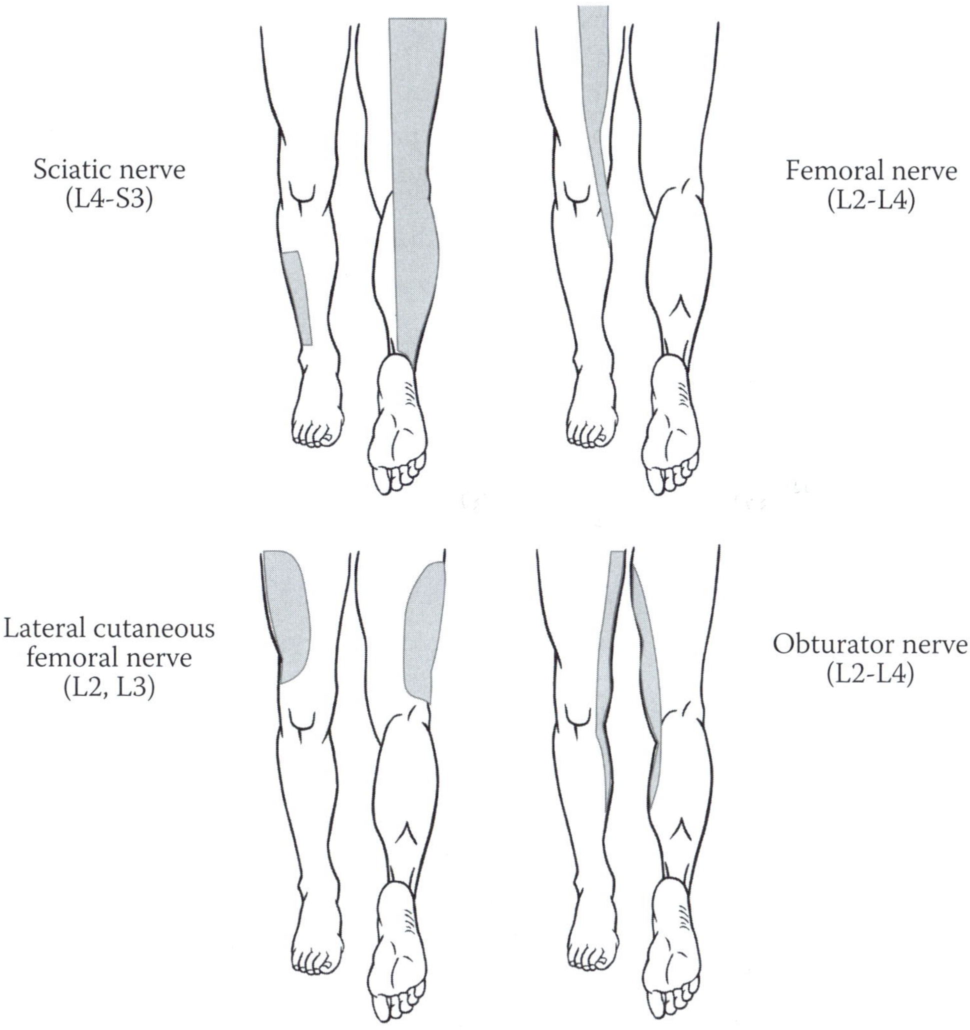

Fig. 4-2 Nerves of the legs[3]

6. Obturator neuritis

With this condition patients often complain of pain in the medial thigh. There are two different types. The first type of pain occurs at the attachments of the pectineus muscle (origin and insertion), and usually occurs in middle-aged women. There is pain when the tight and protruding part of the muscle is pressed toward the bone. Since this area is quite private and difficult to examine and treat directly, I give a root treatment and treat points like Onodera's point and GB-29. Sometimes this isn't enough to make

---

3. Adapted from *Monshin Shinsatsu Handobukku (Handbook of Questioning and Examination for Acupuncture)* by Debata Akio, Ido-no-Nippon, 1987.

the pain go away. In such cases, I needle 5mm into the most tender point, remove the needle, and then place a small press tack (Seirin Pyonex) on the point. When the key tender point is treated precisely, the symptoms can resolve in just one treatment.

The second type of pain is spontaneous pain (pain at rest) in the medial thigh. The pain is usually between the middle of the thigh and the top. Pinching and pressing the medial thigh reveals thickened areas and indurations. Treatment consists of needling these reactive points directly and retaining intradermal needles in the most sensitive points. You can also treat GB-30 and reactive back associated points in the lumbar area.

The course of the obturator nerve overlaps with the Liver meridian. This is where Ogawa Harumichi discovered some special points. He used these points on the medial thigh, which he called Ogawa points, for whiplash (see Fig. 4-3).

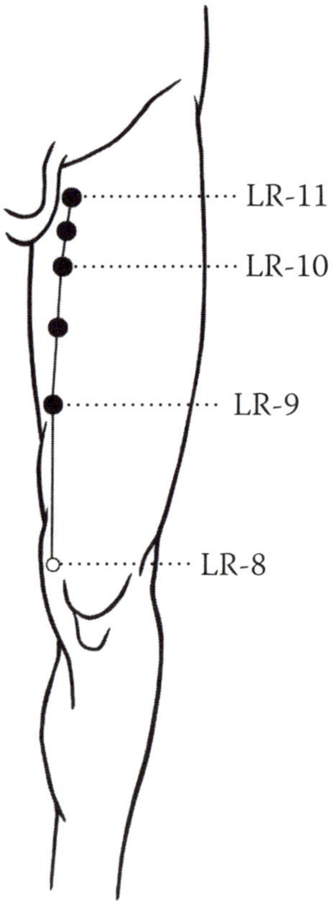

Fig. 4-3 Ogawa points

Case Study 68

PATIENT: Female, 61 years old

FOC: June 1, 2010

MAIN COMPLAINT: Pain in the posterior right leg. There is pain at rest.

Pulse Diagnosis: Liver deficiency

Treatment: I applied SRT on LR-8, KI-10, ST-36, LI-11, SP-21, Gluteal point, BL-25, BL-37, and BL-58.

Progress:

(**3rd**) There is spontaneous pain at rest in left hip.

(**5th**) Spontaneous pain recurs in the posterior right leg.

(**7th**) Used teishin instead of SRT.

(**8th**) Spontaneous pain in the medial right leg.

(**9th**) No pain while in bed at night for the first time after the previous treatment. Pain returned the next day.

(**12th**) Pain okay for three days.

(**16th**) No pain for two days.

(**27th**) No more pain.

Comments: Judging from her symptoms, this patient had both sciatica and obturator neuralgia. She was told at a hospital that it was a minor problem, but her general hypersensitivity made it difficult to make a clear diagnosis. The pain did not resolve after several treatments using SRT so I tried using a gold teishin only, and that night she was pain free. After hearing that she was pain free for a day, I was encouraged and continued with treatments using only teishin. The results were good after that. The location of her pain moved around, but there was no more spontaneous pain at night and the patient was pleased.

Summary

- Try using teishin when pain does not diminish with repeated SRT treatments.

7. Spinal stenosis

I would like to begin this section with a case study. A few years ago, a 65-year-old woman came in, and she had low back pain only when she walked. The pain had started three months ago, and she could only walk for 2-3 minutes at a time. The pain was on the right side only. After an exam at a hospital she was told that she had spinal canal stenosis. The doctor recommended surgery and she was put on pain medications. Someone recommended acupuncture, so she decided to give it a try first. She wanted to avoid surgery, but she said that she would have surgery if that proved to be the only alternative.

She had no problems with sleep, appetite, bowel movements or urination. The orthopedic tests I did on her were all negative. Her pulse showed Liver deficiency. I did SRT on the standard points including LR-8, KI-10, and CV-12. On the right side only, I treated only the right side on the Ischial point, Iliac point, BL-58, BL-59, and ST-36. I also inserted needles (30mm, 0.12mm) superficially about 5mm into BL-25 on both sides. I continued rotating the needle briefly after feeling the arrival of qi at BL-25. I also inserted the needle a little in the Ischial point. I concluded the treatment with five small cones of moxa on BL-59 and the Ischial point on the right, and ST-36 and BL-25 on both sides.

I gave this patient exactly the same treatment in subsequent visits; even the pattern was the same. It was quite unusual how little my treatments changed. This patient came for treatments once a week, and in about three months, after 10 treatments, she was able to walk 20-30 minutes at a stretch. In four months, after 13 treatments, she was able to walk for a whole hour. It seemed that she would be able to avoid surgery. Her pain had disappeared, but she said she wanted to continue the treatments. Walking also served as therapy for claudication. Her condition should improve as she continues with her acu-moxa treatments and regular walking. Her spirits also improved, and she has been looking younger. When people tell her this, she feels even better.

Two years had passed since she first came for treatment, and she was having no problems. But she had injured her leg recently and had an X-ray taken at the same hospital that gave her the original diagnosis. She asked the radiologist to compare that X-ray with the original one, and there didn't seem to be much change in the stenosis. Since there were no symptoms, even when the subject of surgery was raised, she simply declined. Her doctor said he supposed that would be alright.

7.1 Thoughts on difficult cases

How could pressure on a nerve caused by narrowing in the spinal canal be cured or improved with acu-moxa? Common sense would say this is unlikely. Yet things that cannot be explained by present-day medical science happen every day. It can be said therefore that whether acupuncture or moxibustion will actually work cannot be determined until these therapies are attempted.

In advanced cases of spinal canal stenosis with bladder and colon dysfunction, however, the condition is way beyond the scope of acu-moxa, and we have to concede defeat. Simple orthopedic tests cannot ascertain such abnormalities. About the only sign that indicates spinal stenosis is thigh pain with standing extension of the lumbar spine, but this is not definitive. So we have to rely on diagnostic imaging, which means the view of the orthopedic specialist. Often they recommend immediate surgery for cases of spinal stenosis. What happens if one goes without surgery? They say that gradually the patient will be unable to walk.

In the case of those who seek acupuncture for this condition, there are those who say they will never have surgery and those who say they want to try acupuncture and have surgery only if it doesn't have an effect. In an earlier era when diagnostic imaging was undeveloped, such cases were often treated as "lumbar disc herniation," or "sciatica." And in some cases these patients still recovered, so it is worth the attempt to see whether acu-moxa will help. When acu-moxa is continued over time there are cases, such as I have just mentioned and more to come, where patients experience substantial improvement.

Even though surgical techniques have advanced in recent years and the invasiveness has been reduced, this still doesn't change the invasive nature of surgery and naturally it is better to go without it if possible. I would recommend trying acu-moxa first, if possible, for six months. One could give up (and have surgery) if there is no effect. When there is an effect, it tends to happen gradually rather than suddenly, so one can get some idea of the effect before six months.

My treatments these days consist mostly of SRT, but in cases of spinal stenosis, I believe that it is better to insert needles next to the spine in local points like BL-25 and BL-27. I don't have a successful case using only SRT, and it's hard to say, but this is something I need to investigate further. When it comes to palpating the back associated points, it is better to look for indurations rather than depressions. I use my middle finger to palpate the points. I like to treat the normal side along with the affected side, especially with back associated points.

One more thing: direct moxibustion at home is highly recommended. I prescribe points like BL-25, ST-36, and BL-58. When the patient is enthusiastic about moxibustion, I add reactive points on the thigh like BL-37.

The patient mentioned just above sustained a fracture in her lateral malleolus during the course of her treatments. We were concerned that this might set her back, but it never exacerbated her condition, and two years later she is still leading a normal life. She walks at least an hour every day. She comes in for treatment a few times a month, and she says she isn't thinking about surgery anymore. Her orthopedic doctor at the university hospital now says, "Surgery should be the last resort. It's better not to have surgery if you can avoid it." Looking at my medical reference text, it states that surgery is not always the first or the only option. Just one successful case may not be convincing, so I'll describe a few more.

7.2 More cases where surgery was avoided

Case Study 69

Patient: Male, 72 years old

FOC: April 19, 2010

Symptoms and Condition: He is diabetic and has glaucoma, gastroesophageal reflux, and low back pain. The back pain caused difficulty in walking. The cause of his back pain was diagnosed as spinal stenosis. We began intensive treatments for his back pain.

Pulse Diagnosis: Liver deficiency

Treatment: Standard treatment including insertion (5-10mm with 5-minute lifting and thrusting movements) in BL-26 and the Iliac points, which was followed by moxibustion. The patient also applied five cones on the above points every day at home.

Progress: After 10 treatments, 100 days later, he was able to walk quite a bit.

Comments: He told me he is advertising his improvement to others with the same diagnosis. This means that there are quite a few people with the same diagnosis around him. So it's obvious that it's wise to put off surgery until after carefully monitoring the patient's progress. There is another issue here, however, and that is the reliability of the diagnosis.

Case Study 70

Patient: Male, 74 years old

FOC: January 29, 2011

Main Complaint: Pain in the right lower back at rest and with movement. There is little pain while sitting.

History: Myocardial infarction 12 years ago, gallstones

Situation: He went to two different orthopedic doctors who both gave him the diagnosis of spinal stenosis. He was placed on a pain killing suppository and also received transcutaneous electric stimulation. He was told to avoid activity and to rest as much as possible. He can walk if he bends over, but the numb sensation is too great when standing if he tries to walk while standing straight.

Assessment: Among the orthopedic tests, straight leg raising (SLR) test was positive on the right side.

Pulse Diagnosis: Liver deficiency

Treatment: Teishin used LR-8 and KI-10. SRT on ST-36. I repeated the straight leg raising (SLR) test on the right and it had become negative. I found an induration at the right Ischial point and BL-25, as well as a depression at M-BW-25 *(josen/shí qī zhuī xià),* so I applied SRT on these three points. Direct moxibustion was applied on ST-36, BL-25, the right Ischial point, and M-BW-25 *(josen/shí qī zhuī xià).*

Progress:

(2nd) Feb 2 – There is pain with movement but no more pain at rest. He can walk without bending over. Pain caused by SLR test. After SRT on LR-8, KI-10, and ST-36, there was no more pain with the SLR test. After the treatment he got up and moved around but felt no more back pain.

(3rd) Feb 7 – SLR test negative. He had discomfort in his right gluteal region. SRT and moxibustion on the induration at BL-25.

(4th) Feb 14 – SLR test negative. His back feels 90% better.

(5TH) Feb 21 – He is 100% better. Treatments concluded.

COMMENTS: So what are we to make of this case? Two different hospitals diagnosed this patient with spinal stenosis, so there is no doubt that the diagnostic imaging reveals a constricted area in his spine. Yet there doesn't seem to be a direct relationship between this and the patient's pain. So some question remains about the diagnosis. No doubt there could be some thickening in the ligamentum flavum with aging, which could narrow the spinal canal, but then not all elderly people have intermittent claudication. In any case, this case gives more support to attempting acupuncture before more invasive procedures.

Now, I have been saying that insertion at BL-25 is necessary, but this conclusion may be premature given the following case.

Case Study 71

PATIENT: Female, 52 years old

FOC: November 1, 2010

MAIN COMPLAINT: Numbness in left leg when standing. She received the diagnosis of spinal stenosis.

PULSE DIAGNOSIS: Liver deficiency

TREATMENT: SRT on LR-8, KI-10, CV-12, left Ischial point, BL-25, left BL-58, and ST-36. Direct moxibustion on BL-25.

PROGRESS:

(3RD) Nov. 30 – A week ago her back pain got so bad, she went to the hospital and got an injection. I decided to use only teishin for her treatment. I used only teishin for all subsequent treatments, including at BL-25.

(4TH) Back pain persists.

(5TH) No more spontaneous pain at rest.

(7TH) Heavy sensation in low back.

(8TH) Some pain in center of low back.

COMMENTS: This patient had a delicate build, and even on her low back and hips, needle insertion was contraindicated. Once I switched to teishin, her back pain gradually diminished and now she is completely pain free. The question still remains, however, if one can cure real spinal stenosis with only teishin.

As I accumulated more cases of spinal stenosis, I came to the conclusion that acu-moxa is effective in many cases. So I suggest attempting treatment without being intimidated by the diagnosis. When there is no effect after 3-6 months, it is still not too late to go to the surgeon. In cases with bowel or bladder dysfunction, however, it is better to have surgery without delay.

Case Study 72

Patient: Male, 63 years old

FOC: February 29, 2012

Main Complaint: Diagnosis of spinal stenosis with pain on anterior right thigh region, numbness in big toe of right foot. Pain after 10 minutes of walking.

Pulse Diagnosis: Liver deficiency

Treatment: Standard treatment for Liver deficiency. SRT on LR-8, KI-10 CV-12, right Ischial point, right BL-25, BL-58, and ST-36. Direct moxibustion on ST-36 and the right BL-25 and Ischial point.

Progress:

(6th) Apr 7 – Able to walk 15 minutes without pain.

(7th) Apr 14 – Able to walk one round of golf (10km) without pain.

(13th) June 11 – Able to walk quite a distance without any pain.

Comments: This patient didn't do moxibustion at home, but he still recovered nicely. So moxibustion at home is not always necessary for recovery.

Summary

- Differentiate from occlusive arteriosclerosis. (Pulses in foot can be palpated in spinal stenosis.)
- Insertion (5-10mm with 5-minute sparrow pecking movements) at BL-25 and reactive Gluteal or Ischial points on affected side.

8. Osteoporosis and spondylosis deformans

I'm not sure about the validity of this category. I am referring to the low back pain of elderly women with spinal deformities (usually bent forward). The pain is not chronic but starts suddenly. Often the complaint is that the pain started after picking something up. The underlying cause is osteoporosis. The bones become weak after menopause with inadequate hormone secretion. Those with osteoporosis are at risk for compression fractures, and it is difficult to differentiate this from the pain of myofascial back pain. Differentiation requires an orthopedic doctor, but they have no good treatment beyond pain medications.

Cases like this are extremely hard to treat. First of all, you can't press points on the back. Even slight pressure can make things worse. That is why palpation must be done very gently, like stoking over the back. Primarily I look for depressed points, and I consider myself lucky if I can find an induration this way. The treatment must also be very gentle, and SRT treatments are best. Often things get worse if needles are inserted in local points.

Also, the treatment must be done in the side-lying position. Lying prone will make things worse. Elderly patients don't respond to acu-moxa as quickly as younger patients. You need to explain to the patient in the beginning that recovery will take time and one has to proceed at a leisurely pace. It's an extra bonus if they just happen to recover quickly.

There are no secrets to treating back pain from osteoporosis, but of course it is important to treat the Kidney and Bladder meridians. Often the cause of the fracture is lifting things without holding it against the torso. It is important to advise patients about safe lifting.

The above is my conclusion after making many mistakes. Even if you are aware that you must be careful, often you still go overboard (inserting needles). When the pain is extreme it is best to advise patients to get an orthopedic exam first. Usually such patients are hospitalized for observation or advised to say in bed.

8.1 A case of osteoporosis

This was an 82-year-old woman who has been coming to me for back pain over the last four years with symptoms of numbness in the right leg and pain in the hip, and then pain in the posterior aspect of the left thigh. For the first year she received treatments once a week, and the next year she received one or two treatments a month. This May she lifted a potted plant and suddenly experienced low back pain. The pain was all over the low back, not in any specific place. I treated her for Liver deficiency and also treated BL-23, BL-25, and the Iliac point for local treatment. We continued treatments once a week for 11 weeks and finally she returned to her normal state.

People with back problems should not lift or hold heavy objects. It seems in this case, the patient was trying to keep her clothes clean and held the pot away from her body. It would have been better to hold it against her lower abdomen. Many people make this mistake. The expression on this patient's face when she was in pain, and her expression when the pain resolved, was very distinct. Even though she doesn't have all the signs of inflammation, my charts show that she has slight heat in her joints from time to time. So there is some doubt that she actually had arthritis. Also, a year ago she had been told that there was a 1cm shadow in her left lung, but there has been no change in her condition. Treatment of this type of back pain takes a long time. It is really a test of patience for both the practitioner and patient. The patient is well aware that she needs to be careful, but tends to forget when she's feeling good.

9. Low back pain from unknown cause (depression?)

I have a male patient who claims to have had low back pain for 25 years. He is 48 years old and appears sturdy. No abnormalities were found in an examination at a hospital. His other symptoms include insomnia, upper back pain, abdominal distention, and general fatigue. All the orthopedic tests I did on him were negative, and abdominal palpation revealed nothing out of the ordinary. All I found was some induration and tenderness at BL-59. His pulse showed Liver deficiency. It is amazing that he had low back pain for 25 years and there were no local findings! He is an electrical contractor and has been able to keep working.

I suspected a psychological issue based on his insomnia and general fatigue. But his appetite was normal and it was clear that he didn't have Lung deficiency (which is common in depression). Anyway, I used only SRT for the entire treatment. I did some direct moxibustion on BL-59 and, even though there wasn't a reaction, on a slight depression at BL-52.

He said the back pain was a bit better on his third visit two weeks later. He continued to come in about every other week. I didn't inquire much about his condition, but just quietly administered my SRT treatment. By the 11th treatment he told me he was doing much better. There was some hope... Two weeks later, on the 12th treatment, he had Lung deficiency, and he told me working in a bent forward position was still painful. Nevertheless, overall he was doing much better.

Note: Masked depression is a term used to refer to physical symptoms that mask depression. It has been controversial, but the idea that unpleasant or intolerable emotions can be somaticized as various symptoms is becoming more accepted. Commonly somaticized symptoms include generalized fatigue, sleep disorders, weight loss, digestive disorders, sexual dysfunction, upper and low back pain, neck and shoulder stiffness, palpitations and discomfort in the chest, and respiratory problems. The key feature is the lack of objective findings that correspond with the symptoms. Somaticized symptoms are not hard to identify once the underlying affective disorder and loss of motivation is recognized, along with the cyclical fluctuation of the symptoms.

10. Back stiffness in the morning

One variety of low back pain that I encounter from time to time is pain with movement in the morning, which gradually diminishes as the person continues to move. It takes 30 minutes to an hour at the most, and I view this as a rheumatic pain. Among the symptoms of rheumatoid arthritis there is "stiffness in morning," and this low back pain is similar in nature. In contrast, low back pain that is related to neuralgia tends to be okay when getting up in the morning but gets worse as the day goes on. With back stiffness in the morning, you cannot find indurations or tender points in specific places, and the pain seems to be distributed over a broad area.

In cases like this, real needle insertion is not good, and after trying various low back treatment protocols with insertions, I've found that SRT or superficial retained needles works best. Stick to SRT when the patient doesn't have much energy or strength. If there is some strength, I retain needles superficially (1mm) for just five minutes in points like

BL-27, Iliac point, BL-23, BL-52, BL-18, and BL-59.

Be sure to check for problems in other joints with patients like this.

11. Back pain in the morning

This is a unique type of low back pain. These patients wake up in the morning because of low back pain. It is difficult to sleep so they get up, but soon thereafter the pain goes away like magic. The pain dissipates much faster than the above-mentioned back stiffness in the morning. Even if patients consider getting an acupuncture treatment when they wake up, they forget about it because the pain goes away by itself.

You can palpate local findings in such cases, but they are not pronounced. In the beginning, I used to treat these like any other case of low back pain, but I had no success. The more I tried using deeper needles and thicker needles, the more the body seemed to resist healing. Once I had an idea and used only superficial insertion and the pain in the morning ceased after that. Nowadays I think that SRT is enough. The main thing is not to insert the needle. This is the best approach.

Then what causes this back pain in the morning? Some authors attribute it to blood stasis (*oketsu/xuè yū*). According to *A Precious Record of Acupuncture and Moxibustion,*[4] "Mild [low back pain] during the day and intense [pain] at night is blood stasis." The *Guide to Essential Techniques of Acupuncture and Moxibustion,*[5] from the same period, says exactly the same thing, as does *Gathering of the Blossoms of Acupuncture*[6] from China in the Ming Dynasty. Further, the *Handbook of Pulse Diagnosis*[7] states, "The pulse [for low back pain] is rough, and it indicates blood stasis." So what is blood stasis? According to the *Compendium of Sino-Japanese Herbal Medicine,*[8] it refers to "various symptoms which arise from persistent hyperemia or congestion primarily in the pelvis." Does this mean that reproductive hormones are involved? The cause of this type of low back pain is difficult to understand, but the right kind of acupuncture works well. The reasoning does not matter that much.

12. Pain over spinous processes

Patients with this type of back pain complain of pain right on the spine, but often,

4. Hongo Masatoyo 本郷正豊, *A Precious Record of Acupuncture and Moxibustion (Shinkyu chohoki* 鍼灸重宝記), 1718. Considered to be among the three great acupuncture texts of the Edo Period (1611-1868).

5. Iwata Risai 岩田利斎, *Guide to Essential Techniques of Acupuncture and Moxibustion (Shinkyu yoho shinan* 鍼灸要法指南), 1720. Also among the three great acupuncture texts of the Edo Period.

6. Gao Wu 高武, *Gathering of the Blossoms of Acupuncture (Zhen jiu ju ying* 鍼灸聚英), 1529.

7. Yama Nobutoshi 山延年, *Handbook of Pulse Diagnosis (Myakuho tebikikugusa* 脈法手引草), 1770.

8. Tatsuno Kazuo 龍野一雄, *Compendium of Sino-Japanese Herbal Medicine (Kampo igaku taikei* 漢方医学大系), 1905, p. 263.

reactive points cannot be found. For cases of low back pain related to damage to interspinous ligaments (see section 3 above), I have a habit of palpating around the spine, but I don't often touch the top of the spinous processes themselves. This type of pain can occur in any spinous process, but it seems to occur most often in the lower thoracic and upper lumbar vertebrae, that is, between T10 and L3. Touching the affected vertebra is painful. That is why patients become aware of the pain when they sit down and lean against a backrest. Often there are no other symptom. Palpation also tends to reveal little besides tenderness on the spinous processes.

I have found that retaining intradermal needles works the best for this type of back pain. I place the needle right on the most tender point and insert it horizontally at a right angle to the spine. I replace the intradermal needles once a week. I also give a root treatment and apply SRT to some abdominal points as well as a few points around the tender spinous processes. The pain usually goes away with 1-3 treatments.

There are exceptions, of course, and once the pain didn't go away even after three treatments. So I had the patient have someone at home apply five cones of direct moxibustion right over the affected spinous process every day. The pain resolved in three months. Some patients with this condition ask me what causes this pain. I tell them that the spine is a joint, just like the knee, so it could be a type of osteoarthritis, but I'm not really sure. I wish I had a better answer.

13. Back pain from kidney stones (ureteral calculus)

Since the main complaint of kidney stones is usually low back pain, I have included this in this chapter on back pain. It could very well be put in the chapter on diseases of internal organs. Back pain from a kidney stone occurs quite suddenly, the pain is excruciating, and can be severe enough to make the person pass out. The face of someone in throes of this pain looks washed out and it is obvious that the situation is dire. The pain is mostly in the low back and flank regions, but sometimes the pain is felt in the lower abdomen. The pain occurs when the kidney stone becomes stuck in the ureter. The pain goes away when the stone goes back to the renal pelvis, or if it passes down into the bladder. A stone that has descended past the bladder to become lodged in the urethra engenders a different kind of pain. This is called urethrolithiasis and the pain radiates along the urethra to the lower abdomen and sacral region.

Acupuncture and moxibustion are indicated for low back pain caused by kidney stones. As long as the pulse diagnosis is done correctly, it can have dramatic results. One needle in a root treatment point makes all the difference. That is, either SP-3 for Spleen deficiency, LR-1 for Liver deficiency, KI-7 for Kidney deficiency, or LU-9 for Lung deficiency. Fortunately in my case, my first patient with this problem got pain relief when I needled SP-3 for Lung deficiency. (Along with LU-9, SP-3 is a standard tonification point for Lung deficiency.) After that, I had patients with this problem who had Liver deficiency, Kidney deficiency, or Spleen deficiency, and they all got relief from the root treatment.

In textbooks, it says that stones that are less than 10mm in size can pass naturally. Of course, those stones that are rounded can be passed easier. Even small stones are difficult to pass if there are sharp edges. With acupuncture, instead of physically forcing the stone to pass, we just facilitate the innate physiological release of the stone, so in some cases the pain cannot be stopped. Fortunately, these days kidney stones can be broken up by ultrasonic lithotripsy so that they are more easily passed. This greatly reduces the strain on the patient.

13.1 Diagnosis and treatment

Gently strike BL-23 or -52 with the ulnar side of your fist, and the pain will be aggravated if it's due to a kidney stone. This is the easiest method, but be careful not to strike with too much force. It is easy to identify this type of low back pain when you take into account the low back pain coupled with pain in the lower abdomen or groin.

As I have said already, the root treatment is the best approach. I find that Spleen deficiency is the most common pulse presentation found. The pain subsides as I do SRT on SP-3 or apply rotations after I superficially insert the needle. I retain the needle on both sides and rotate the needle alternately. You can also leave the needles in for the duration of the treatment. In one case this treatment on SP-3 didn't relieve the pain, so I found an induration on SP-8 and needled it and that stopped the pain. I don't have any experience with it, but potentially SP-1 could work too.

I treat LR-1 in cases of Liver deficiency, but why don't I use the standard tonification point LR-8? Can't the pain be relieved with LR-8? In my practice, I've seen quite a few patients who didn't have any back pain when they came in, but had a sudden onset of kidney stone pain on the treatment table. Once a patient like this had a transposed radial artery that makes pulse diagnosis difficult, so I retained needles in SP-3 since many patients with kidney stones have Spleen deficiency. I observed the patient for a while, but the pain did not diminish at all. I decided he had Liver deficiency instead and as soon as I put a needle in LR-1, the pain subsided. Ever since then I have used LR-1 for Liver deficiency patients with kidney stones. In critical moments like this in my clinic, I don't have the time to experiment with points like LR-8.

As I said above, I treat KI-7 for Kidney deficiency and LU-9 for Lung deficiency. Putting needles in the right points causes abdominal sounds. I will say, however, that I haven't seen many cases of Kidney or Lung deficiency with kidney stones.

Is there any effective symptomatic treatment other than the above root treatment? Putting needles in BL-22, BL-23, and BL-52 causes a sensation in the most painful place, but there is not as much effect as the root treatment points. It is also risky when you consider the patient moving while the needles are inserted that causes sensations in the back. Once I did see my teacher manage to stop kidney stone pain by inserting a long needle into a point around M-BW-19 *(romanji/pǐ gēn)*, which is located 3.5 units lateral to the lower border of the spinous process of the first lumbar vertebra.

13.2 Some cases of kidney stones

A. A case of Lung deficiency

I had a call from a friend who could not move due to low back pain. He couldn't come for a treatment, so I made a house call. This was 28 years ago, and he had been my classmate in elementary school. At that time he was 50 years old. I found him lying on his side with his right side up. His face was the characteristic mask of deep distress. I asked him where it hurt, and he grabbed his side around GB-26 saying, "Here!" The pain was mostly in the right waist area but he had some pain in the abdomen as well. He said the pain was beyond words. I tapped on BL-52 and he experienced intense pain.

I tried inserting a needle (50mm, 0.2mm) in BL-52, but this did not change the pain. I took his pulses with him still lying on his side. It was a rapid pulse and felt like Spleen deficiency/Liver excess. I did a superficial insertion in left SP-3 and retained it after rotating it a while. I noticed that his groaning had lessened, so I asked him to lie on his back and took his pulse again. Both the Spleen and Lung positions were weak. I placed another needle in right SP-3. When I put a needle in LU-9, his abdomen began to make sounds, and the pain stopped. I checked the pulse again and found that the Spleen and Lung positions were stronger, and the excess in the Liver position was gone.

I had him lie on his stomach, and I inserted needles into the most tender points: right BL-20 and BL-23. I used a 50mm, 0.2mm needle in BL-23. My friend gave a small grunt as the needle sensation reached the part of his back that had been the most painful. The next day he went to the hospital where he had to stay for observation. X-rays did not show anything. On the third day of hospitalization, small stones came out in his urine. He actually had a history of gout, and the stones were from uric acid so they didn't show up in X-rays. This was my first patient with kidney stones.

B. A case of Spleen deficiency

This treatment took place in one of the annual summer seminars of the Meridian Therapy Association. I was teaching and giving demonstrations on the treatment of low back pain. About halfway through my presentation someone brought in "a real patient." He was an acupuncturist about 60 years old with back pain on his right side. He was drenched in sweat and holding a towel over his right hip and lower abdomen. This was no ordinary back pain, and I suspected a kidney stone. His pulse was floating and tight on the left, and the pulses on the right, especially the Spleen and Stomach positions, were weak and soft. I decided he had Spleen deficiency. I had him lie on his left side and inserted a 30mm, 0.12mm needle superficially in left SP-3 followed by another needle retained in right BL-52. I went back to the needle in SP-3 and continued rotating it. In a short while his pain began to diminish so I removed the needle in BL-52 and had him lie supine. I resumed the rotation on SP-3 and soon thereafter his pain stopped. As I was doing the treatment, the students observing made comments like, "His complexion is better." "His abdomen is filling in." "His skin is gaining luster." "His face is softening." The face of those with pain from kidney stones becomes drawn and gaunt, and as the pain improves, so does their facial appearance. His sweating stopped and I took his pulse and confirmed that the Spleen position had become stronger and the tight Liver position had softened.

This man came to the Meridian Therapy summer seminar the following year and his face looked plump and happy. He told me he had been very healthy. It appeared he was also doing well financially.

C. A case of Kidney deficiency

I once had a 48-year-old man come in with low back pain who reported he also had blood in his urine. I think of something like renal tumor when there is hematuria. I inquired into his medical history, and he had had surgery for bladder stones. Of course, the kidney also had stones and later he had to have kidney surgery. He told me quite a few stones were removed. Unfortunately, he got an infection in the surgical scar and he had to have his left kidney removed. But that wasn't the end of his problems. The right kidney also had stones and caused him pain from time to time. It wasn't acute and severe pain, but a deep dull pain. The reason he came for acupuncture was to see if I could do something about this dull pain. He had also experienced diseases of other internal organs, including chronic hepatitis and pancreatitis.

Pulse diagnosis showed weakness in all positions on the left side at the deep level (Heart, Liver, and Kidney), but the pulses were all strong at the superficial level (yang meridians), especially the Gallbladder, Bladder, and Stomach. The pulse quality was very slow and rough. I examined him in the prone position. There was pain with percussion over BL-52 and the spinous process of the first lumbar vertebra. I inserted but did not retain needles in BL-20, BL-23, and BL-52 on the right side. I had him lie supine and checked his pulse again. I palpated tenderness at CV-12 and KI-16, while CV-6 was deficient. Based on this I decided to treat him for Kidney deficiency. I rotated the needle at KI-7 on the right and felt the arrival of qi. His abdomen made a loud sound. I left the needle in the left KI-7 and treated the right KI-7 in the same way. I felt a similar sensation of arrival of qi and the abdomen made a sound again. I left the needle in on the right side as well. I needled LU-5 on each side and again there were abdominal sounds. The patient started to sleep around this time. His pain had stopped. There were also abdominal sounds when I tonified CV-6.

I gave this treatment 30 years ago. After that I treated this patient from time to time for the same symptoms. With the advent of shock wave lithotripsy, this patient finally found permanent relief. People each have their unique fortune. If they are lucky, they find good therapy that extends their life, just like my acupuncture teacher came across streptomycin for tuberculosis. It is a mystery whether we have any control over such fortune.

Summary

- Acupuncture works for kidney stones.
- One root treatment point can make the difference.
- Patients with kidney stones often have Spleen deficiency; treat SP-3.

Q&A

QUESTION AND ANSWER NO. 3

(From a Gensai Jyuku study group in 2007)

What does it mean to put your spirit into it?

Q. I have heard you say that you "put your spirit into" points that are important. What is the difference in your awareness when you are doing SRT when you "put your spirit into" a point and when you don't? Are you clearly envisioning how the qi is working in the patient's meridian? Or are we only to pay attention to the speed of rotation and the fine details of our technique?

A. Even when the same person inserts needles in the same point at different times, there is difference in the outcome when one does it in a distracted way or pays close attention and puts his spirit into it. It is a mysterious thing, but this is where we are different from machines. Putting your spirit into it refers to mental states like doing the needling technique seriously, not allowing distracting thoughts to interfere, not letting your attention wander, staying focused, paying attention to your lower abdomen, and keeping silent. It is a state in which even if someone speaks to you, you cannot answer. No matter what comes up, you can respond instantly. I think we can call this the ultimate state of consciousness. It is difficult to describe, but the main thing is to pay attention. Acupuncture is serious business. You aren't going to get good results in your ordinary state of mind. As you get more clinical experience you will come to understand what I'm saying. Keep it stored in your head somewhere until you do.

CHAPTER

5

Leg Problems

1. Gastrocnemius spasms (leg cramps)

This section covers all leg cramps represented by the common term "Charley horse" that usually occur in the gastrocnemius muscle. The pain of leg cramps is excruciating and only those who have had them know what it's like. In my case, I tend to get leg cramps especially over the whole left leg. My knee bends and the knee cap comes up to my belly. It is the pose of a high diver bent forward fully getting ready to jump off the board. It is a powerful cramp, and it's not easy to move my leg. I am usually awakened at night with a cramp and sometimes can't help yelling out "Owww!" My beloved dog Ranko upstairs hears me and starts barking and runs down to see what's going on.

So what can be done to quickly relieve the pain of a leg cramp? This question was posed in a medical advice column in the Asahi daily newspaper. A 71-year-old woman asked about occasional leg cramps in her calf muscles. Two months ago while sleeping she suddenly got a strong cramp that caused a wrenching pain up the thigh all the way to the abdomen. This sounds similar to the cramps I get. The answer of the neurologist featured in the column was as follows: "It will resolve quickly when the contracted muscle is stretched. Stand up in a posture that stretches the Achilles tendon. It is effective to bring your toes up toward your shins. There are several kinds of muscle relaxing drugs. The Kampo formula Peony and Licorice Decoction *(sháo yào gān cǎo tāng)* is also said to be effective in preventing cramps."[1]

Orthopedic doctors use the same approach of stretching the muscle in cases of cramps and put the foot into strong dorsiflexion. So their answer to cramps is the same as the above newspaper column. This approach, however, doesn't always work so well,

---

1. Asahi Shinbun (daily paper) medicine section, December 23, 2010. Answer by Takahashi Masaki, M. D., assistant professor of neurology in stroke department of Osaka University Hospital.

and it is also a very painful method for the patient. Probably it's not likely that you would be able to do this when you are in the middle of a terrible cramp.

1.1 Needling the Onodera's point

The cause of leg cramps is attributed to imbalances in electrolytes like calcium and magnesium, but taking these as supplements doesn't seem to completely eliminate cramps. And it certainly is no help when you are trying to get relief from a cramp you are having right now.

So getting back to my own experience, I thought with my sleepy brain that since cramps have to do with muscles and tendons, they must be associated with the Liver. This could mean LR-8 would work, so I needled LR-8, but the cramp didn't go away. Well points are supposed to be good for acute pain, so I tried LR-1, but that didn't help either. I could have inserted needles in the local area, but since in my case the cramp is over the whole leg, that would have been a problem. Since both my knee and hip were in flexion, I tried needling Yanagiya's GB-30. The depth was 5mm to 1cm. The pain and cramping began to soften as I continued small sparrow-pecking movements. It was a very painful cramp, and this method worked very well. I've had a few cramps since then, but each time they are relieved by the same method. I haven't had that many cramps recently, but the secret seems to lie in the lateral hip area.

When I examine patients with a leg spasm in the clinic, I usually find a hard point (induration) around Onodera's point. This point is close to GB-30. So I tried inserting a needle in Onodera's point on the affected side. The spasm starts to dissolve in less than a minute. So my treatment for leg spasms is to insert a needle 2cm into Onodera's point and adding 3-5 sparrow-pecking motions, but I actually keep manipulating the needle until the spasm is relieved. Then all you have to do is retain the needle for another minute. It works even better to do a few cones of direct moxibustion on the point. After I use this method on myself, I don't have any spasms that night. When treating patients, I don't forget to do a root treatment first and some treatment on the low back and leg. Often one treatment is all it takes and the patient doesn't have any more leg spasms. Even if they do recur, the same method works to relieve the spasm. When the patient is unable to lie prone, you can treat them on their side and needle Yanagiya's GB-30 instead.

So, then, what causes such spasms? Since there are indurations in the muscles of the lateral hip, the cause seems to be an abnormality in this area. It must be from compromised blood circulation, but this doesn't help with treatment. The cold pathogen could be another cause. In this case, it's often an abnormality in the Kidney and Bladder and the symptoms appear on the Kidney and Bladder meridians. Another cause could be blood deficiency or abnormalities in the Liver and Gallbladder.

1.2 Yanagiya's GB-30

Let me explain about Yanagiya's GB-30, which was so dramatically effective in relieving my leg cramp. Why did I happen to find and treat this point? In Yanagiya Sorei's text on effective points, *Guide to Secret One-Needle Technique,*[2] under "acupuncture for diseases of the lateral leg," he explains his location and needling technique for GB-30:

Point location: Have the patient lie on his side with the affected leg up, and have him flex his hip. In this case it is even better if the thigh comes up against the torso as much as possible. There is a big muscle in the crease lateral and inferior to the anterior superior iliac spine. There is a ropy, tense band in the posterior aspect of this muscle. Pressing this band, there is a point that causes a radiating sensation down the lateral thigh. This is the point we call GB-30 [Fig. 5-1].

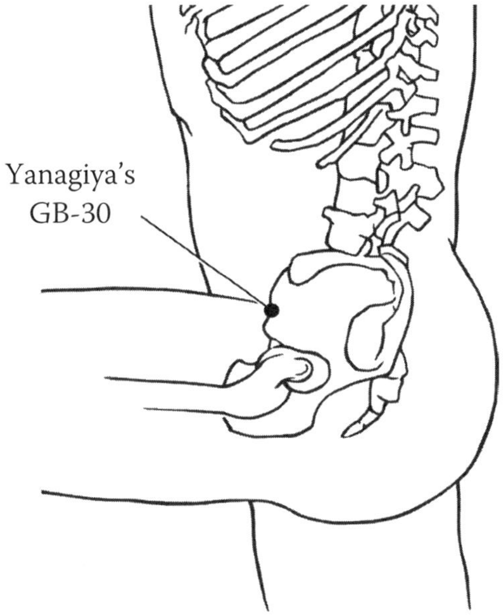

Fig. 5-1 Yanagiya's GB-30

Needle: I use a 3-inch #2 (0.18mm) or #5 (0.24mm) silver needle, or a #2 (0.18mm) or #3 (0.20mm) steel needle of the same length.

Posture of patient: Lie on side with unaffected side down. Grasp the knee of the affected leg up to the abdomen so the thigh comes as close as possible to the abdomen.

Angle of needle: Place the needle so that it is perpendicular to the skin.

Technique: Insert the needle and gently lift and lower the needle to work the needle in deeper.

So I located and treated Yanagiya's GB-30, just as explained in this text. Probably this information was sleeping somewhere in my head. As I said, cramps in the gastrocnemius quickly resolve by inserting a needle in Onodera's point. When the cramp is ongoing, I insert a needle in Yanagiya's GB-30 or Onodera's point and apply sparrow pecking until the spasm subsides. When there is no spasm at the moment, I retain needles (at a depth of 3-4cm) in these points. There was no cramping that night after this acu-moxa

2. *Guide to Secret One-Needle Technique* (*Hiho Ippon-shin Densho*), 1955, Ido-no-Nippon.

treatment. Cramps cease to occur after the treatment below is continued on a regular basis.

Root treatment: (Liver deficiency) SRT on LR-8, KI-10, and ST-36

Branch treatment: Insert needle in Yanagiya's GB-30 or Onodera's point. SRT on BL-18, BL-25, BL-58, and BL-59.

Direct moxibustion: Five cones on Yanagiya's GB-30 or Onodera's point ST-36 and BL-58

The *Systematic Classic of Acupuncture and Moxibustion (Zhen jiu jia yi jing)* suggests BL-65, BL-60, and BL-58 for "binding in the leg" and searing pain in the calves.

Summary

- Insert a needle in Onodera's point and apply sparrow pecking until the spasm is relieved.
- As an alternative, use same technique on Yanagiya's GB-30 with patient in the side-lying position. Retain the needle after manipulation.

2. Osgood-Schlatter disease

Osgood-Schlatter disease is seen in children during their growth phase. It is a characteristic form of osteochondritis (degeneration in the articular surface of bones) that occurs most often in children in their early teens. Pain is caused by pathology on the epiphyseal cartilage of the tibia. In the extension movement of the knee, the quadriceps contract and pull on the tibial tuberosity. In the growth phase, there is a lot of soft cartilage here, so repeated stress on the tibial attachment causes inflammation. This condition is said to resolve naturally when the growth in bones is complete.

As described in the case below, this condition can be alleviated quickly with acumoxa. The trick is to find the most tender point, but the knee must be palpated gently. Too much pressure is quite painful. I palpate the tender point with my right index or middle finger with stroking motions. An intradermal needle in the tender point is usually enough, but 80% moxibustion[3] is also effective. The intradermal needle should be left in place until it comes off by itself. Along with treating the tender point on the knee, whole body treatment including a root treatment and points on the legs and low back are indispensable.

Case Study 73

Patient: Male, 15 years old (9th grader)

3. 80% moxibustion is direct moxibustion that is not burned all the way to the skin. Each cone is removed after it burns down 80% so that just a little heat is felt.

FOC: January 17, 2009

Main Complaint: He is a first baseman on his school team. For a week, both his knees have been hurting with physical activity.

Examination: Extreme tenderness at the highest point of the tibial tuberosities, especially marked on the left knee. There are no other findings.

Pulse Diagnosis: Liver deficiency

Treatment: Root treatment – SRT on LR-8 and KI-10

Branch treatment: Needles inserted superficially in the middle of the most tender point on each knee. This was followed by 80% moxibustion and then an intradermal needle. In addition, ST-36, BL-40, and Onodera's point were needled superficially.

Progress: (2nd) Jan 31 – There is no more knee pain, and no more tenderness on the knees.

Comments: The acu-moxa on the tender points was probably responsible for most of the effect. This patient came in just a week after the pain began; treatment at a very early stage probably had a great deal to do with the good outcome.

Summary

- For Osgood-Schlatter disease, locate tender points on tibial tuberosity.
- Palpate gently and retain an intradermal needle.
- Shin splints.

The medical term for shin splints is medial tibial stress syndrome or tibial micro fractures. This is a general term for a condition caused by stress or overuse of muscles of the leg including the soleus, tibialis posterior, tibialis anterior, extensor digitorum longus, flexor digitorum longus, extensor hallucis longus, and flexor hallucis longus. It also often occurs during the teenage years with overuse of leg muscles by repeated jumping or long distance running. Pain usually occurs from the inflammation in the medial calf on the bottom one third of the tibia.

Case Study 74

Patient: Female, 13 years old (team handball player)

FOC: March 28, 2011

Main Complaint: Calf pain in both legs R<L (shin splint). Dizziness, hay fever, rhinitis, coughing, stiff neck and shoulders, low back pain, heaviness over entire body.

Examination: Temperature 37.3°C, SP-6 and SP-8 extremely tender

Pulse Diagnosis: Rapid, Lung deficiency

Treatment: Direct moxibustion on SP-6. SRT followed by direct moxibustion on SP-

8, with intradermal needle retained afterward. SRT on LU-9, SP-3, BL-25, Onodera's point, BL-58, BL-59, BL-13, and GB-21.

Branch treatment: Needles inserted superficially in the middle of the most tender point on each knee. This was followed by 80% moxibustion and then an intradermal needle. In addition, ST-36, BL-40, and Onodera's point were needled superficially.

Progress: (2nd) Apr 4 – Liver deficiency. No more knee pain. No tender points on calves.

Comments: Reactions (tenderness) appeared on the posterior border of the tibia along the Spleen meridian. Tender and indurated points can be located by sliding a fingertip along the posterior border of the tibia. Treating reactive points between SP-6 and SP-8, with retained or non-retained needles, moxibustion, and intradermal needles all are effective. In extreme cases there is risk of stress fractures, so advise against heavy workouts. Treatment can take months and needs to be continued until relief is obtained.

Summary

- Locate reactive points along tibia.
- Intradermal needles on SP-8.

4. Occlusive arteriosclerosis

Intermittent claudication is often seen with this condition. One cannot walk at all when it gets really bad. Since it is caused by arteriosclerosis in the legs, it usually occurs after middle age. There is a condition called Buerger's disease in which there is a complete loss of pulse in the foot. One must be careful when a circulatory obstruction is suspected and advise immediate medical attention. The first place to feel the pulse is the dorsal pedal artery (just proximal to LR-3) and the second place is the posterior tibial artery (around KI-3). When these pulses are strong, there is no problem with circulation in the legs. A problem is likely when they are faint or you have trouble palpating them. When a pulse cannot be felt at these points at all, there is likelihood of arterial occlusion.

What is the effect of acu-moxa on arterial occlusion? Unfortunately, I can't get any effect at my skill level. In this case I refer the patient to a vascular surgeon. Be sure to refer pulseless patients with cold and numb feet to a vascular specialist. Otherwise they may end up wasting time making the rounds of different doctors. If they go to any hospital, they are likely to be sent to an orthopedic specialist and probably be tested and told there is no problem. Be sure to refer them to a hospital with a vascular surgeon. If it is in fact arterial occlusion, they will receive balloon therapy, or a stent if it's more advanced. Therefore, refer patients whose foot pulses are absent or very faint right away. Sometimes the results come back with the ABI index normal and the CT scan also showing normal vessels, and the tests do not match the results of our palpation. When arterial occlusion is refuted or when surgery is not indicated for various reasons, acu-moxa is highly recommended. It seems that acupuncture, and especially moxibustion, can actually facilitate the formation of new vessels.

Bear in mind, however, that when patients have this condition, they will also have arteriosclerosis in other places. How is their heart? What about their brain? We must inquire and avoid getting in over our heads.

The treatment of occlusive arteriosclerosis is similar to other leg problems, but always include LR-3 and KI-3. Home moxibustion treatments are highly recommended. Moxibustion on ST-36, LR-3, and KI-3 is especially useful.

Root treatment: Liver deficiency is common.

Branch treatment: LR-3, KI-3, ST-36, Ischial point, BL-25, BL-58. Direct moxibustion on the most reactive points.

5. Leg pain (neuralgia)

Case Study 75

Patient: Male, 69 years old

FOC: March 4, 2009

Main Complaint: He started having spontaneous pain (at rest) in his leg a month ago and went to an orthopedic doctor who told him he had herniated his lumbar vertebrae. The pain has diminished with treatments at the hospital, but he still has some pain and numbness.

Examination: Dorsiflexion in the big toe of left foot is slightly weak.

Pulse Diagnosis: Liver deficiency

Treatment: SRT on LR-8, KI-10, ST-36, and BL-23. SRT on the left side only – BL-25, Ischial point, BL-37, BL-58, and BL-59.

Direct moxibustion on the left side only – BL-25, ST-36, BL-58, and BL-59.

I had the patient apply moxibustion on the last three points on his leg, five cones every day.

Progress: For two months he came in once a week for treatment. After that, he came once every other week.

(9th) Dorsiflexion in the left big toe became normal.

(20th) No more leg pain.

Seven months later, he had no more symptoms.

Comments: You want to cure the patient as quickly as possible. One month would be ideal, but many cases take 3-6 months. This is why it takes resolve on the part of the patient as well as the practitioner. At first the above patient applied moxibustion diligently, but he stopped once the pain eased. So he just received acu-moxa in the clinic.

Case Study 76

Patient: Male, 70 years old

FOC: September 30, 2005

Main Complaint: Pain in the right leg. All of a sudden on Sept 7 he was unable to walk, with pain in his right leg. There was constant pain, day and night, even at rest. Examination at a hospital yielded a diagnosis of sciatica. He had numbness all the way down to below his right ankle.

History: Prostate surgery

Pulse Diagnosis: Lung deficiency, Liver excess

Treatment: SRT on LU-9, SP-3, LR-2 (dispersion), GB-21, GB-20, and LU-7 on healthy side. SRT on the affected (right) side – ST-36, BL-23, BL-25, Ischial point, BL-37, BL-58 (dispersion), and BL-59 (dispersion).

Direct moxibustion on BL-25, ST-36, BL-58, and BL-59 on the right, and LU-7 on the left.

Progress:

(2nd) Oct 3 – Leg pain persists.

(3rd) Oct 5 – A little better. He can sleep. Liver deficiency.

(6th) Oct 26 – No pain. Liver deficiency.

Comments: The ideal is for the patient to get at least a little relief with the first treatment. This motivates the patient to get more treatments. Clinical reality is more difficult. Perhaps this corresponds to the advice given in chapter 35 of *Basic Questions* to avoid acupuncture during a raging fever.

6. Numbness in legs

Case Study 77

Patient: Male, 61 years old (driver)

FOC: January 15, 2011

Main Complaints: Numbness in both legs since six months previously. He also has pain in his hips that is worse on the right. Sometimes he has pinprick sensations that go down his lower legs (Stomach meridian) for 10 seconds at a time.

Examination: Orthopedic exams all negative

Pulse Diagnosis: Liver deficiency

Treatment: Mostly SRT treatment (similar to Case 75) with some insertion in BL-25 and the Ischial point on both sides. Direct moxibustion also applied on the above points.

Progress:

(7th) Pinprick sensation occurs 2-3 times a day.

(10th) No more pinprick sensation, but the numbness remains.

(12th) Symptoms are almost gone.

Comments: There are many causes for numbness in the legs, but sometimes it is unclear, even with Western medical exams. I see it quite a bit in my clinic. If you know the cause or source, you can treat it and also attempt SRT on the points in the center of the numb areas.

7. Other leg problems

7.1 Sports injuries

Athletic injuries usually heal easily. This is natural when you consider that what heals an injury is the patient's own body. We need to be careful because sometimes we fall under the illusion that acupuncture, moxibustion, or medicines heal the body. Athletes' powers of recovery are simply amazing. I recall a rugby player with anterior thigh pain who was carried into my clinic by his coach and teammates. The day after treatment he was back to normal and competed in a match. The secret to a good treatment is determining exactly what has been injured and precisely locating tender points. Sports acupuncture is all the rage these days in Japan, and this growing knowledge base is a great help.

7.2 Achilles tendonitis & peritendonitis

When the Achilles tendon is swollen and red, you can press it anteriorly and it is tender. When the inflammation is minimal, you can pinch it from both sides, and pain will be felt. Those points that are sensitive will often have a catch when you stroke over it. Treat those tender points that catch your finger. This feeling of going over a nodule occurs not only over BL-59 but elsewhere, such as ST-36.

When the inflammation is extreme, there is greater chance of a tear in the Achilles tendon, so one must be careful. When you palpate the Achilles tendon carefully with the foot in dorsiflexion, occasionally you will find a fissure. Sometimes the patient and even their doctor is unaware of it. Surgery is the best solution for tears in the Achilles tendon.

CHAPTER

6

Joint & Connective Tissue Diseases

1. Overview of joint pathology

In ancient China the symptoms of pain, swelling, and deformity in the joints came under the heading of "body heavy joints painful."[1] The body feels heavy and joints hurt all over. This is a very apt expression. This was designated as symptomatology of the Spleen, and it makes clinical sense. Aside from joint symptoms, the symptomatology of the Spleen includes the following: lack of appetite or excessive appetite, a craving for sweets, poor sleep, and a heavy feeling throughout the body. Rheumatoid arthritis (RA) is one of the representative diseases where there is pain in many joints. Even specialists can be at a loss when it is acute and pervasive. It is no easy condition to treat. Even when anti-rheumatic or steroidal drugs are used to alleviate the acute symptoms the arthritis often transitions to a chronic disease and continues to plague the patient.

What about acupuncture and moxibustion? They work quite well, but acute cases are quite difficult to treat. Nevertheless, sometimes we can get patients through the acute phase with just acu-moxa treatments. When it doesn't work after several treatments, however, it's hard to bear witnessing patients suffer day after day. So we have to refer them to a specialist. Judicious use of drugs will get them through the acute phase and calm their symptoms. Acu-moxa treatments have a complementary effect in this stage. The symptoms go away almost completely as weekly treatments are continued. Doctors don't talk about complete cures when it comes to rheumatoid arthritis. They call it amelioration or remission. The root of the disease doesn't go away and it can recur at any time. Recurrence is prevented by continuing acu-moxa treatments. They are truly ideal forms of treatment.

---

1. Body heavy joints painful (体重節痛): One of the five-phases classification of symptoms in chapter 68 of the *Classic of Difficulties*.

Aside from RA, simple arthritis is a common joint disease. The joint becomes warm and swollen. As long as it's not RA, it can be treated pretty effectively with acu-moxa. What about other joint diseases? Often they don't feel warm. Nevertheless, the joint slowly becomes deformed. Such joint problems come with overuse or aging. Acu-moxa treatments don't have an immediate effect because we are dealing with an aging process, but steady improvement can be obtained when treatments are continued patiently. Acu-moxa treatments can be recommended as an effective treatment for such conditions.

Summary

- Acupuncture and moxibustion are indicated for acute rheumatoid arthritis, but refer the patient to a doctor if there is no immediate improvement.
- In chronic cases symptoms can be alleviated when treatments are continued.
- Regular treatment is the ideal approach.

1.1 Examination and treatment

Examination: First examine closely and note the condition of the joint(s). How swollen is it? Is it flushed or red. Especially note whether there is edema. Next palpate the joint(s). Feel for warmth, coolness, tenderness, indurations, and the presence of edema. Chart your findings and remember them. We must track how these finding change with treatment. Finally, move the joint(s). Confirm its range of motion. With any improvement, naturally the range of motion also increases.

Pulse diagnosis: The basic pattern must be determined for treatment; Spleen deficiency is common.

Tight back associated points: This idea came from Fukaya style moxibustion,[2] but when there is rheumatoid arthritis in the upper limbs, indurations appear around BL-13, LB-14, and BL-15. When an induration appears on the right, it indicates the arthritis is in the upper right extremity. When it appears on the left, it indicates the arthritis is in the upper left extremity. The symptoms disappear or are alleviated when this induration is accurately located and moxibustion is applied. The size of this induration is directly correlated to the severity of the pain. One can also gauge the progress of treatment based on the size of this induration.

In Fukaya style moxibustion, arthritis in the lower extremities is said to produce indurations between BL-23 and BL-26, but this reaction doesn't seem to appear as clearly as with arthritis in the upper extremities. In the case of arthritis in the lower extremities, I just narrow the target down to BL-25 or BL-26 and locate and treat the most reactive point.

---

2. Fukaya style moxibustion : An approach to direct moxibustion therapy developed by Isaburo Fukaya 深谷伊三郎 (1900-1974).

To summarize, when there is systemic rheumatoid arthritis, determine the pattern based on the pulse and give a root treatment. Then apply direct moxibustion on indurations around BL-13 and BL-25. These two steps form the foundation for the treatment of arthritis.

Summary

- Observe, palpate, and move the joint.
- Take the pulse and determine the pattern.
- Find indurations around BL-13 and BL-25.

1.2 Basics of joint treatment

Once the above foundation of treatment is established, specific joints must be addressed. What kind of attention is required? When many joints are affected, the number of points treated increases. This is why the points for each joint must be kept to a minimum. Palpate the joints before the treatment to confirm how much heat is in each. The warmer the joint is, the higher the priority for treatment. After confirming the severity of symptoms in each joint, decide which one gets acupuncture. When there are few affected joints, the number of points treated on the joints can be increased a little.

The points over the joints must be palpated with the most sensitive finger. Experience counts here. Can you find the best points without asking the patient? This is where your expertise shows. The affected joints must be palpated with very light pressure because it hurts the patient and it can aggravate the pain. Be very gentle. The super-rotation technique (SRT) is the best approach. Inserting the needle can fatigue the patient and it is easy to over-do the stimulation. More moxibustion can be used instead. Apply stronger moxibustion on indurations around BL-13 and BL-25 and apply smaller cones on the affected joints. The cones don't have to be burned all the way to the skin (80% moxibustion). It is best if the patient is able to apply moxibustion at home. The same points, indurations around BL-13 and BL-25, and points on affected joints can be used, but mark just a few points for home treatment. Refer to the sections below on individual conditions for how to treat different joint conditions.

Continue treatments as described above, and if possible give treatments once a week. The patient's condition will improve little by little. Give it at least three months. When you patiently give treatment over a year or two, the patient will reach a satisfactory condition. Even when their symptoms are almost completely absent, they should not stop getting treatments. It would be ideal to continue treatments once a month. In some cases, the RA factor disappears. I am convinced that acu-moxa is really an ideal form of treatment.

Summary

- Find the warm spots on joints and apply SRT.
- Keep the number of points to a minimum.
- Continue monthly treatments even after the symptoms resolve.

2. Knee joint pathology

Knee pain is the most common condition in my clinic after neck and shoulder stiffness and low back pain. It is to be expected since it is rare (as we age) for the knees that support all our body weight to remain problem free. I have passed my whole life without doing heavy labor, yet even so I began to feel some pain in my knees after age 70. When it gets bad, they swell and become warm. It must be the so-called geriatric osteoarthritis. Given that my grandmother and both my parents had knee pain, it must be my inherited constitution.

The knees of my older patients who continue to participate in sports and those who make a practice of walking tend to be in great shape without any sign of deformity. I call these "sports knees." When I palpate these knees using the base of my thumbs, the bone is firm and there is no sponginess. (See below for a method of checking the knees.)

2.1 Osteoarthritis of the knees

The most common knee joint disease is osteoarthritis. Some even say aging begins in human beings in the knees. Supposedly this is followed by occlusions in the vertebral arteries. Even though I'm not convinced about this sequence, rounded backs, hunching forward, and limping from knee pain is a typical image of the elderly.

The first thing is to examine the extent of deformity. How much does the knee bend? Can the medial sides of the knees touch each other? If not, they have genu varum or bow legs. Can the ankles come together? If not, they have genu valgrum or knock knees. Do the back of the knees come close to the treatment table? If not, it's a flexion deformity. Also examine the position of the patellas and their perimeter. How swollen are they? How much fluid is in the joint? Can you feel any heat?

Confirming the amount of heat is important. Sometimes it is warm over the entire knee. In cases of localized pain you can compare the temperature of that spot with the normal side. Always recheck the amount of heat after treatment. If the treatment goes well, the heat diminishes or subsides.

Next palpate the areas with deformity. My method is to use the anterior surface of the thumb joint[3] (Fig. 6-1). When you move the thumb back and forth (knead) over the bone in small movements, you can clearly distinguish the problem areas. Once you become used to this method, you can even find these areas over clothing (like a pair of jeans). You will be able to quickly pinpoint the problem area. Using this method, you will find that not all parts of the knee are affected. With medial knee issues, often the problem spot is found slightly medial to M-LE-16 *(xī yǎn)*, just under the patella. Reactions also often appear at ST-34. In cases of genu valgrum (knock knee), a reaction appears at M-LE-16 *(xī yǎn)*. In cases of genu varum (bow leg), a reaction appears at ST-35. When there is

3. Palpation with thumb joint: This method of palpation is my preferred method for many hard areas. Even when doing Anma massage, it feels better for the patient when I use the base, rather than the tip, of the thumb.

flexion deformity, the reaction tends to appear around BL-40.

Locating the reactive points precisely over the joint will determine the outcome, and this is true in the treatment of all joints. You can use SRT, simple insertion, or retain needles superficially. Deep insertion isn't good. The most common treatment points are M-LE-16 *(xī yǎn)*, ST-35, and ST-36. Sometimes ST-34 is also useful. If possible, have the patient apply moxibustion on these points at home. The results are better with home moxa treatment. When there is heat or swelling, I often treat the patient for Spleen deficiency using SP-3. If there is no inflammation, only deformity, I often treat for Liver deficiency using LR-8.

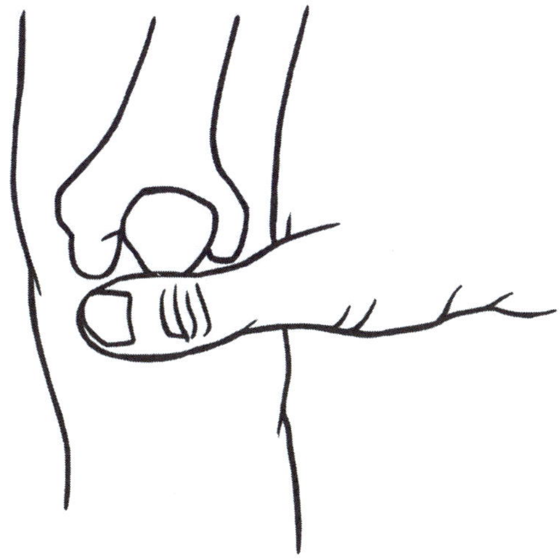

Fig. 6-1 Using thumb joint to palpate knee

Summary

- Use the anterior surface of the thumb joint to palpate the knee.
- Move the thumb back and forth (knead).
- Treat M-LE-16 *(xī yǎn)*, ST-35, and ST-36

2.2 Rheumatoid arthritis of the knee

Note the condition of other joints, treat around M-LE-16 *(xī yǎn)*, and keep the number of insertions as few as possible. Focus on the places with the most heat. (See section 1.2 Basics of joint treatment, above.)

2.3 Bursitis of the knee[4]

With this problem the area around SP-9 will exhibit tenderness along the tibia. It begins with pain while walking, but there is no pain when sitting. In acute cases the

4. Bursitis is inflammation of bursa, small fluid-filled sacs that reduce friction and cushion contact points between bones, tendons, and muscles near joints. The condition referred to here is a common complaint for athletes located at the insertion of three muscles on the medial condyle of the tibia.

patient cannot walk without limping and requires some support. Yet because there is no deformity or changes in the joint, it doesn't show up on X-rays. Orthopedic doctors thus often make light of this condition.

Needle the most tender points. It is good to place intradermal needles in these points afterward. It takes time to heal, but it can heal completely. Often there is no heat in the affected area, but sometimes it gets warm when aggravated or it begins to hurt in tandem with ST-35 and M-LE-16 *(xī yǎn)*.

2.4 Osgood-Schlatter disease (see p. 148)

2.5 Sports injuries (see p. 153)

2.6 Baker's cyst

Lumps like rubber balls form in the popliteal fossa on and below BL-40. These are known as Baker's cysts. These cysts are full of a viscous clear fluid. Home moxibustion is the best treatment for this. Have them do direct moxibustion on ST-36 if possible. The viscous fluid will be absorbed and the cysts will disappear.

2.7 Patellofemoral pain syndrome

In this condition there is knee pain with walking, but no pain when standing or sitting. Unlike bursitis of the knee mentioned above, there are no tender points whatsoever in the surrounding area. It is caused by loss of glide between the patella and the femur. This syndrome comes on suddenly without any provocation and patients are surprised. Many orthopedic doctors in Japan don't know what to do about it.[5]

I discovered the way to identify this condition and treat it. Great discovery! Place the distal joint of the thumb on the inferior margin of the patella, and gently press upward (Fig. 6-1). If there is pain, it's patellofemoral pain syndrome. When the knee joint is intact, it is firm and there is not much movement of the patella up or down. This condition tends to occur when the patella becomes loose and moves too much. Acupuncture is the only way to treat it. The needle must be inserted to work. Insert a needle horizontally under the patella from where the patellar tendon attaches to the tibia. After inserting about 1cm, gently sparrow peck the needle about three times. You can think of it as cleaning the joint surface that has become gunky. In mild cases, just one needle can eliminate the pain. Even in severe cases, the pain can be alleviated with a series of treatments. Sometimes, in elderly patients, this condition presents itself along with other joint pathology.

Case Study 78

Patient: Male, 78 years old

5. In the United States, orthopedic doctors offer arthroscopic smoothing of the back of the patella and front of the femur, although this is not always possible.

FOC: Jan. 26, 2004

Symptom and Condition: Pain in right knee for the last two months. Pain with movement from hips down to lateral thigh and knee. It especially hurts when walking. There is no pain at rest. He cannot sit on the floor. No abnormalities were found at the hospital, so a neurological problem was suspected, and he was referred to a neurologist, but no abnormalities were found.

History: Surgery for prostate cancer 15 years ago. His prostate was removed. He hasn't had a good appetite for years, and he has lost 25kg in that time. He blames the drugs he takes for his cancer. He only has one bowel movement a week.

Examination: Patrick's test positive on right. Tenderness over knee (+), heat (–), upward movement of patella (+). His lower abdomen is hard. Tenderness and sensitivity to pinching along medial thigh (Upper LR-9, see Fig. 6-2), also induration and tenderness at Onodera's point. From the above I deduced that this patient had a combination of knee and hip joint pathology, patellofemoral pain syndrome, and neuralgia of the obturator nerve.

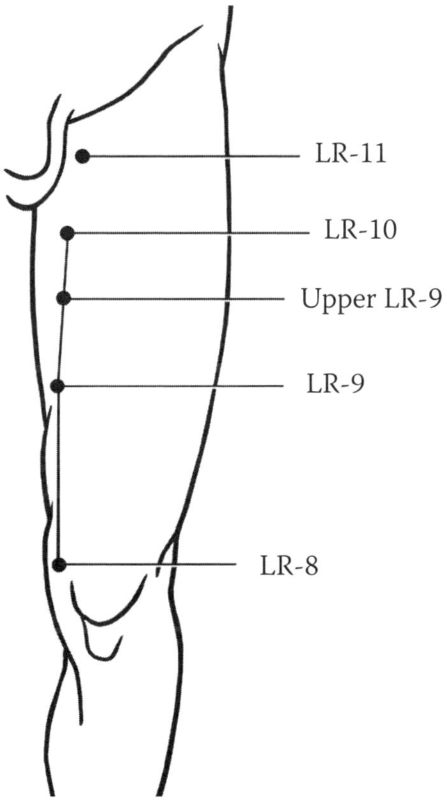

Fig. 6-2 Upper LR-9

Pulse Diagnosis: Liver deficiency

Treatment: Only the affected side was treated. SRT on LR-8, KI-10, LI-11, CV-12,

CV-6, ST-35, M-LE-16 *(xī yǎn)*, ST-36, BL-58, BL-59, BL-37, Ischial point, BL-27, and BL-52. A needle was retained in Onodera's point; direct moxibustion applied after removal. A needle was inserted 1cm under the patella from below, accompanied by sparrow-pecking motions.

Progress: Walking became easier after the first treatment.

(2nd) Feb. 2 – Pain has eased, and patient can walk without cane. Acupuncture and direct moxibustion applied on Upper LR-9 for pain in the medial thigh.

Comments: This case of leg pain was a combination of many conditions. The most difficult symptom, however, was pain when walking. Needling directly into the patellofemoral joint brought instant relief. It would have taken a lot longer without this technique.

Many things can cause leg pain with walking. Arteriosclerosis obliterans is well known for causing difficulty in walking, but it is often mistaken for something else because X-rays don't show it. Check the pulsation in the dorsal pedis artery (LR-3) and posterior tibial artery (KI-3). Suspect arteriosclerosis obliterans if these pulses are weak or absent. In cases of bursitis in the knee, often there is tenderness at SP-9. Leg pain from herniated discs can be determined by orthopedic tests, tenderness over the lumbar vertebra, and imaging studies when available. You can't give the appropriate treatment unless you know what you are treating.

Summary

- When there is pain only when walking, rule out arteriosclerosis obliterans.
- Push the patella upward to confirm patella-femoral joint syndrome.
- Insert a needle about 1cm under the patella from below.

2.8 The limits of treating knee pathology

Acu-moxa can completely resolve knee problems when there is just some tenderness and heat but no deformity. Swelling (edema) can also be treated in this way, but it's difficult for the patient when there is severe edema. Sometimes it is better to have the fluid extracted. In some cases, the swelling returns even after fluid extraction. Deformity from osteoarthritis depends on the degree, but recovery is unlikely once deformity sets in. The best we can do is to relieve the pain. When there is deformity, but no tender points, there is no hope for improvement with acu-moxa treatments.

Advanced cases end up requiring knee replacement. Orthopedic specialists do fluid extraction, cortisone and hyaluronic acid injections, and micro-surgery with an arthroscope, before the final step of replacement with an artificial joint. In mild cases, applying moxibustion at home regularly will prevent the need for knee replacement. Unfortunately, these days not that many people can stand the heat and have the patience to apply moxibustion year after year. It's really too bad!

Case Study 79

Acute Leg Pain

Patient: Male, 40 years old (acupuncturist)

FOC: April 9, 2010

Main complaint: Pain in left knee after going to gather seaweed. Pain is around the medial left knee, but it also hurts behind the knee, on the anterior and posterior thigh, and in the hip and lower back. There is pain with movement, especially when walking.

Examination: There is heat all over the knee, especially on the medial side. Even light touch is painful. It seems that there is some discrepancy between the condition of the knee and the pain the patient is experiencing. I find tenderness in points like GV-22, CV-17, GV-11, GV-10, and GV-9.

Pulse Diagnosis: Liver deficiency

Treatment: Needle retained at GV-22. SRT on LR-8, KI-10, and ST-36. I found a marked depression at ST-43 of the affected leg, so I also retained a needle there.

When I palpated the left knee again, the extreme sensitivity was gone. I found one tender point just medial to M-LE-16 *(xī yǎn)*. I applied SRT and then placed an intradermal needle. I followed this up with SRT on BL-40, GV-11, GV-10, and GV-9. I ended the treatment with direct moxibustion on M-LE-5 *(shitsumin/shī mián)*. The patient was able to walk without pain after the treatment.

Progress: I examined and treated this patient three hours later, and the tenderness and pain were 80% better. I could not feel any heat over the knees. He was able to walk without pain after the same treatment.

Comments: The patient had a very sensitive constitution that belied his sturdy build. From the extreme sensitivity when I first palpated the knee, I suspected that the pain may be amplified several times over in his brain. This suspicion was borne out when I put together all the tender points on other parts of his body related to stress and the mind (GV-22, CV-17, GV-11, GV-10, GV-9). It is apparent that his sensitivity returned to a normal level with some root treatment and some branch treatment on a few reactive points. One must first calm the system down when treating pain because trying to treat everything that shows up with the patient in a hypersensitive state is confusing.

By coincidence, this patient got the same taxi driver for his first and second visits to my clinic, and the driver was amazed at the difference. I heard about this from the driver who happened to give me a ride sometime later. This patient, who was an acupuncturist himself, lived far away, but he drove six hours each way after that for a year to get two treatments a month until he completely recovered.

Summary

- View the patient objectively when there is extreme pain and consider its cause.
- Determine which positions and which movements aggravate the pain.
- Learn and practice how to palpate the most tender point.
- Remember the importance and benefits of distal treatment.

Case Study 80

Acute Arthritis

Patient: Female, 76 years old (acupuncturist)

FOC: March 5, 2010

Symptoms and Condition: Pain in various places around the body beginning 10 days ago. She had pain in the neck so she saw a neurologist, but was told there was nothing abnormal. Her joints became suddenly painful from the day before, and movement is difficult. The pain is worst in the knees, left lateral elbow, and the shoulders. She cannot sleep well due to the pain.

Examination: The above joints are warm and swollen. Heat and tenderness found as follows: knee —LR-8, ST-35, M-LE-16 *(xī yǎn)*; elbow—lateral epicondyle of humerus; shoulders— medial to LI-15.

Tongue: Thick dark-yellow coating

Pulse Diagnosis: Rapid, Spleen deficiency

Treatment: SRT on SP-3, PC-7, CV-12, and reactive point on each joint

Direct moxibustion on BL-25, M-LE-5 *(shitsumin/shī mián)* and BL-17

Progress: Movement became easier after treatment.

(**2nd**) Mar 6 – Spleen deficiency; symptoms are the same. Intradermal needles placed in tender point on knees and shoulders on both sides.

(**3rd**) Mar 10 – Spleen deficiency. Pulse is not rapid but it's still not normal. Tongue coating is thinner.

(**4th**) Mar 16 – Lung deficiency. Pulse is slightly rapid. Less tenderness at medial LI-15, but there is a nodule lateral and inferior to LI-15. Intradermal needle placed here. The heat and tenderness on joints reduced.

(**5th**) Mar 24 – Spleen deficiency. Left shoulder feels better, but all other joints are the same. No appetite.

(**6th**) Mar 31 – Spleen deficiency. Elbow pain gone. Pain remains in knees and right shoulder. Appetite has slightly improved. Tongue coating is thinner.

(7TH) Apr 7 – Spleen deficiency. The pain was light so she went shopping. Appetite is still not good.

(8TH) Apr 14 – Spleen deficiency. No pain experienced. Left shoulder has some pain when the arm brought around the back in internal rotation. Tongue coating is not normal. Treatments concluded for the time being.

COMMENTS: This is a case of acute arthritis in multiple joints. The patient was told she didn't have rheumatoid arthritis, but the pain in many joints starting with her neck is suggestive of rheumatoid arthritis. I was hoping that the symptoms, especially the heat in the joints, would diminish with one treatment, but it took two. For the patient these were hellish days. The joint pain, lack of appetite, and tongue coating all indicate the connection with the Spleen. Her improvement was slow after her acute symptoms were resolved. It would have been ideal to treat her for two more months. That would have made her feel even better, but people have different ways of concluding treatment. People are different, and their treatments are different. Still, a year later she had no more pain, and she was leading a normal life.

Summary

- When there is pain in multiple joints, find just a few key reactive points.
- The importance of giving a root treatment for Spleen deficiency.
- Treat acute symptoms intensively; take your time with chronic symptoms.

Case Study 81

OSTEOARTHRITIS OF THE KNEE

PATIENT: Female, 65 years old

FOC: March 29, 2010

MAIN COMPLAINT: Pain in left knee beginning nine days ago. The knee is warm and she has difficulty walking.

PULSE DIAGNOSIS: Spleen deficiency

TREATMENT: SRT on SP-3, PC-7, CV-12, ST-36; on just the left side, BL-27, BL-40, medial and ST-35.

Direct moxibustion on ST-36, medial and ST-35 on left leg. Patient started applying moxibustion on these points at home after third treatment.

PROGRESS: Movement in left leg became easier after first treatment.

(3RD) Apr 26 – The knee is still warm.

(5TH) May 28 – Lung deficiency. Patient had fluids extracted from knee three times.

(8TH) Jul 5 – Heat over the knee diminished.

(9TH) Jul 21 – Patient caught a cold and has throat pain.

(16TH) Nov 8 – Heat over the knee diminished.

(17TH) Nov 29 – Heat over the knee gone.

Comments: This patient had always been a strong walker, so this debilitating knee pain really got to her. The results were not good in the first few treatments with just occasional acu-moxa. So I had her apply moxibustion at home on three knee points every day. Eventually the heat went away, the knee was no longer tender, and it became as good as before. She continues to apply moxibustion at home, and this is to be desired. She is really motivated to keep her knees in good shape!

Summary

- Small cones of direct moxibustion on local points applied regularly at home speeds recovery.

3. Elbow joint pathology

In cases of rheumatoid arthritis (RA) of the arm, refer to Overview of Joint Pathology, above. The most common condition I see in the elbow is pain on the outside, or so-called tennis elbow (lateral epicondylitis). The second most common condition is pain on the inside of the elbow, called baseball or golf elbow (medial epicondylitis). In the case of real tennis elbow, a tennis player has hit too many balls, which has caused inflammation in the lateral epicondyle of the humerus. In the case of athletes, all they need to do to alleviate it is to take a rest from practice. Nevertheless, it does take a while to heal completely. The same applies to non-tennis repetitive stress injuries. In medical clinics they give cortisone shots, but this treatment cannot be repeated over and over. Acu-moxa can be very effective for repetitive stress injuries of the elbow. The most important thing is to find the point of greatest inflammation (usually on the lateral epicondyle). If you pinpoint the exact spot, you are halfway to solving the problem.

To palpate the exact spot, when the left elbow is affected, lightly grasp the patient's left wrist in your right hand and use the base of the thumb of your left hand to probe the lateral epicondyle. This is the same technique as described above to palpate for osteoarthritis in the knees. Press above and below the bone with a back and forth movement. You are in luck if you can find a depressed point that is tender. Often it only takes only a little pressure to elicit tenderness. The point will move a bit depending on whether the elbow is straight or slightly flexed. Since you're taking the time to locate the point precisely, be sure to apply acupuncture and or moxibustion with the arm in the exact same position. If patients are going to do moxibustion at home, be sure that they learn the right position for the elbow. When it comes to acupuncture, SRT, superficial insertion, and retaining needles all work fine.

While you are at it, be sure to look for reactions at LI-10, LI-11, and Sawada's TB-9. If these points are tender or tight, there is generalized strain and pain in the elbow from overuse. Be sure to treat these reactive points as well. If possible, have the patient apply moxibustion at home on the one most reactive point. If this isn't possible, retain an intradermal needle.

3.1 Two types of medial elbow pain

There are two common types of medial elbow pain. The first is pain in the medial epicondyle. This usually corresponds to HT-3. Just as with tennis elbow, use the base of your thumb to palpate the point. It is usually quite tender, so be sure to use light pressure to find the point. Pain in the medial epicondyle is tenacious and doesn't go away so quickly. It is best if the patient applies moxibustion at home on the most reactive point. Unlike on the lateral epicondyle, however, the inside of the elbow is sensitive and many patients are unable to consistently do moxibustion there. The condition will improve faster, however, if patients are able to persist with moxibustion at home.

The other kind of pain in the medial epicondyle is so-called baseball elbow. The pain is close to PC-3 (this is on the medial border of the biceps, but it is best to palpate its tendon.) Light pressure on this area with the base of the thumb will reveal hard bulging fibers. The harder the induration, the worse the problem. Baseball pitchers sometimes throw curves. The finger placement for gripping the ball is different for throwing curves than for throwing straight balls. Baseball elbow is especially common in grade school and middle school pitchers whose muscles and bones are still developing. They really should forbid grade school and middle school pitchers from throwing curve balls. Treatment outcome depends on whether you are able to locate and needle the reactive point accurately. This is true for other elbow problems as well. It would be best to have the patient receive moxibustion at home on the reactive point, but often this is not possible due to sensitivity and age of the patient. You can place an intradermal needle instead. Naturally, other points related to the repetitive strain of a pitcher such as LI-10, LI-11, SI-9, SI-11, GB-21, and LU-1 need to be examined for reactions of stress or fatigue and treated.

Case Study 82

ACUTE LATERAL EPICONDYLITIS

PATIENT: Female, 70 years old

FOC: October 9, 2009

MAIN COMPLAINT: Sudden pain in left elbow started the previous day. There is pain without movement. The slightest touch or movement aggravates the pain. It was caused by overuse in farming. She also has some low back pain.

EXAMINATION: The elbow is swollen and warm. Body temperature: 37.6°C.

The pain and heat is along the Large Intestine and Triple Burner meridians. Induration found around BL-15 on left.

PULSE DIAGNOSIS: Lung deficiency, floating and rapid

Treatment: SRT in supine position: tonification of LU-9 and SP-3, dispersion of LI-10 and HT-8. SRT in side-lying position with left side up: GB-20, GB-21, and SI-11. Direct moxibustion was also applied on these points. Also some SRT on low back points.

Seated position: 20 cones of direct moxibustion on induration at BL-15 on left. The last five cones were made slightly larger to increase heat.

Local treatment: 3 cones of heat-sensing moxibustion[6] over the most tender point on the elbow. An intradermal needle was placed in this point afterward.

Progress: The pain was alleviated by the above treatment. The pain resolved quickly because it was in the early stages of inflammation. I told the patient to avoid bathing and using the left arm. If the pain was not better the next day, she should come back the following day, and if the pain was better, she should come back in four days. Her elbow was relatively pain free the next day and she was able to resume farm work.

Comments: In this case I attempted dispersion of the fire points of the Lung and Heart meridians, LI-10 and HT-8. Sometimes I use this dispersion technique of Yanagiya Sorei[7] when I have trouble getting the pulses to come up with the standard treatment for Lung deficiency. This patient returned for treatment two months later complaining of difficulty raising her left arm, but interestingly enough, her elbow was just fine.

4. Temporomandibular joint dysfunction (TMJ)

It wasn't so long ago that it became recognized in medicine that problems in the temporomandibular joint can affect the brain, not to mention the whole body. With this in mind, when I examine anyone with TMJ issues, I gently press the eyes (to check for abnormally high ocular pressure) and I press BL-2, LI-20, and GB-5 to look for signs of tension. While I'm at it, I also press ST-7. When the muscles below ST-7 are tense, I assume there is some TMJ issue and apply SRT technique on that point.

This is in the realm of subclinical diseases, but occasionally there are patients who come in with the chief complaint of jaw pain. They find it hard to chew, it hurts them to chew, and in extreme cases they can't open their mouth. Jaw problems can lead to many problems down the line. I am one of those who believes that chewing each mouthful 50 times is one condition for good health. The main thing in treating conditions like this is to assess the condition of the jaw muscles and grasp the condition of the jaws. To be specific, have the patient open their mouth as wide as possible and measure the distance. This distance will increase as they improve with treatment.

4.1 Treatment of TMJ

6. Heat-sensing moxibustion: The moxa cone is burned directly on the skin but removed as soon as the patient feels the heat.

7. Yanagiya Sorei 柳谷素霊 (1906-1959): A leader in the traditional acupuncture movement in Japan who inspired the creation of the Meridian Therapy style.

ROOT TREATMENT: There is no typical pattern for TMJ dysfunction, but if you are not sure, you can treat for Spleen deficiency pattern. Also, based on the flow of the meridians over the jaws, check and treat the *yáng míng* meridians, especially the Stomach meridian. I like to use points like ST-36 and ST-43.

LOCAL TREATMENT: Palpate the jaw area, pressing gently with the middle finger. It is easiest to position yourself above the head of the patient and palpate both sides at once. Of course, this works when the jaw problem is on one side, but comparing the sides does not work when both sides have a problem. Insert needles in the tightest points. When there is strong pain or pain without movement, it is better to use just SRT. Inserting needles can aggravate the pain when it's strong. Insertion is fine when the problem is chronic. Stop the insertion and rotate the needle when the needle tip reaches the hardest point. It also works to retain the needle.

In severe cases, follow this up with direct moxibustion, or heat-sensing moxibustion. When the point is sensitive you can apply direct moxibustion but let it burn just 80% of the way down. It can also be effective instead to place an intradermal needle on the tightest point, but this leads to an issue of the person's appearance, especially with women.

Also check and treat other local points with SRT such as ST-7, GB-5, GB-20, and TB-16. And don't forget to look for tight points on the shoulder and back such as GB-21 and BL-13. For direct moxibustion on indurations at BL-13 on the affected side, the more severe the symptoms, the greater the number of cones.

Apart from this, when the jaws feel tired or the mouth is heavy, it can be viewed as a jaw problem. Treat it as a disease yet to manifest and it will serve as preventative treatment.

Summary

- Acu-moxa works well for TMJ problems.
- Treat Spleen deficiency, Stomach meridian (ST-36), and moxa on BL-13.
- Local treatment: SRT on ST-7.

5. Shoulder joint disorders

Of all the joints, the shoulder joint has the greatest range of motion. This is why it has problems. It's really inconvenient to have a shoulder problem. Until recently, I have had no personal experience of "frozen shoulder," commonly referred to in Japan as "50-year-old shoulder." However, just recently my right shoulder started to feel uncomfortable. When I tried to reach for something in front of me, there was a sharp pain. There was also pain when I reached my hand behind me. Since my "frozen shoulder" came after age 80, I braced myself for a one-year course of recovery, but I received acu-moxa and it resolved in about a week. The point that seemed to work best was SI-9, and especially when the tip of the needle reached to the tight spot I felt deep in there. In terms of muscles, it must be a point in the deltoid. I think that the motion of typing on my computer was the cause of the problem. So it wasn't anything to worry about after all, just a phenomenon of aging.

The important thing in treating shoulder problems is distinguishing adhesive capsulitis (frozen shoulder) from other shoulder pathologies. Middle-aged people with shoulder pain tend to be quickly diagnosed as adhesive capsulitis when there is pain reaching behind, but this is not appropriate. In medical clinics they give you a blood test, and if the rheumatic factor is negative, it is automatically adhesive capsulitis, not arthritis. Why must we be careful to clearly distinguish adhesive capsulitis? It is because the treatment required with acu-moxa is different. In cases of adhesive capsulitis, the shoulder can withstand strong treatments using thick needles, deep insertions, and even moving the arm after insertion with the needle in place. If you give such strong treatment to an arthritic shoulder, however, it will immediately get worse. It takes more time to recover. If one always uses shallow insertion with thin needles, of course, there is no real need to clearly distinguish the shoulder problem.

5.1 Frozen shoulder (adhesive capsulitis)

This condition is sometimes referred to as bursitis or "periarthritis." The cause varies, but often it is attributed to diminishing hormones. That means people who are middle-aged or older. When we explain to patients that they are approaching middle-age they often laugh and agree. It's not so wise to bluntly say, "You're getting old."

The first thing to check for is indurations on the first Bladder line between BL-11 and BL-14. If you find an induration, especially on the affected side, you can assume that it is arthritis or a combination of arthritis and adhesive capsulitis. If the two conditions are combined, the symptoms of arthritis-like pain will eventually subside and loss in range of motion, a hallmark of adhesive capsulitis, will remain. It takes at least a year to recover from adhesive capsulitis once it sets in. It is good to measure the range of motion. That way you can see how well your treatments are working. Before each treatment, record the angle of flexion, extension, abduction, and extension with internal rotation (how far back the hand goes behind).

What we must bear in mind here is that shoulder pain can originate from pathologies other than in the shoulder. Most commonly it is secondary to cervical syndrome and thoracic outlet syndrome. If the shoulder pain is related to either or both of these syndromes, they must also be treated. Of course, this would not change the root treatment, only the branch treatment.

5.1.1 Treatment of frozen shoulder

When the pain is in the anterior shoulder, an active point shows up around the origin of the biceps where a tendon attaches to the scapula. The chances are greater for the active point to appear on the lateral side, around the attachment of the long head. This is M-UE-48 (*mae kengū/jiān qián*), which I often call "anterior LI-15" (see Fig. 1-7).

When the pain is in the posterior shoulder, there is a point that shows up, usually at SI-9, but occasionally at SI-10. Restrictions in ROM can be approached by choosing both anterior and posterior active points. In addition, SI-11 is an important point in these situations; it is especially good for relieving pain.

What about the standard LI-15? It doesn't often show up as a reactive point, but it is good for increasing the ROM, especially abduction. Insert a needle medially toward the centerline between the bones (humerus and scapula) and lift and thrust gently several times. This has an effect on the supraspinatus muscle. Have patients reach around behind with the affected arm before doing this technique. Have them do it again after performing the above technique, and they will be amazed how much easier it is. The problem is, the next day the ROM will go right back to where it was. Still, the effect is dramatic.

Other points to check include LI-10 and -11 on the Large Intestine meridian, TB-5 and Sawada's TB-9 on the Triple Burner meridian, and SI-11 on the Small Intestine meridian. The effect is even better when whichever points you select receive regular direct moxibustion at home. The cones of moxa can be rather big. In some cases, the effect is better with bigger cones. If the pain comes from arthritis, however, moxibustion will make it worse so we must be careful to differentiate. Beware of heat or redness in the shoulder area. If it is adhesive capsulitis, three months of weekly treatments should do the trick. When the pain is extreme, some patients ask for more than one treatment in a week. This is just fine in the acute phase; you can even treat them every day.

No more treatment is necessary once both pain at rest and pain with movement are gone and all that is left is some limitation in ROM. The pain will go away by itself with moderate movement in about one year. So it is true that it takes about a year for adhesive capsulitis to resolve completely, no matter who gives the treatment. It's not advisable to tell this to a first-time patient, however. They might say, "If it takes that long anyway, I may as well forget about acu-moxa." Tell them, "It will take about a year for the restriction in ROM to resolve completely. This is true no matter who treats you. Once the throbbing pain and the sharp pain with movement goes away, it will heal naturally." They might ask, "How long will that take?" You can reply, "It will be about three months." There is an old saying in Japan, "one hundred days of moxa." It means most chronic diseases start to resolve in about three months with regular moxibustion. It also means it won't get better unless you persist for three months. In any case, when the pain is relieved and eventually goes away with the help of acu-moxa, people also notice that it makes them feel great and become regular customers.

Summary

- Determine if it is only adhesive capsulitis, or if there are other causes.
- Recommend a three-month course of treatment; after that, let the patient decide.
- Needle M-UE-48 *(mae kengū/jiān qián)*, SI-9, SI-11, and do horizontal insertion in LI-15.

5.2 Arthritis in the shoulder

There is a saying in Japan, "First eyes, second legs." It means the most difficult disease is of the eyes, and this is followed by disease of the legs. The rest may not be as debilitating, but what about severe pain in the shoulder and arm?

When treating arthritis, first you have to get a feel for where the heat is coming from. The most common hot spot is around M-UE-48 (*mae kengū/jiān qián).* Sometimes it can be felt at the joint of the clavicle and the scapula. Palpate the shoulder carefully to make sure. The hot spots should be treated gently with contact needling or SRT. When the heat is intense, avoid retaining any needles, which means that even intradermal needles are contraindicated. Once the heat subsides after several treatments, intradermal needles can be retained. Multiple cones of direct moxibustion on back associated points around BL-13 is very good for arthritis. But don't forget to do a root treatment, and on the affected arm use points on the affected yang meridians. Inflammation usually resolves relatively quickly. Until then, instruct the patient to avoid hot baths.

Case Study 83

ACUTE INFLAMMATION OF SHOULDER

Patient: Female, 63 years old

FOC: March 11, 2008

Situation and Symptoms: She was playing with her grandchild when he jumped onto her left shoulder. He was quite heavy. There wasn't any pain then, but the next day it felt uncomfortable. The pain intensified during the night two days after the injury. She can't sleep.

Examination: She cannot move her left arm. The shoulder is swollen and feels very hot. The swelling is around LI-15, about the size of the hand placed over it. There is extreme tenderness in the anterior shoulder such that just placing an insertion tube on it causes her to cry out in pain. It is swollen and tender all around the affected area.

Comments: This was obviously a case of an acute injury. There is another condition that resembles this called calcific tendonitis of the rotator cuff. This also causes sudden and intense shoulder pain, but the location is slightly different. This case was on the anterior shoulder and the cause was clearly due to an impact, so I ruled out calcific tendonitis. Now what to do? If I referred her to an orthopedic doctor, he could resolve the pain with a cortisone shot in the shoulder. Yet I often have good results with cases like this so I wanted to take care of it with acupuncture if I could.

Temperature: 37°C

Pulse Diagnosis: Floating and rapid, Lung deficiency

Treatment: I did the branch treatment first, applying 30 cones of direct moxibustion on an induration at BL-13 on the left. I left the reactive point at anterior LI-15 alone and performed SRT on LI-11, SI-9, and SI-11 on the left, followed by five small cones of direct moxibustion on these points. I concluded with the root treatment with SRT on LU-9, SP-3, LU-10, and HT-8.

Usually I suggest treatments once a week, but this case was acute so I treated her the next day.

(2ND) Mar 12 – She was able to sleep, but the pain persisted. The shoulder was still warm. Her temperature was 37.1°C. Lung deficiency. I added heat-sensing moxibustion on the painful shoulder and retained an intradermal needle. I also did multiple cones of direct moxibustion at BL-14.

(3RD) Mar 15 – The shoulder pain had subsided beginning the day after the last treatment. Her temperature was 36.1°C. The shoulder is no longer warm, but it is still tender. She can lie on her back. Kidney deficiency. Used the root treatment points KI-7, LU-5, SP-3, and KI-3.

(4TH) Mar 21 – Kidney deficiency. The tenderness of her shoulder is all gone.

Comments: I thought this patient's pain could be resolved with one treatment, but it took two. This case is not a real success in that sense. Thinking back, I did not tonify LU-9 enough. I may have lost my composure because the patient was in so much pain. I also could have placed an intradermal needle in the first treatment, which might have helped. In cases of acute inflammation, the pain must be relieved as soon as possible. It doesn't do to make the patient wait.

There are three keys in treating acute inflammation in the shoulder:

1. Find an induration in the upper back associated points on the affected side and apply multiple cones of direct moxibustion. Ten cones is just a start. The more you can do, the better.
2. Give the root treatment of Meridian Therapy. This is the distal treatment.
3. For the local treatment, find the most reactive point. You need to find an induration the size of a soybean. You can ask the patient and use heat, protrusion, and tenderness as a guide. When there is heat in the shoulder, apply heat-sensing moxibustion, never direct moxa. The area around the heat-sensing moxa cone can be lightly pressed to reduce the heat sensation, but it might be too tender to press. An intradermal needle over the most reactive point is also effective.

Case Study 84

Inflammation of the shoulder

Patient: Male, 54 years old

FOC: March 1, 2010

Main Complaint: Pain in the left shoulder joint that started 10 days previously

Examination: The left shoulder joint was hot and generally swollen. There was severe pain with movement of the arm, including internal rotation and extension. Careful palpation revealed extreme sensitivity over the acromion.

Pulse Diagnosis: Liver deficiency

Treatment: SRT on LR-8, KI-10, BL-18, GB-20, GB-21, LI-11, ST-36, and LR-11 on the affected side only. SRT on the most tender point on the shoulder right at the acromioclavicular joint followed by direct moxibustion and an intradermal needle. Direct moxibustion (left side): 10 cones on BL-17 and 5 cones on LI-11.

(2nd) Mar 5 – The heat on the shoulder decreased and pain diminished. The most tender point on the shoulder moved medially 2cm. Another intradermal needle retained in this point.

Comments: This was a case of inflammation over the entire shoulder joint, but the tender point was right on the acromion, where reactions rarely appear. The key is to find this most tender point. If you can't locate it, it takes longer to treat.

Summary | • Find the tender point within the warm area.

Case Study 85

Inflammation of the Shoulder

Patient: Female, 70 years old

FOC: June 9, 2008

Situation and Symptom: Cannot raise left arm due to pain. She thinks she did too much weeding, as waking up the day after this work she found she could not raise her left arm. That was the day before her visit and she still could not raise her arm because of the pain. She can lift her arm with her right hand. She had not had a medical exam.

Examination: Both the Jackson and Spurling tests were negative. Pain with 30° abduction, 80° of flexion (arm just below horizontal), and internal rotation with extension. Some heat in the shoulder joint around the acromion. Tender point on the anterior shoulder about 2cm inferior to LI-15 and the origin of the biceps. Induration found at left BL-15.

Temperature: 36.9°C

Pulse Diagnosis: Rapid, Lung deficiency, pulse rate: 96/min

Comments: She didn't have severe pain at night so it didn't seem like calcium deposits in the rotator cuff. I suspected damage in the supraspinatus tendon because of the pain with abduction, but I decided it was inflammation affecting the entire shoulder joint.

Treatment: Simple insertion to tonify LU-9, SP-3 and LI-11, followed by the same to disperse LU-10. SRT on local points on left side: M-UE-48 *(mae kengū/jiān qián)*, SI-9, and SI-11. Horizontal insertion in left LI-15 to a depth of 1.5cm with five sparrow-pecking motions before withdrawing. Direct moxibustion (left side only) on M-UE-48 *(maekengū/jiān qián)*, SI-9, LI-11, BL-15 (20 cones), and BL-14. Intradermal needle retained in left M-UE-48 *(mae kengū/jiān qián)*.

Progress:

(2nd) June 10 – Pain was much better. She could abduct her arm without pain. She can flex her arm 120 degrees, but there is a little pain. Pulse rate normal. Temperature 36.7°C. Liver deficiency. SRT on LR-8, KI-10, ST-36, and LI-11. Same local treatment as before except for no direct moxibustion on BL-15.

(3rd) June 17 – The pain was completely gone, like a miracle. Liver deficiency. The induration at BL-15 has diminished.

Comments: I suspected damage in the supraspinatus tendon because of the complaint of not being able to raise her arm, but it ended up being inflammation in the shoulder joint. The key points for this case were the intradermal needle in M-UE-48 *(mae kengū/jiān qián)*, horizontal insertion in LI-15, and multiple cone moxibustion on BL-15.

5.3 Calcium deposit in rotator cuff (bursitis)

This condition is similar to arthritis in the shoulder, but the etiology is different. It often occurs in middle-aged women where they feel sudden intense shoulder pain at night. Of course, there is some restriction in the range of motion. These signs give you a clue. The reactive point appears about 3cm below LI-15, but it is slightly swollen and feels warm. The heat is not extreme, but you can tell by comparing it to the surrounding area. To treat this condition, find reactive points on the upper back associated points. In extreme cases, there is a strand of hardened muscle about 5cm in length from approximately BL-12 to BL-14. In such cases, locate 2-3 points over the induration and apply multiple cone moxibustion. As you apply 20, 30, and even 50 cones, the heat sensation diminishes, so apply as many as you can.

For local treatment, use SRT; apply a few small cones of direct moxa or an intradermal needle.

For the root treatment, the patient often has Lung deficiency, but not always. Treat for Lung deficiency when you are not sure and needle LU-9 and SP-3.

If possible, continue the above treatment every day. The symptoms should diminish in 2-3 treatments.

There was, however, one patient whose symptoms did not improve. It was an 80-year-old woman, and I had treated her for arthritis in the shoulder repeatedly. Since my treatments were not working, I told her to go to an orthopedic doctor and have the offending calcium deposit removed. She came back a few days later and said her shoulder was still in pain. It seems she was only given physical therapy and massage after consulting an orthopedic doctor. I told her to go to a different doctor. Sure enough, after taking an X-ray, calcium deposits were confirmed and these were removed by a hypodermic needle. She looked 100% better when she came to me the next time. Nevertheless, she continues to come regularly for treatment. I examine her joints and continue to treat those that feel warm, but these days she rarely experiences any pain. She seems to be under the illusion that I was the one who cured her shoulder pain.

Summary

- In cases of sudden pain in the shoulder, look for heat, tenderness, and induration 2cm below LI-15.
- If not sure, treat for Lung deficiency.
- Multiple cone moxibustion on induration on back associated point on same side.

5.3.1 Discriminating frozen shoulders from other pathology

We tend to think of frozen shoulders when a middle-aged patient presents with shoulder pain in which arm movement causes severe pain. In hospitals and medical clinics also, usually this is the diagnosis. Yet as an acupuncturist we must learn to more carefully discriminate frozen shoulders from other pathology. Let's consider this issue by reviewing a couple of case studies.

Case Study 86

Patient: Male, 56 years old

FOC: March 17, 2009

Symptoms and Situation: Pain in the left shoulder. Severe pain with arm movement. Twenty days ago the shoulder began to hurt with arm movement for no particular reason.

Examination: Pain with internal rotation and extension of shoulder (moving arm behind to back). Range of motion of left shoulder: 85 degrees flexion, 100 degrees abduction, 45 degrees extension. When arm was brought around behind the back in internal rotation, the thumb of the left hand did not reach as close to C7 as that of the right. Slight warmth and extreme tenderness at the origin of the biceps on the scapula.

Pulse Diagnosis: Liver deficiency

Treatment: Root treatment – SRT on LR-8, KI-10, LI-11

Branch treatment (on left side) – SRT on M-UE-48 *(mae kengū/jiān qián)*, SI-11, and SI-9

Direct moxibustion (on left side) on M-UE-48 *(mae kengū/jiān qián)*, SI-11, SI-9, and BL-13 (30 cones)

Intradermal retained in left M-UE-48 *(mae kengū/jiān qián)*

Needle inserted in left LI-15

Comments: From the patient's age, it might seem like frozen shoulder, but still there is some doubt. The painful side felt slightly warm compared to the normal side. Also the tenderness is marked, where even slight pressure is painful. This is clearly different from the tenderness found in frozen shoulders.

I applied 30 cones of moxibustion on BL-13, which is one of my strategies for arthritis. I also inserted a needle about 1cm in LI-15 and applied three sparrow-pecking motions and had the patient move his arm. The pain was reduced. So this seemed more like arthritis in the shoulder. If that was the case, the pain would resolve more quickly. The range of motion should also improve. Even if the pain resolves, it is possible that the condition could transition to frozen shoulder or adhesive capsulitis. I told the patient that we would decide and establish a treatment plan based on the progress noted in the next treatment. He was satisfied with this.

The next day, another patient came in with similar shoulder pain, so I will detail his treatment for the purpose of comparison.

Case Study 87

Patient: Male, 65 years old

FOC: March 18, 2009

Symptom and Situation: Pain in the right shoulder. One month ago when he was practicing hitting golf balls, he felt a sudden pain in the right shoulder when swinging. Ever since then, pulling his pants up with his right arm is painful.

Examination: No heat or swelling in the right shoulder, but there is tenderness at LI-15. Pain with internal rotation and extension of shoulder (moving arm behind to back).

History: Gout

Pulse Diagnosis: Liver deficiency

Treatment: Root treatment – SRT on LR-8 and KI-10.

Branch treatment (on right side) – SRT on M-UE-48 (*mae kengū/jiān qián*), SI-11, SI-9, and LI-11. Direct moxibustion (right side) on M-UE-48 (*mae kengū/jiān qián*), SI-11, SI-9, and LI-11. Needle inserted in right LI-15.

Progress: Moving his right arm after the treatment, the pain was almost gone.

Comments: This case seems to be slight damage to the tendon by hitting golf balls. When things go well, it only takes one treatment to resolve. When not so lucky, it can transition to frozen shoulder. I told this patient to wait for three days to see if any pain remained, and give me a call.

Comparing this case with the previous one, we notice a very clear difference in the pathological condition. The location of the lesion is exactly the same, but the presence of inflammation and the amount of tenderness is quite different. So the treatment must be subtly varied. The previous case with inflammation must be treated with utmost care. It will get worse if you carelessly over-stimulate. So it's important to get rid of concepts like frozen shoulders and just treat the patient.

5.4 Rheumatoid arthritis in the shoulder

Patients will have a positive rheumatoid factor with a laboratory exam. Arthritis in the shoulder is just one of the joints affected by this condition. The shoulder becomes hot and swollen, and at times an increase in synovial fluid causes the joint to become unstable. The reactions appear most often on the anterior shoulder, then on the lateral shoulder, and least often on the posterior shoulder. My standard treatment is root treatment, followed by SRT on local points, concluding with multiple cone moxibustion on the back associated points (around BL-13) on the affected side.

5.5 Damage to tendon of supraspinatus tendon

This is a lesion in the shoulder that I have seen quite often in my practice. It occurs when a middle-aged or elderly person takes a fall and stops the fall with their hands. Suddenly the arm cannot be raised by itself. It can be raised with help from the other arm or another person. There is no pain. It is caused by a tear or lesion in the tendon of the supraspinatus muscle, which abducts and raises the arm. There isn't much that can done with acupuncture if the tendon is completely severed. If the tear is small, however, acupuncture can work wonders.

The point to treat is LI-15. I insert a needle horizontally and medially toward the midline, between the humerus and the acromion. It is easy to locate the point when there is space between bones in the joint, but when the space is closed you need to palpate carefully to find the right point. I use a 30mm, 02 gauge (0.14mm) Seirin needle that I use for SRT applications. Insert the needle about one centimeter and do about three sparrow-pecking motions if possible. Remove the needle and have the patient try to raise their arm both in flexion and abduction. If it works well, the arm goes right up. Some patients are able to raise their arm only about 90 degrees. When this technique has no effect at all, the tendon is severely damaged. For elderly patients, recovery is slow so even if this technique only has a little effect, give 2-3 treatments to see if there is any change. Refer them to an orthopedic doctor when there is no change at all.

Of course, it is important to also give a root treatment as well as other local treatment. Among elderly patients, loss of ability to raise an arm often occurs without a fall. It is due to aging, or degeneration of the muscles. Inserting a needle in LI-15 can be beneficial, but it doesn't work all the time.

Summary

- Sudden inability to raise arm.
- Insert about 1cm horizontally in LI-15, sparrow-peck three times.

Case Study 88

Patient: Male, 75 years old

FOC: October 31, 2005

Main Complaint: Inability to raise right arm. Problem began after taking a fall and landing on right hand.

Pulse Diagnosis: Lung deficiency

Treatment: Insertion into LI-15. SRT on LU-9, SP-3 and ST-36, LU-10, GB-20, GB-21, BL-13, BL-43, CV-12, and SI-11 on the right. Direct moxibustion on GB-21 both sides, and SI-11 and BL-13 on the right.

Progress: (2nd) Right arm can be raised slowly.

(3rd) Able to raise arm normally.

5.6 Sternoclavicular arthritis

Sometimes a patient comes in with severe shoulder pain, but the source of the pain cannot be found by examination of the shoulder. When you ask them to point to the painful spot, they point broadly to GB-21 or the shoulder in general and a specific problem area cannot be located. When you move your palpating fingers to the anterior side to feel the clavicular region, you might find an extremely tender point around KI-27 that almost makes them jump. Careful examination reveals swelling, redness, and heat. This is arthritis in the sternoclavicular joint.

Only one in ten patients with this condition is able to point right at the inflamed area, so even in medical clinics the location causing the pain is not usually discovered and patients are given pain killers and plasters to place on GB-21. Acu-moxa on KI-27 works quickly when there is inflammation. When the inflammation has gone and there is deformity in the joint (it protrudes prominently) and some tenderness, it takes longer for the treatments to work, but acu-moxa is still indicated.

People who tend to get arthritis in the sternoclavicular joint often have Heberden's nodes on their fingers. This condition seems to be inherited. The pattern is usually Lung or Spleen deficiency. In addition to treating the tender point in the inflamed area, look for reactions at the Scalene point, GB-21, and LI-11. There will be a marked induration around BL-13 on the affected side, so be sure to apply multiple cones of direct moxibustion there. It is also good to suggest home moxibustion on the most tender point and on the induration around BL-13. Otherwise, retain an intradermal needle at these points when patients are unable or unwilling to do moxibustion at home.

Summary

- Lung or Spleen deficiency common.
- Needle the most tender point followed by moxibustion, or an intradermal needle.
- Multiple cones of direct moxibustion on induration around BL-13.

Case Study 89

Patient: Male, 83 years old

FOC: June 11, 2012

Symptom and Situation: Pain in the right shoulder that began 10 days ago. There is pain with movement in all directions. The examination at the hospital was inconclusive. The doctor said they could shave off some bone if the problem persisted.

Examination: Slight warmth in the anterior shoulder. Induration at BL-15 on the right. Examining the sternoclavicular region, the right side protrudes markedly, and is slightly red and tender. The patient was completely unaware of it, but it was inflammation in the right sternoclavicular joint.

Pulse Diagnosis: Liver deficiency, not rapid

Treatment: SRT on LR-8, KI-10, BL-18, GB-20, and GB-21. Needle inserted and retained in the most tender point close to KI-27. This was followed by 15 cones of direct moxibustion on the tender point and BL-15 on the right. In addition, SRT and five cones of direct moxa were applied to right SI-11, LI-11, and M-UE-48 *(mae kengū/ jiān qián).*

Progress: (2nd) June 13 – No more pain. The area of tenderness at KI-27 shrank to one small point. Intradermal needle retained in the tender point. This will probably eliminate the pain. After a treatment similar to the first except at the tender point, I told the patient to contact me if he ever felt anything odd around the right sternoclavicular joint.

Comments: I was able to locate the inflamed joint causing the shoulder pain. Experience is everything. If I hadn't found the source, I would have focused on treating the shoulder, but I don't think we would have gotten good results. We did one more treatment just to be sure, and then concluded after three treatments.

Case Study 90

Patient: male, 53 years old

FOC: July 2, 2012

Main Complaint: Chest pain on left side. The pain was so intense that it was even uncomfortable to talk. He had to take leave from his work (as a teacher).

Examination: Warmth over the sternoclavicular joint. Marked tenderness over a large area. Temperature: 37.7°C.

Pulse Diagnosis: Kidney deficiency

Treatment:

Five cones of direct moxa applied on SI-11 on the left, and 15 cones were applied on BL-15 and BL-16 on the left. Intradermal needle retained in the most tender point in the vicinity of KI-27.

SRT on KI-7, LU-5, CV-12, LR-8, CV-6, BL-23, and SI-11.

Progress:

(2nd) July 3 – He ran a fever of 38°C the night after his first treatment. Pulse was rapid, Liver deficiency. He has some low back pain.

(3rd) July 7 – Liver deficiency. Temperature 37.7°C. Pain in the sternoclavicular joint is mild. Tenderness has diminished, but his low back pain is severe. The improving condition of his inflamed joint did not correspond to his continued fever. A continuation of the fever could possibly be due to a kidney infection, so I told him to get examined by a urologist if his temperature remained high.

(4th) July 11 – Liver deficiency. Temperature 36.7°C. Went to hospital for exam on July 8. X-ray showed 1cm stone in bladder. Tenderness at BL-32. This patient is sensitive, but needles inserted 5mm in BL-32 with five small sparrow-pecking movements. Sternoclavicular joint 90% better.

(5th) July 21 – Temperature 36.6°C. Low back pain gone but a little chest pain remains.

Comments: This patient's condition had a convoluted progression from inflammation in sternoclavicular joint and fever to low back pain and bladder stones, but the treatment was on target. This is an unusual case.

6. Hip joint disorder

There are many women who suffer from hip joint disorders in their middle and advanced ages, although of course it can also affect men.

The symptoms in the early stages of hip joint disorders are pain when walking and limping. There is pain when stepping onto the foot, and also when one sits cross-legged, but in the case of Japanese women, they usually sit in seiza or on chairs so they seldom notice the last symptom. Of course, the young women today sit cross-legged without thinking anything about it, so this will change.

Hip joint disorders are quickly identified with the Patrick's test, in which the supine patient's hip is placed in flexion and external rotation (cross-legged position). The extent of deformity in the hip joint is inferred by whether the leg with flexed knee and hip (leg up with feet on the treatment table) cannot go into external rotation (90 degrees) or it can go halfway down to the table (45 degrees) or the knee comes close the table. If hip rotation is limited to 90 degrees by deformity, there is not much that can be done with acu-moxa. It is better to have surgery. Sometimes, however, the ROM restriction to 90 degrees of rotation is caused by tension in muscles around the hip joint. When the cause of pain is in soft tissue, acu-moxa treatments are highly recommended. We don't have any way of assessing the condition of the hip joint beyond the Patrick's test, so if you are not sure, have the patient receive an orthopedic examination. Decide whether the patient should continue acu-moxa treatments after you find out the results of this exam.

6.1 Treatment of hip joint

The primary points for hip joint disorders are two points on the front and back of the hip joint. The anterior point is Shudo's GB-29 *(kyoryō)* and the posterior point is Onodera's point. Shudo's GB-29 *(kyoryō)* is the tightest and most tender point on the inguinal ligament, just medial to the ASIS. Onodera's point should be located on the induration in the upper region of the gluteus maximus. I use simple insertion on Shudo's GB-29 *(kyoryō)* (needle not retained) and for Onodera's point I retain the needle at a depth of 2cm after applying some sparrow pecking at the induration.

As for other points, there are BL-25 and BL-27. Also palpate around the greater trochanter with the patient in the side-lying position, and if you can find a hard or indurated point, it can serve as a good treatment point. Apply direct moxibustion on the two primary points on the front and back, and you can also moxa other points like BL-27 and LR-3. The results will be even better if the patient is able to have someone apply direct moxibustion on these points at home. Treat for a three-month period and think about surgery if there is no effect.

Case Study 91

Patient: Female, 74 years old

FOC: July 28, 2010

Symptom and Situation: Pain in left hip joint. She has had osteoarthritis in this hip and pain when walking. Today she felt sudden shooting pain in her left hip as she got out of the car and is unable to walk. She was examined at a hospital and told that she needed surgery, but they didn't have room in the hospital, so she was asked to wait for a while. This patient had been coming to me for the previous three years for hip pain. It was not getting any worse, but her condition was not improving either.

Pulse Diagnosis: Liver deficiency

Treatment: SRT on LR-8, LI-11, ST-36, GB-20, GB-21, BL-18, and BL-23. Needle inserted and retained on the left side in BL-27, Onodera's point, and Shudo's GB-29 *(kyoryō)*. Direct moxibustion on both BL-23 and Onodera's point, Shudo's GB-29 *(kyoryō)* and ST-36 only on the left.

Progress:

(3rd) Aug 8 – Palpating carefully around the left greater trochanter, I found quite a few indurations in the muscle. I retained five needles around the greater trochanter at a depth of 5 – 10mm. The patient was able to walk without pain after this treatment.

(5th) Sept 8 – She is much better and there is no problem with her daily activities.

Comments: It is very unlikely that the hip joint could become damaged all of a sudden. I had suspected that the muscles around the hip joint were the problem. But the pain was so bad she couldn't walk, and the orthopedic surgeon showed her the image of her hip and suggested surgery. She told me she didn't want surgery but thought there was no alternative given the level of pain. Her pain resolved dramatically by retaining needles in points around the greater trochanter. She feels no pain with normal movements. Since she didn't want to have surgery to begin with, she decided to postpone it. It has been two years since this episode and she is still doing fine.

7. Wrist joint disorders

Arthritis is the most common among disorders of the wrist joint. The initial onset of arthritis is often on the wrist along the Small Intestine meridian, close to SI-6. When it is arthritis, there is a characteristic sheen of the skin over the inflammation and response to light pressure, so it is easy to tell once you have some experience. Even if blood tests do not reveal rheumatoid factors, you can presume the patient is very close to developing this disorder when there is this finding.

We must determine which part of the wrist is affected. It is fine to ask the patient where it hurts the most. I like to press around the wrist with the base of my thumb. Once you have some experience, you can find the exact spot. Based on the texture, temperature, and extent of inflammation, you will be able to locate the spot more accurately than the patient. The main points I use are TB-4, SI-5, SI-6, LU-9, and Sawada's HT-7 (Fig. 6-3). I find that reactions don't appear very often at PC-7 or the standard HT-7.

With wrist joint disorders, it is difficult to twist the wrist as when wringing out a hand towel. The treatment is a success if patients can do these movements without pain.

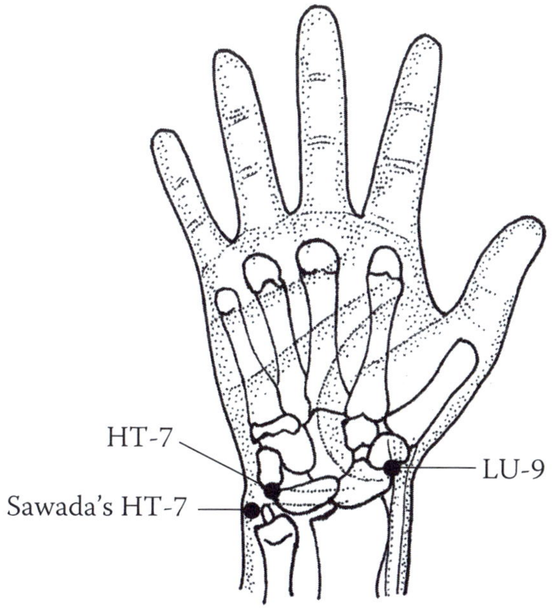

Fig. 6-3 Sawada's HT-7

7.1 Examination and treatment of the wrist joint

First examine the degree of swelling and sheen of the skin. Next feel for heat over the wrist. The higher the temperature, the worse the problem is in that place. This will become the main target of treatment. Keep these places in mind. As you continue treatments, the heat will diminish. I mark the points with a red pencil. Usually around three points get marked, but sometimes it's as many as six.

The acupuncture should be left at SRT, as inserting needles tends to make it worse. In cases of arthritis, often other joints are involved, so keep the number of points treated to a minimum. In extreme cases (where there are many joints involved), besides treating whatever points show up on the wrist, limit yourself to just the two most tender points elsewhere. Don't needle any other points. For moxibustion also, limit yourself to just two points per joint when other joints are involved. When just the wrist is affected, direct moxibustion can be applied on all the reactive points on the wrist. Keep the moxibustion mild by applying three cones of thread-like moxa.[8] Also, for arthritis in the wrist, don't forget to look for indurations in the upper back associated point on the affected side, and apply multiple cones of direct moxibustion over any induration you find.

8. Trigger finger

I see trigger fingers quite often in my practice. Stubborn cases require surgery, but the vast majority of cases resolve with just acu-moxa. You can set a goal of three months for treatment and then refer for surgery if there is no improvement. I press the palmar aspect of the metacarpal bones and look for tender and hardened points. There are some who claim to fix trigger fingers with only SRT, but I insert needles in these points. It takes some practice to insert needles in the palm painlessly. I use a very thin needle (30mm, 0.12mm). The key is to press the tube into the point with some force. When you flick your index finger onto the upper corner of the tube as intensely as you can, even if you don't hit the handle of the needle, the needle goes in slightly due to the strong vibration. I find that a stainless steel tube works better than the plastic tube for this technique. Next remove the tube and insert the needle a bit more and retain it. This is then followed up with a few small cones of moxibustion. It is best to have the patient apply moxibustion at home. I generally recommend five cones.

There have been some amazing cases that resolved with just one treatment. These are usually younger patients, however, so rather than being a real case of trigger finger, it could have been more of a joint pathology. For most cases of trigger finger, it takes one treatment a week for three months.

---

8. Thread-like moxa: The smallest and mildest form of direct moxibustion in which the cone is made as thin as possible. Even though the cone is burned all the way down to the skin, the minuscule size of the cone keeps the heat sensation to a minimum.

Summary
- Find reactive point on palm along tendon.
- Be careful to avoid causing pain with insertion.
- Ask patient to apply moxibustion at home.

9. Ankle joint disorders

Ankle sprains are the most common condition among all ankle joint problems. In acute cases we find swelling and heat on the ankle along the Gallbladder, Stomach, or Liver meridians. Sometimes we find internal bleeding and bruising. When the swelling, bruising, and pain are severe, we suspect a fracture even though I have been told that is this is not a reliable differentiation. If it's just a sprain, acu-moxa can alleviate or resolve most of the symptoms, but refer the patient to an orthopedic doctor right away if the ankle continues to hurt while in bed at night.

9.1 Treatment of ankle sprain

Locate the five most tender points on the ankle and retain needles superficially in these points. Remove the needles after about five minutes. If there is a little bleeding with the removal, that is a good thing. This is natural blood-letting. Check the tender points again, and you will find some are no longer tender, while others remain tender. Apply five small cones of direct moxibustion on the remaining tender points. Check the tender points after moxibustion, and you will find one that is least diminished. This remaining most tender point is over the injured site; apply 10 more cones of direct moxibustion on this point and finally retain an intradermal needle in this point.

The root treatment is also important. I often treat for Liver deficiency. Aside from LR-8 and KI-10, I suggest palpating and needling reactive points at ST-36, GB-34, GB-38, BL-59, BL-27, or Onodera's point. In acute cases, even severe symptoms can be resolved with one treatment. Even if symptoms persist, two or three treatments are enough for complete recovery. Moxibustion on a few points at home is recommended to prevent any after-effects.

When an acu-moxa treatment is not given early on, and the ankle is left to heal on its own, sometimes it doesn't heal completely and can turn into chronic arthritis in the ankle. In cases of incompletely healed ankle sprains, it is important to skillfully palpate tender points around the ankle and treat them. Often the reaction appears along the Gallbladder meridian on the foot between GB-41 and GB-43. It is ideal if the patient can apply moxibustion on the most tender point on the foot. Occasionally the reactive point appears more on the medial side of the foot around ST-41, LR-4, or even KI-6.

Case Study 92

Patient: Male, 37 years old

FOC: March 29, 2010

Symptom and Situation: Pain in the left lower leg. He had pain above and below his left ankle. Despite this he kept on working and the pain spread to his whole lower leg.

Pulse Diagnosis: Lung deficiency

Examination: Orthopedic tests for sciatica were negative. Comparing the right and left ankles, the lateral aspect of the left ankle seems slightly swollen. I looked for a reactive point, but without much success. Even though the ankle seemed swollen around GB-40, I felt nothing there. Palpating with more attention, I found a reaction on the posterior side of the lateral malleolus.

Treatment: SRT on LU-9, SP-3, LI-11, ST-36, GB-21, BL-13, and BL-25. SRT on left side only on Onodera's point, BL-58, and BL-59. Needle retained shallowly in the reactive point on left lateral malleolus. Direct moxibustion was attempted on this point after removing the needle, but it was too sensitive, so I retained an intradermal needle instead.

Progress:

(2nd) Apr 3 – The symptoms resolved completely. The reactive point on the ankle was still tender, so I replaced the intradermal needle and told him to keep it on until it fell off. Treatments were concluded.

Comments: This patient is the grandson of the only surviving elementary school teacher of mine. When her grandson (my patient) said he was going to a hospital to have his leg looked at, this elderly former teacher of mine said, "Have Mr. Denmei look at it instead!" I'm relieved to have gotten it right in the first treatment. It goes to show how important it is to carefully palpate the reactive point.

10. Other joint disorders

10.1 Sacroiliac joint disorders

Dysfunctions in the sacroiliac joint, which is between the sacrum and ilium, often go unnoticed. About the only time it comes to our attention is when a patient comes in with acute low back strain. The best acupuncture point for treating the sacroiliac joint is the Iliac point. Refer to the section on back strain in Chapter 4 for treatment.

10.2 Pain in the big toe

The most common condition that causes pain in the big toe is osteoarthritis. There is deformity and tenderness on the medial and lateral aspects of the big toe. If possible, have the patient continue direct moxibustion treatment on the toe at home. The toes are sensitive to heat and some patients may be reluctant, but the pain and deformity only get worse without treatment.

When there is redness and signs of inflammation in addition to tenderness, suspect gout. In cases of gout, insert needles superficially in the tender points like SP-2 followed by small cones of direct moxibustion. Also treat points like ST-36, SP-6, BL-23, and BL-27. Be sure to suggest a medical exam for patients who aren't already under the care of a doctor. To get better, the patient has to adhere to a health regimen in addition to receiving acu-moxa treatments.

10.3 Pain in the calcaneus (plantar fasciitis)

Pain in the heel is another condition I see quite often in my practice. In severe cases the whole heel becomes red and swollen. When this happens, the patient cannot walk with their heel on the ground. The key for treatment in mild cases is to find the tender points on the heel. If the points are hard to find, work together with the patient to find the most sensitive points. Direct moxibustion works best. The pain resolves naturally when patients are able to apply moxibustion at home every day.

10.4 Pain in the finger (DIP) joints

When there is pain and swelling in finger joints other than the distal interphalangeal (DIP) joints, we must suspect rheumatoid arthritis. Pain is felt when the joint is pinched from the sides (radial and ulnar sides). Pinching the top and the bottom of the joint seldom causes much pain. Often there is heat and swelling over the joint. I like to quickly prick the most painful point with a medium-sized needle. I follow this up with one small cone of direct moxa.

CHAPTER 7

Respiratory Diseases

I have joined and benefitted from the acupuncture profession because I was exposed to it at a young age due to often being ill from a weak respiratory system. I am very careful about my respiratory health and have a deep personal interest in the treatment of respiratory conditions. Nevertheless, when my own respiratory system acts up, sometimes I am at a loss about what to do. The times have changed, and nowadays many of us are saved from an untimely death by the use of antibiotics.

1. The common cold

It is ideal if a cold can be warded off before it really takes hold. For this purpose I suggest multiple cone moxibustion on GV-14. You must apply at least 20 cones, and you can apply as many as 50. The cold will clear right up if it's in the early stages. Direct moxibustion on BL-12 also works well. I also recommend contact needling and skin needling (see Fig. 1-9) in the upper back area around these points.

Those patients who tend to catch colds often have excess hair growth in their upper back. This hair goes away if they continue to receive acu-moxa.

1.1 Treatment for common colds

The usual pattern for patients with colds is Lung or Kidney deficiency. KI-7 and LU-5 are the tonification points for Kidney deficiency. SP-3 and LU-9 are the tonification points for Lung deficiency. It is also good to use LU-8, the metal point of the Lung meridian, instead of LU-5 or LU-9. Other points that need to be checked and treated if reactive include LU-1, CV-12, CV-6, BL-13, GV-10, and GB-20. As for direct moxibustion, I use LU-5, LI-10, and GV-10 in addition to the above mentioned GV-14. When the patient is running a fever, I only apply direct moxibustion to GV-14. Regardless of whether the patient has a fever, the acupuncture should be limited to contact needling or SRT. Inserting needles is not wise, especially if the patient has a fever.

If the patient starts to sweat with the treatment, you can wipe it off with a dry hand towel; this also stimulates the skin.

Sometimes, the patient has the precursor symptoms of neck and shoulder stiffness. The tension is felt around points like BL-41, BL-42, and BL-10. A few days later they get upper respiratory symptoms and realize the neck and shoulder tension had been the early symptoms of a cold.

If the patient has coughing or phlegm, retain an intradermal needle in the axillary point on the side that is the most tender (Fig. 7-1). If the patient has a sore throat, insert a needle in LU-11. It works best when the point bleeds a little when the needle is removed.

For headaches, use the auricular vertigo point and the five-phases points on the arms and legs. Treatment of the head and neck area will make the patient feel worse unless you are careful. Some colds manifest as abdominal symptoms like pain and diarrhea without any respiratory symptoms. Do not try to stop the diarrhea. Sometimes the cold symptoms resolve when the diarrhea comes to an end. Needling SP-3 is helpful.

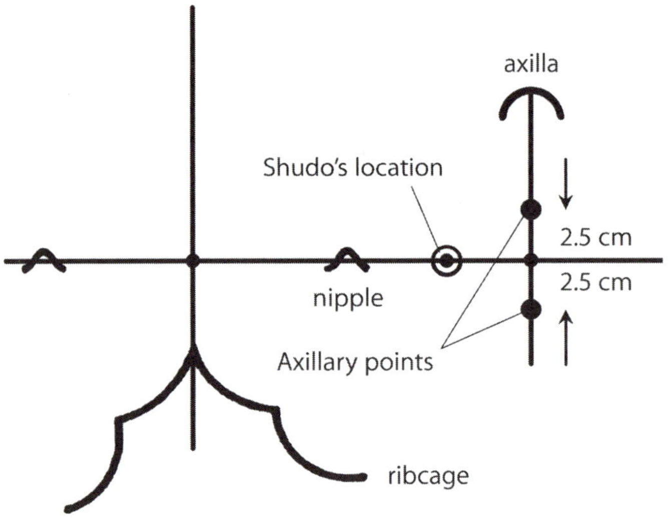

Fig. 7-1 Axillary points

Sometimes a patient feels pain all over their body. When they have neuralgia or arthritis, the fever causes these areas to ache. I do SRT directly on the places that hurt. Do not insert the needle in these painful places.

1.2 Strategy for preventing colds

1. Take care of your gastrointestinal system.

2. Strengthen your skin. Especially recommended is applying friction on the upper half of the body with a dry towel, or a cold wet towel.
3. Preventative moxibustion on GV-14.
4. Keep body in balance with acu-moxa.
5. Avoid cold foods and drinks.

Concerning the last item, there is an explanation in the classics about what causes a cough. When cold drinks or cold food is digested, it reaches the Lungs as cold qi. When the pathogenic cold attacks from outside the body, there is both external and internal cold and this causes coughing. That may mean that drinking beer is contraindicated for those who are sensitive to cold, and who tend to catch colds easily. Does that mean they should drink warm beer?!?

1.3 One case of cold treatment

Once I saw a two-year-old boy with a fever of 38°C. He was coughing up a storm. The doctor said there was danger of his catching pneumonia. He received an injection, but his coughing continued unabated. His mother and grandmother who brought him in seemed distraught.

The boy's pulse was rapid with Lung deficiency. Except for not being able to hear any wheezing, he reminded me of other asthmatic patients I had seen. The moment I placed an intradermal needle in the tender axillary point, his coughing eased up. I followed this with contact needling on LU-8, SP-5, and CV-22. Then I did some skin needling along the Lung meridian and on the upper back. His coughing became much better, and the boy began to sleep.

This boy's coughing subsided two hours after treatment, but his temperature went up. The next day he came in again for treatment, and both the coughing and fever were gone. I treated him for Liver deficiency.

In cases like this, it is safest to follow the doctor's treatment. Nevertheless, the power of acupuncture should not be underestimated. The injections and medications can work even better with acupuncture. The fact that this boy's cough subsided with each needle was clearly the effect of acupuncture.

For nasal symptoms, refer to the section on rhinitis in Chapter 8.

2. Tonsillitis

Tonsillitis can begin with throat pain during a cold or there can be a sudden onset of fever and throat pain along with pain when swallowing. The latter case is more common, and it occurs often in children and young people. When you look down their throat, the redness and swelling is evident. In severe cases a yellowish white membrane forms. The temperature climbs to almost 40°C. While the symptoms are acute, acu-moxa is indicated.

I treat for Lung deficiency and tonify LU-9 and SP-3. Also bleeding a few drops from LU-11 is good. If there are objections to bloodletting, simply dispersing LU-11 will do. The dramatic effect of this point can be seen in the case studies that follow. It is also possible to disperse LU-10, the fire point of the Lung meridian, with the idea of dispersing the controlling phase of the Lung. The above treatment will achieve the desired outcome, but it is also good to do SRT to gently disperse other points like LU-5, KI-27, and BL-13.

The symptoms will resolve in one or two treatments in most cases. Direct moxibustion on GV-14 and LU-5 is also good. My cousin suffered from tonsillitis every year but this came to an end with just one acupuncture treatment. Another man was hospitalized for one week with acute tonsillitis, but his mother couldn't stand it any longer and had him come back home to her from another prefecture. She brought him to me for acupuncture and his tonsillitis resolved in one treatment. Compared to acute tonsillitis, however, chronic cases with enlarged tonsils are difficult. The inflammation and enlargement doesn't go away even with repeated acu-moxa treatments. In most cases, I end up recommending surgery.

Case Study 93

Patient: Female, 21 years old

FOC: April 16, 2002

Main Complaint: Acute tonsillitis

Symptoms and Condition: Medications haven't helped. She also has a headache, dizziness, nausea, and swelling in her throat.

Examination: Both tonsils are red and enlarged and the left tonsil has a white membrane (white exudate).

Pulse: Floating, rapid, and deficient; Lung deficiency

Temperature: 38°C

Treatment: SRT on LU-9, SP-3, KI-27, GB-21, BL-12, BL-13, BL-20, and on submandibular lymph nodes (Fig. 7-2). Few drops of blood let from LU-11. Direct moxibustion on LU-5 (5 cones) and GV-14 (10 cones).

Progress:

(1st) The symptoms resolved after treatment.

(2nd) A feeling of pressure and pain behind her eyes since yesterday. Dizziness. Liver deficiency.

Comments: The tonsillitis resolved in one treatment. This patient has had no more symptoms in her throat for 10 years. There are many cases in my experience where one treatment at the peak of the acute phase prevents recurrence for the rest of one's life.

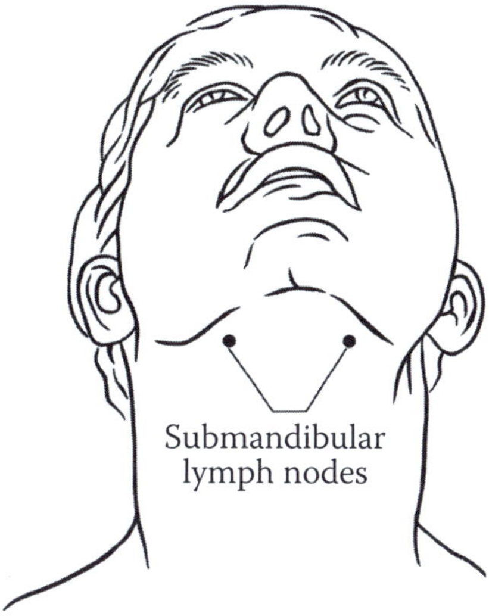

Fig. 7-2 Submandibular lymph nodes

Case Study 94

Patient: Male, 5th grader

FOC: August 12, 2010

Main Complaint: Acute tonsillitis

Symptoms and Condition: In the season when heat strokes became common, he was driven five hours to my clinic. He has a temperature of 39.9°C. He has no appetite. His face is visibly swollen on both sides from ST-9 up to the lower jaw.

Pulse: Floating, rapid, and Lung deficiency

Temperature: 38°C

Treatment: Gold teishin, for maximum tonification, used on LU-9, SP-3, GB-21, BL-12, BL-13, and BL-20.

Needle inserted in right LU-11 and finger was squeezed to release some blood. This point bled quite a bit.

Progress: This boy wanted to go swimming in a pool the next day. I said the fever should have subsided by the next day so he should have been able to go swimming. That evening his parents thought he had wet his bed because he sweated copiously in bed twice. The next morning his fever was gone and he was able to go swimming as he had hoped. His grandmother told me, "It worked like magic."

Comments: I also gave this boy's younger sister a treatment. She had a fever and nausea. At a hospital she had received a diagnosis of emesis and diarrhea due to viral infection. But she didn't have diarrhea; in fact, if anything she was constipated. I gave her a Liver deficiency treatment using the gold teishin and placed an intradermal needle in the right axillary point. She too was back to normal the next morning and had a ravenous appetite. A little treatment goes a long way for young patients.

3. Asthma

Around New Years with my 80th birthday only about a month away, I had an outbreak of herpes zoster on my head and face. Thanks to an infusion of antiviral agents, I avoided complications such as meningitis, but for a while I suffered from cold symptoms and herpes simplex (cold sores) around my mouth. The cold going around that winter was not the usual kind, and it seemed more like the whooping cough. I once again had the breathing difficulties I used to experience when I was young. I tried sitting down to recover and also gave myself the root treatment for Lung deficiency, but once the wheezing subsided, I began coughing. I was coughing to expel phlegm, but the phlegm wouldn't come out. It was stuck deep inside. This symptom was new to me and I thought, even as I was suffering, this must be what it was like for asthmatics whose wheezing just got worse as they were unable to expel their phlegm. I could breathe in, but I couldn't breathe out. This is a common symptom in asthma.

3.1 A story of asthma treatment

I once saw an old man in his mid-80s who had bad asthma attacks that started in the morning. He received injections at the hospital but the wheezing hadn't stopped by the evening. He was told that they couldn't give him two injections in one day, so he came in for acupuncture hoping it might help. The asthma attack continued and he couldn't lie on his back or side, so I examined him in the sitting position. Listening with the stethoscope, I heard wheezes on both sides of the chest. The pulse was rapid, and although it was hard to tell, it seemed to be Kidney deficiency. I applied SRT on KI-7 and LU-8,[1] and placed intradermal needles in the axillary points. Then I used a teishin on BL-13, BL-17, BL-23, CV-14, and CV-6. I followed this with three cones of direct moxibustion on BL-13 and GV-10. I could tell that he was doing a little better from his breathing.

On his way home he felt better and better, and he slept deeply that night. When he came to see me the next day he was completely better, and he didn't even seem like the same person.

In times past, I had a lot of opportunity to treat asthmatic patients, but their number seems to have diminished. This is probably because the idea that asthma is an allergic inflammatory process has taken hold, and treatment with steroidal inhalers has become common. In the above case, the terrible side effects of steroids was avoided by not having to receive so many injections.

---

1. The standard tonification point for Kidney deficiency is LU-5, but LU-8 was used here, applying the principle in chapter 68 of the *Classic of Difficulties:* "The river points control wheezing, coughing …" See p. 198 of *Introduction to Meridian Therapy.*

3.2 The treatment of asthma

❶ Reduce the needle stimulation

The secret to treating asthma is light stimulation. It is easy to make a mistake by giving a strong treatment. It will aggravate the problem. Observe the suffering of the patient and treat them carefully with the intention of relieving their suffering even just a little. This paradoxically will yield the best results.

Light stimulation means fewer points and more superficial insertions with thinner needles. When the results are good, patients will understand. Moxibustion also can make the patient worse if overdone. Stick with a few small cones.

❷ Intradermal needle in axillary points (Fig. 7-1)

Placing intradermal needle in the axillary points as a branch treatment is effective for the symptom of wheezing. I like to compare the tenderness on the right and left side and retain an intradermal needle on the more tender side, but you don't always have to treat only one side. If there is a strong reaction on both sides, retain an intradermal needle in both sides.

With the patient lying supine, find the intersection between the horizontal line between their nipples and the vertical midaxillary line. Akabane[2] designated the tender point above or below this point as the axillary point. The axillary point I use is found by palpating toward the nipple with my middle finger. It is rare that the most tender point is right on the midaxillary line. Most often I locate the tender point at the midpoint between the nipple and the midaxillary line. Place an intradermal needle in the most tender point.

Be careful to insert the intradermal needle horizontally just a millimeter or two so that it does not go under the skin. In the case of children, I find that improvement can be obtained with the very small press tacks (Pyonex orange 0.3mm or yellow, 0.6mm) and even the silver spheres on round adhesive used for auricular acupuncture. Sometimes an intradermal needle gives too much stimulation.

❸ Treatment of epigastric region

When a person has asthmatic coughing, often the epigastric region from CV-14 to CV-12 becomes hard. In contrast, the lower abdomen is weak. The chest starts to feel better and coughing subsides when the epigastric region is softened. I have personal experience of stopping my own asthmatic coughing with just one needle at CV-12.

Of course, when the root treatment or other methods are used to reduce coughing without treating the stomach, the epigastric region also softens. So you can gauge the severity of the coughing by the hardness in the epigastric region.

2. Akabane Kohei (1895-1983): An acupuncturist from Tochigi Prefecture who is credited with inventing and popularizing the use of intradermal needles in Japan.

❹ Reactive points on upper back

All tight, tender, or abnormal points on the upper back need to be treated. Common reactive points for asthma include GV-10, BL-17, and the Asthma associated point (Fig. 7-3).

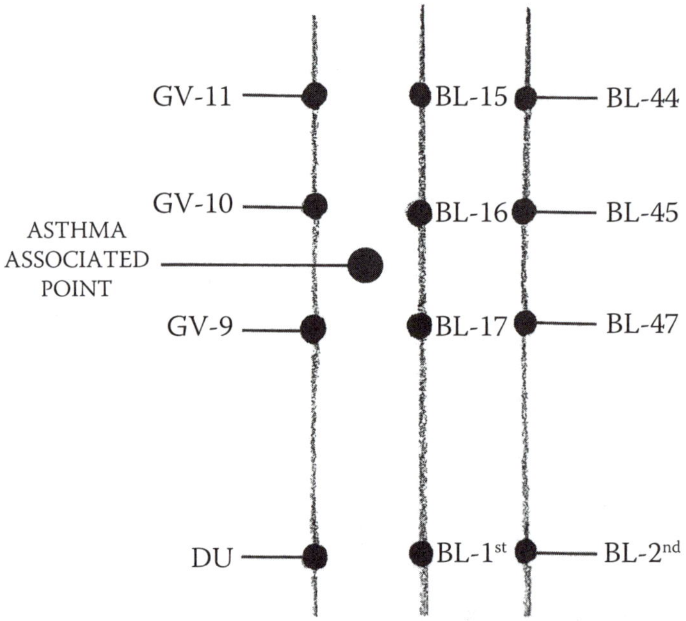

Fig. 7-3 Asthma associated point

❺ Treat affected meridians

In *Basic Questions (Suwen)* the character for asthma (喘 *zen/chŭan*) appears in 83 places. In eight instances the character refers to the pulse quality, and in all other instances it refers to the symptom of wheezing. Among the meridians associated with this character, the Lung meridian is the most frequent. The Kidney and Stomach meridian come after the Lung.

In chapter 34 of *Basic Questions* the causes of asthma are described as follows:

1. Those who can't lie down and breathing is noisy have counterflow qi of the *yáng míng* meridians.
2. Those who have no difficulty lying down but have noisy breathing have counterflow qi of the Lung meridian.
3. Those who can't lie down and lying down causes the wheezing have fluid (stagnation) so the problem is in the Kidneys.

The reference to the Kidneys makes me think of fluid metabolism and the function of the adrenals. In any case, pay attention to these meridians and treat the patient according to their pattern. I suggest using the metal points of the meridians (since metal is associated with Lungs and tonifies the Kidneys).

Case Study 95

Patient: Female, 60 years old

FOC: November 7, 2008

Main Complaints: Dizziness and asthma that began a month ago. Currently she is not wheezing.

Pulse: Liver deficiency

Treatment: Treatment directed primarily at dizziness. SRT on LR-8, KI-10, LR-4,[3] CV-12, CV-6, GV-10, BL-18, BL-23, GB-20, and GB-21. Intradermal needle retained in left axillary point. Direct moxibustion on LR-4, BL-10, GV-10, and BL-23.

Progress: I treated this patient regularly twice a month until the present (March of 2012). She has had occasional outbreaks of asthma and coughing. I retained an intradermal needle in the axillary point with the greatest reaction. I treated GV-10 and BL-17 whenever there was a reaction. I started using the teishin in addition to SRT, but I continued to use direct moxibustion. I continued for some time with SRT and moxibustion on BL-23. Her physical condition continues to improve.

Case Study 96

Patient: Female, 6 years old

FOC: June 30, 1976

Main Complaint: Chronic asthma. She receives an injection or medication every time she has an attack. She has been taking medications for about six months now, but she still has attacks about twice a week.

Pulse: Liver deficiency

Treatment: Intradermal needles retained in both axillary points. Contact needling on KI-7, LR-4, BL-17, and GB-21.

Progress:

(2nd) July 1 – No more asthma, just a little coughing.

(3rd) She had an attack for an hour last evening. Parents had taken her off the medications.

July 21 – She had a little asthma on the 17th. Her appetite is better and she has gained weight. After this, she had occasional bouts of asthma, but each time one treatment was enough to end it.

Comments: This patient lived far away, and I suggested to her parents that they should go to a nearby clinic or hospital for acupuncture, but they insisted on coming the long

3. The standard tonification point for Liver deficiency is LR-8, but LR-4 was used in addition to apply the principle in chapter 68 of the *Classic of Difficulties.* See footnote 1, p. 194.

distance to my clinic. Because there was an effect from the very first treatment, even the little girl trusted me. In a year's time she became healthy and sturdy.

(*Translator's note*: Mild stimulation is appropriate for pediatric cases so contact needling was used. This case occurred before the author had developed SRT, and now he also uses SRT to treat children.)

Case Study 97

Patient: Female, 67 years old

FOC: November 28, 2011

Main Complaints: She had bronchial asthma since July of that year. She had recurrence of asthma 10 days ago and has difficulty breathing. She also has allergic rhinitis. Listening with a stethoscope, I could not hear wheezing sounds. She is anxious and has trouble sleeping.

Pulse: Liver deficiency

Treatment: SRT on LR-8, KI-10, CV-14, ST-21, CV-6, GB-20, TB-15, BL-18, and BL-23. Direct moxibustion on LR-4, LU-5, GB-21, GV-10, and BL-18. Intradermal needle retained in left axillary point.

Progress:

(2nd) Liver deficiency. She had palpitations the day of the first treatment and her pulse rate went up to 100. She didn't have any asthma.

(3rd) Liver deficiency. No palpitations. Some coughing, but she feels much better.

(4th) Treatment frequency changed from once a week to once every 10 days.

(6th) Lung deficiency. No symptoms. The dosage of steroids from the hospital remains unchanged.

(9th) Dosage of steroids reduced by half. Frequency of acupuncture treatments also changed to once every 20 days.

(11th) She has stopped taking steroids. She appears much happier.

Comments: When I first saw this patient, the drawn look on her face made me concerned. She must have been really desperate because she even seriously considered going to see the doctor outside this prefecture that had referred her to me. I caught her expression and told her that the condition would improve, but she had symptoms other than asthma that troubled her. It took her about 100 days to get off of steroids after beginning acupuncture.

Case Study 98

Patient: Female, 60 years old

FOC: January 20, 2012

Main Complaints: Asthma for two years. She cannot lie supine because she starts coughing. She sleeps sitting at the *kotatsu*.[4] There seems to be an issue with having to also look after her husband. She doesn't get enough sleep because she has to tend to his illness. Her appetite and eliminations are normal. There is no wheezing.

Pulse: Kidney deficiency

Treatment: Intradermal needle retained in left axillary point. Direct moxibustion on LU-5, GB-21, GV-9, GV-10, and BL-23. SRT on KI-7, LU-8, LI-11, BL-23, GB-20, GB-21, CV-6, and CV-12.

Progress:

(2nd) Jan 25 – Lung deficiency. Mild wheezing. Patient can lie on her side without coughing.

(6th) Feb 22 – Lung deficiency. No wheezing. She can lie on her back at night to sleep.

(9th) March 12 – Coughing much less. Intradermal needle retained on right axillary point also.

(11th) April 2 – No more symptoms. She feels much better.

Comments: I was surprised to hear from this patient that she had not been able to sleep in a bed (futon on floor) for two years. I had to ask her to repeat herself just to be sure. She said life was much easier once she could lie on her back. Of course! Even if one uses steroidal inhalers, the effect is not always so good. In contrast, acu-moxa can do wonders. This is why people sometimes say about my treatments, "You do fantastic work!"

Summary

- Retain intradermal needle in reactive axillary points.
- Use metal points like KI-7 and LU-8.
- SRT and direct moxibustion on GV-10.
- Keep the stimulation light.

4. Other respiratory problems

4.1 Intercostal neuralgia

Strictly speaking this is not a respiratory problem, but this is a convenient place to mention it. At one time intercostal neuralgia was a respectable disease classification in Japan, but these days it is no longer considered a single disease. In many cases this condition is secondary to various other pathologies such as rib fractures, spondylosis deformans, spinal compression fractures, and spondylolisthesis. For acupuncture treat-

4. A low table used in Japan with a heater attached to the bottom. It is covered with a quilt to warm the legs of those seated on the floor at the table with their legs under the table.

ment, one must look for reactions along the sides of the spinous processes, Hua Tuo *jiá jĭ* (M-BW-35), the back associated points, and on the Kidney meridian next to the sternum. Skillfully located tender points become good treatment points. Intradermal needles can be retained in reactions around the axillary point. What is important in dealing with intercostal pain is not to overlook a far more serious cause such as heart disease. In general, be very careful with chest pain, have a low threshold to refer to a specialist to rule out heart problems.

4.2 Rib fractures

It's not unusual to see patients with rib fractures in my practice. In many cases a hairline fracture develops while playing golf. The orthopedic doctors don't seem to have any treatment other than fixing the ribs with tape and bandaging. Movements cause pain in the chest and this stimulates healing. Carefully palpate the damaged area and retain intradermal needles in the most tender points. If there are more than three fractured ribs, however, it is beyond the scope of acupuncture because serious complications such as pulmonary atelectasis and pneumothorax can occur.

4.3 Intercostal muscle injury

Sometimes people bruise the intercostal muscles by doing things like leaning over to clean a deep bathtub. (*Translator's note*: Japanese bathtubs are two to three times as deep as western tubs and have high sides.) Injury to intercostal muscles causes chest pain. When you carefully palpate the intercostal spaces, you can find the most tender point. A few cones of direct moxa followed by retaining an intradermal needle works better than plasters and compresses.

4.4 Bronchitis

An upper respiratory tract infection can go deeper to cause inflammation in the bronchi. Some are bacterial, but most cases are acute viral bronchitis. It can persist and turn into chronic bronchitis. There is fever, coughing, and expectoration of phlegm. Treatment is more complicated than for colds, but the foundation is the same. In the root treatment, skillfully select fire points and metal points. The foundation is the root treatment, which works well for a whole spectrum of yin and yang organ diseases. The back associated and front alarm points can be the branch treatment. For the Lung, BL-13 is the back associated point and LU-1 is the front alarm point. Use these back associated and front alarm points according to the basic pattern. However, it is important to locate the points based on the palpable reactions, not their predetermined locations. That is, check such back points as BL-12 and BL-14 and needle those that are reactive. Sometimes this corresponds exactly to what is supposed to be treated for that pattern and sometimes not. Still, it is really amazing how often the points that are reactive are the points that are supposed to be treated. Just remember that branch treatment is a double-edged sword. Too much stimulation is good for nothing. You must be extremely careful about inserting needles or else you could aggravate the condition. It's better to stick with contact needling and SRT. Be especially careful when the patient has a temperature.

4.5 Pneumonia

I advise hospitalization and taking antibiotics. Acu-moxa treatments are recommended as supplementary treatment. You can expect a combined effect. Of course, acu-moxa is excellent for improving health after the pneumonia has cleared. SRT is immediately effective for generalized symptoms like fatigue and soreness. Inserting needles doesn't work as well.

I experienced pneumonia once. I remodeled a storehouse (for farming supplies) and built a library on the second story. I helped with the clean-up of the interior, but I was careless enough not even to wear a mask. Right after that I ran a high fever and had coughing with phlegm. I got the diagnosis of pneumonia at the hospital and was put on intravenous fluids and antibiotics, then slept for three days. Relieved that my fever was gone, I left the hospital to attend the annual meeting of our prefectural acupuncture association (I was president at the time). I remained discharged from the hospital and began to work in my clinic. But I felt so heavy and exhausted. It made me appreciate what it might be like to have chronic fatigue syndrome. Even I, who prided myself in being hardworking, settled for just seeing patients in the morning. A week went by like this, but there was no sign of improvement. All this time I had been giving myself acupuncture using superficial insertion. I switched to all SRT and the effect was dramatic. By that evening my heaviness and fatigue were gone.

4.6 Pulmonary tuberculosis & pleurisy

Refer to the question and answer section on tuberculosis, following this chapter.

4.7 Lung cancer

Refer to discussion undern "Cancer and acupuncture" in Chapter 14.

Q&A

QUESTION AND ANSWER NO. 4

Response to inquiry from founder of *MoxAfrica*[1] about treatment of tuberculosis.

Tuberculosis and moxibustion

Q. I would like to use moxibustion to treat tuberculosis, but I'd like some advice.

A. Moxibustion is highly recommended for the treatment of conditions involving tuberculosis, but there are some things one needs to be careful about. One must give treatments with utmost care. Be advised that I have never treated tuberculosis. Personally, however, I suffered for 10 years with tuberculosis for which I received both acupuncture/moxibustion and Western medical treatments. I contracted pulmonary tuberculosis, peritonitis, pleuritis, and hemorrhoids. Acupuncture and moxibustion are effective for all of these, and I will discuss treatment beginning with the easier conditions.

1. **Hemorrhoids:** Once after my peritonitis had calmed down, I went to see a baseball game. This was 60 years ago, and the outfield seats were concrete on which I sat for many hours. The next day a swelling appeared next to my anus and it really hurt. I had it cut and drained, but the incision would not heal. The doctor said I would need more surgery, but my acupuncture mentor was against this, saying it would adversely affect my lungs.

   So I continued receiving acupuncture/moxibustion treatments from my mentor and kept replacing the bandage over the wound until it gradually healed and closed.

---

1. MoxAfrica: A charity working to teach medical workers in Africa to treat drug resistant tuberculosis with direct moxibustion. www.moxafrica.org

The thing that was most effective among the things my mentor did to treat me was deep insertion in BL-27. He inserted a two-inch needle until I felt a pleasant radiating sensation in my anus. I'm sure this effect was because my mentor was a master, but we should be able to copy this technique. The next most effective point was from the sacral foramina points, BL-31~34 (八髎 *bā liáo*). I had extreme tenderness over my sacrum that would almost make me jump when pressed, and BL-32 was usually the most tender. He also applied moxibustion to these tender points.

Later my hemorrhoids recurred with the onset of pulmonary tuberculosis, and I got as many as five anal fistulas at once, but these healed naturally. Our natural healing capacity is truly amazing. What is clear from this experience is that recovering health and strength is the foundation of curing hemorrhoids. BL-32, BL-26, LU-6, LI-10 and -11 could be listed as good points for treatment. Of course, don't forget the root treatment of Meridian Therapy.

❷ **Peritonitis:** My mentor cured my peritonitis with acupuncture/moxibustion. It took one year. I had a low grade fever and a month went by but neither my mentor nor my doctor could figure out the cause. Then a hard spot developed on my abdomen, and both of them decided I had peritonitis. My acupuncture/ moxibustion treatments began after that. My mentor made a house call almost every week and did acupuncture and moxibustion all over my body. Between treatments I had direct moxibustion applied at home, and I remember how it burned to receive moxibustion from my inexperienced parents. I especially hated getting it on my abdomen, because there was inflammation inside.

In later years, after I learned about Fukaya style moxibustion, I realized that there is another way. It is distal treatment. Dr. Fukaya wrote that applying moxibustion where the problem is located was the "lower class" approach. To treat peritonitis, Dr. Fukaya uses LI-7 on the Large Intestine meridian. This is a very wise and effective approach that prevents mistakes (overtreatment).

Applying moxibustion on tight spots on the abdomen is risky. And it burns! The thing about distal treatment, however, is that it takes good point selection and careful point location. The points that could be used include ST-36, 37, 38, & 40, LI-10 & 11, BL-52, and KI-3. If points on the abdomen are to be treated, the cones should be burned down only 80%, or use *Chinetsu-kyu* (heat-sensing moxibustion). Also do a Meridian Therapy root treatment and needle corresponding yang meridian points.

❸ **Pleuritis:** I've had both the wet type and dry type of pleuritis. The wet type causes difficulty in breathing and the dry type causes severe pain. The breathing difficulty was helped with acupuncture at BL-17. Acupuncture and moxibustion at LI-11 was effective for the pain. For distal treatment, LU-6, PC-4, and GB-34 were needled.

❹ **Pulmonary tuberculosis:** This condition is quite difficult to treat. The main thing to remember is that it takes a very long time. One must commit to a long term and regular course of treatment. As a rule, one should avoid treating the upper back associated points (above BL-17). This can exacerbate the condition and cause symptoms like hemoptysis (coughing blood). The main focus must be on strengthening the body, for which direct moxibustion should be used to achieve this end. As much as possible give a distal treatment. The basic moxibustion treatment will vary based on the pattern, but the following points are useful: LI-10 and -11, CV-12, BL-20 and -23, and GV-12.

Summary

1. Direct moxibustion is effective for tuberculosis.
2. The disease will go away when physical strength is recovered.
3. Avoid moxibustion on the upper back.
4. Use distal treatment as much as possible.
5. It works even better when Meridian Therapy style acupuncture is provided.

CHAPTER

8

Diseases of the Nose and Sinuses

I've had nasal problems all my life. All diseases are built into our genetic makeup, and they manifest under certain conditions. That is why, in one sense, all diseases can be considered genetic. When I catch a cold it affects my nose. Sneezing, nasal discharge, and nasal congestion make it hard to breathe and is very rough on me. Nasal discharge thickens and becomes phlegm. It is fine when it comes out of the nose, but it's difficult when it comes from deep in your throat as postnasal drip. Sometimes I lose my sense of smell.

Japanese in general are very sensitive to smells and can tell many smells apart. There is even a discipline and performance of discriminating fragrances known as *kodo* (香道) from ancient times. This is an unusual thing in the world. That is why fragrances are an important part of Japanese cooking, and this contributes to the world-renown of Japanese cuisine.

So how much can acu-moxa treat nasal problems? As I said earlier, it is very effective for the early stages of a cold. The progress of the cold can be stopped. It works like the Kudzu Decoction *(gé gēn tāng)* formula in herbal medicine. When the cold cannot be stopped in its early stages and the rhinitis turns into sinusitis, doctors (ENT specialists) prescribe antibiotics. This is a blessing because it allows one to get by without surgery, but in some cases the antibiotics don't resolve the nasal problem. Acupuncture and moxibustion are indicated here. There is a synergistic effect with antibiotics, so it is best when they are used together.

1. Hay fever (allergic rhinitis)

As spring equinox approaches, nasal symptoms begin to appear. The range of people who get hay fever seems to be expanding these days, because even elderly people are getting it. I will begin this section with simple local treatment. In Yanagiya Sorei's

Guide to Secret One-Needle Technique,[1] there is a needling technique which is very useful under the heading "A Needle for All Nasal Diseases." Yanagiya states as follows: "The fingers can feel a V shaped groove at the inferior border between the eyebrows. ... There is a slight depression at the bottom end of the V, just before you go down over edge of the bone. ... This is the extra point M-HN-3 *(yin-dō/yìn táng).*"

This description is not that clear, but the point is to needle M-HN-3 *(yin-dō/yìn táng).* The location of M-HN-3 *(yin-dō/yìn táng)* is "in the depression between the eyebrows," so it's in the groove between the right and left eyebrows. How does Yanagiya suggest needling this point? He says, "Insert with the feeling that you are putting the needle tip through the space between the right and left nasal bones."

This description isn't that clear either, but the needle is inserted inferiorly from M-HN-3 *(yin-dō/yìn táng).* The above can be construed as threading between the skin and the nasal bone. How far is the needle inserted? Until the sensation is felt in the nose.

Yanagiya says, "If the sensation [in the nose] is felt as soon as the needle tip touches the skin, that is enough. Gradually advance the needle if there is no sensation [in the nose] and gently move it up and down [sparrow pecking]. Remove the needle when the needle sensation reaches inside the nose."

When you advance the needle as far as it will go, the tip reaches the start of the ridge of the nose. It won't go any further. I used to like to retain the needle here. The depth is between 1 and 2cm. This insertion technique is not that easy. Even when you use a thin stainless steel needle, sensitive patients can experience pain. Isn't there an easier way? My lazy nature shows its face here. So I focused on the point that the tip of the needle reaches when the needle is inserted in M-HN-3 *(yin-dō/yìn táng).* Sliding the finger down from M-HN-3 *(yin-dō/yìn táng),* it falls into the gap and comes to a stop at the top of the bridge of the nose. What would happen if I just needled this point? I'll just call this point Lower *yìn táng* (Fig. 8-1). The location is on the saddle with clear boundaries above and below and right and left. I put the needle tip on this point and rotate it. I do SRT for quite a while, between 30 seconds and one minute. There is nothing to it. Even children do not complain, and the effect is excellent. While I am rotating the needle, patients usually report that their nose has cleared. This is my recent experience, but I highly recommend this as the local treatment.

The next local point is LI-20. Insertion works for this point, and the needle can be retained. The key is to skillfully locate the reaction. Also I use BL-2. SRT is enough at this point.

Then there is direct moxibustion for local treatment. GV-23 is the best point for this. For this point also, the secret is to accurately locate the tender point. In acute cases I do multiple cones; 10 to 20. A sharp sensation reaches down to the nose. Patients will pull their head in like a turtle. The outcome is even better if they are willing to do about five cones a day at home. Another point for moxibustion is LI-4 or LI-10. Multiple cones also works well here and it's easier to apply.

---

1. *Guide to Secret One-Needle Technique (Hiho Ipponshin Densho),* Yokosuka: Ido-no-Nippon-Sha, 1955.

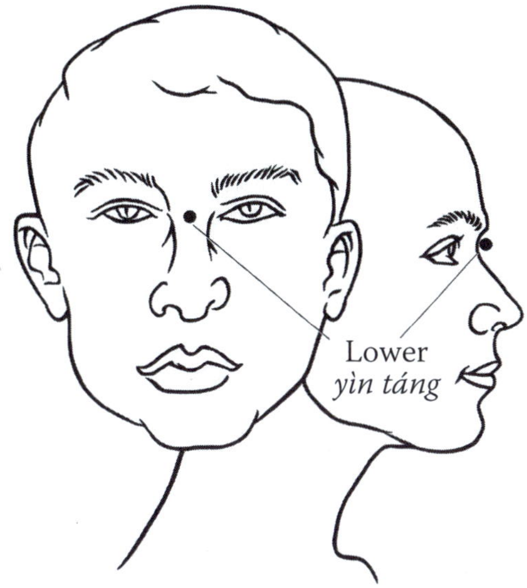

Fig. 8-1 Lower *yìn táng*

Close to the local area is the occipital region. I look for indurations and needle it when there are reactions at points like BL-10 or GB-20. SRT is enough. As for meridians associated with hay fever, I think of the *yáng míng* meridians. On the Large Intestine meridian, I favor points like LI-4, LI-10, and LI-11. On the Stomach meridian, I favor points like ST-36 and ST-43.

In terms of the basic pattern, Lung deficiency is common, but any one of the four basic patterns can occur.

Case Study 99

Patient: Female, 9 years old

FOC: January 7, 2005

Main Complaints: Allergic rhinitis, hay fever, and bronchitis that causes wheezing

History: Pneumonia and then sinusitis

Pulse Diagnosis: Lung deficiency (right wrist had transposed radial artery)

Treatment: SRT on LU-9, SP-3, LI-11, CV-12, LI-20, BL-10, GB-20, GB-21, BL-13, BL-20, and BL-58. Direct moxibustion on GV-23.

Progress: (3rd) March 26 – Coughing. Intradermal needle retained in left axillary point. Direct moxibustion on BL-13.

(4th) July 9 – She is doing well. She no longer misses school. Intradermal needle retained in right axillary point.

2. Sinusitis

With hay fever there is mostly clear nasal discharge, but with sinusitis there is discharge of thick phlegm. Nasal congestion causes great difficulty. Antibiotics work well in acute cases. Surgery was common in years past, but I don't hear about it much these days. When the results are unclear after several months of antibiotics, surgery may be recommended. The acu-moxa treatment is pretty much the same as for hay fever, but more moxibustion is indicated. Multiple cones on a few points like GV-23, LI-10 (or LI-4), and ST-36 can be done twice a day. The moxibustion can cause the nasal discharge to become thicker. The results are better the more discharge there is initially. Acupuncture can also be done on the above points. BL-10 is also effective when there is a reaction at the point.

Case Study 100

Patient: Male, 61 years old

FOC: January 28, 2011

Main Complaints: Sinusitis right > left

Pulse Diagnosis: Liver deficiency

Treatment: SRT on LR-8, KI-10, Lower *yìn táng*, BL-2, LI-20, BL-10, and GB-20. Needles inserted in LI-4 and ST-36. Small sparrow-pecking motions applied five times each. Press tack (Pyonex) retained in right BL-10. Direct moxibustion on GV-23, LI-4, and ST-36.

Progress: (2nd) Jan 31 – He is doing better. The needles at BL-2 feel good. Press tack (Pyonex) retained in right GB-20 (the place that feels most tense to him).

(3rd) Feb 7 – The sinusitis is worse again.

Comments: This patient gets better and then worse again. He continues to come in for treatment, but he is unwilling to do moxibustion at home.

3. Rhinitis

Whether the symptoms of the nose occur with colds, sinusitis, or hay fever, the treatment is all the same. Examining the local area around the nose, there is a strong reaction superior and slightly lateral to the standard location of LI-20.[2] The point protrudes slightly and is boggy. Acute cases have tenderness at this point. Locate this reaction accurately. SRT works on this reaction close to LI-20 and superficial retention of

2. LI-20 variation: See discussion in *Finding Effective Acupuncture Points*, p. 41. This point corresponds to location C.

needles also works. SRT on the margin of the ala nasi is also good. The decisive point for nose problems is Lower *yìn táng*. Slide the finger down from M-HN-3 *(yin-dō/yìn táng)* into the bridge of the nose and locate the lowest point in the center (Fig. 8-1). Apply SRT for over 30 seconds. When it works well the nasal congestion will resolve quickly. GV-23 is the best moxibustion point for nasal problems. It is ideal for home moxibustion treatment because the heat is not felt that much. When more than five cones are applied, the heat sensation penetrates through the head to the root of the nose. The patient will pull their head back when they feel this penetrating heat sensation.

BL-10 and GB-20 can also be needled. Since the face and nose is the domain of the *yáng míng* meridians, treating points on the Large Intestine and Stomach meridians will increase the effect. My favorite points are LI-4, LI-10, and ST-36. LI-4 and ST-36 are good points for moxibustion, and inserting needles and applying sparrow pecking will yield good results.

With patients who get hay fever, give them a preventative treatment when the season arrives. Some get by with light symptoms, some have no symptoms, and others experience the same level of symptoms. The effect varies but usually there is some effect.

4. Sleep apnea

There seems to be a rise in the number of patients who have sleep apnea these days. This isn't a nose problem per se, but snoring is a common symptom of sleep apnea. Usually women who are concerned about their husband's snoring come to me for advice. I did have one case of snoring, which I treated around the nose as described above under rhinitis, and his snoring stopped. I also retain needles in CV-12 and left ST-21 for such cases. These points also have an effect on the mouth and throat.

People who are overweight and those with so-called metabolic disorders tend to snore when they sleep and their breathing stops from time to time. This is a condition that affects the whole body, but I focus on the nose in an attempt to treat it. I start with extended SRT (30 seconds to one minute) on Lower *yìn táng*. This is the same as for other nasal problems discussed above. I also add BL-2, LI-20, and GV-23. I also do SRT on CV-12, left ST-21, and right ST-19 followed by moxibustion. Of course, I do a standard root treatment for the pattern determined from the pulse. This simple treatment has been more effective than expected and I have gotten reports of patients falling asleep less during the day, snoring less, and even having reduced blood sugar levels. This approach is worth trying.

Case Study 101

Patient: Male, 65 years old

FOC: November 29, 2008

Main Complaints: Sleep apnea and diabetes (HbA1c 6.1)

Pulse Diagnosis: Rapid, Kidney deficiency

Treatment: Patient seems to be afraid of needles. SRT on KI-7, LU-5, CV-12, CV-6, left ST-21, BL-13, BL-20, BL-23, LI-11, ST-36, BL-58, Yanagiya's GB-20, BL-10, GB-21, LI-20, BL-2, and Lower *yìn táng*. Direct moxibustion on GV-23, BL-13, BL-23, and GV-6.

Progress: I treated this patient regularly every week, and the typical pattern was Liver deficiency. For diabetes I used CV-12, left ST-21, BL-20, and GV-6. The main points for the nose were Lower *yìn táng*, LI-20, BL-2, GV-23, and BL-10.

Comments: As we continued with treatments, his wife told me his snoring decreased, and he stopped falling asleep around noon. I also treated the wife for depression and her expression brightened and she began to gain a little weight. I gave her a similar treatment as her husband to prevent sleep apnea.

5. Nasal congestion

Case Study 102

Patient: Male, 64 years old

FOC: January 25, 2011

Symptoms and Condition: Right nasal obstruction. Just the right nose is blocked. He doesn't mind it during the day, but it bothers him at night and it's hard to sleep. Examination at the university hospital revealed no abnormality. He was told there was no problem at all and he became even more worried. Aside from his nasal congestion he has glaucoma in the right eye, hypertension (controlled by medication), and borderline diabetic blood sugar levels. He is overweight.

Pulse Diagnosis: Liver deficiency

Treatment: SRT on LR-8, KI-10, ST-36, LI-11, BL-18, BL-23, Lower *yìn táng*, BL-2, right LI-20, GB-20, Yanagiya's GB-20, CV-12, CV-6, BL-58. Needle inserted and sparrow pecking applied to right LI-4. Direct moxibustion on GV-23 and on BL-10, GB-21, and ST-36 only on the right.

Progress: (3rd) Feb 8 – He decided to try losing weight and has lost 3kg. His nose is beginning to clear. His right eye feels irritated from reading. Direct moxibustion on left ST-21 and CV-12. He is instructed to apply moxibustion on these points at home.

(4th) Feb 15 – No more symptoms in his nose. Ocular pressure: right 17mmHg, left 15mmHg.

Comments: He was told that there was no problem with his nose at a hospital. When I had him breath with his left nostril closed, there didn't seem to be any difference from doing so on the other side. So I didn't notice any problem with his nose either. I suspected that there was a psychological issue from his complaints. He started dieting to lose weight and succeeded in losing 3kg, but it's not likely that this caused the sensation of blockage in the nose to disappear. I believe the good outcome was a result of the acupuncture treatments, primarily using SRT.

CHAPTER

9

Circulatory Diseases

1. Overview

The Heart[1] is the foundation of the body. In East Asian medicine the Heart is given a special position among the five yin organs. In the classics the Heart is called the source of life, the transformation of spirit, and the place from which clarity of spirit emerges. Dr. Iemoto[2] attributes the high level integrative function of the brain and the activity of the cerebral cortex to the Heart. In modern medicine, on the other hand, the function of the heart is primarily about blood circulation. There was no association of the Heart with blood circulation in East Asian medicine. I describe the function of this classical Heart as governing all thought and activity, but both classical and modern medicine are in agreement that the heart is the most essential organ.

If the heart stops, all is lost. It is different from all other organs. There is no room for error. There is no backup. That is why when patients come in with symptoms associated with the heart, I always have them get a medical check-up if they haven't already done so. I consider the results of the medical exam to determine the treatment strategy for acu-moxa. One can't be so fearful that one avoids treating patients with heart conditions. Before the advent of modern medicine, East Asian medicine covered every kind of disease. I believe the principle that every disease responds to regulation of the five yin organs is as true now as it was then. You could consider acu-moxa as being supplemental or complementary to Western medicine, and there can be a combined effect. I also

1. Heart and heart: The capitalized organ represents the traditional organ, while the organ in lower case refers to the modern understanding of the organ. In East Asia, the Heart is considered to be the center of mental as well as emotional functions.

2. Iemoto Sei-ichi M.D. (家本誠一): A renowned classical scholar and president of the Chinese Classical Medicine Research Society (中国古典医学研究会) in Japan.

think acu-moxa is very useful for circulatory diseases from the standpoint of improving the quality of life.

In Meridian Therapy, the style of traditional Japanese acupuncture I practice, there is an idea that normally the Heart doesn't get diseased in patients who are still alive. Pathogens do not invade it, because if they do, it's all over. The protector of the Heart, the Pericardium, receives the pathogen, so the Pericardium is treated instead. Does that mean we don't treat the heart directly? One could treat the Heart meridian, but this isn't as good. Often, treating for Spleen deficiency takes care of a Heart problem. (The Pericardium and Spleen meridians—usually PC-7 and SP-3—are tonified for Spleen deficiency.) I am so amazed at the founders of Meridian Therapy who created this treatment system. The theory is great, but the effect of the root treatments is even better.

1.1 Symptoms of the Heart

As for symptoms associated with the heart, there are palpitations, arrhythmia, stifling sensation in chest, and angina. Be especially careful with patients who have angina. Once a patient who complained about pain around left LU-1 fainted while taking a bath later. When the patient is able to point to a rib or intercostal space as the location of pain, it's not a heart problem. The pain that is hard to pinpoint somewhere deep in the chest or left thoracic region is, in contrast, dangerous. This is one way to differentiate the pain from heart problems from other issues, but it's much better when a cardiologist says the problem is not in the heart after a thorough exam. Even so, we can't completely relax just because a doctor says the heart is problem free. It happens quite often that someone dies suddenly after recently being told that there was no problem at an exam. When there are the above symptoms, it is best to treat the patient as if they had a heart problem.

Let's take a look at Heart symptoms and their relationship to the meridians.

The symptoms followed by an asterisk (*) are from Chapter 10 of the *Vital Axis.* Those followed by the pound sign (#) are from the *Moxibustion Classic of the Eleven Yin and Yang Meridians*, excavated from the Mawangdui tombs in Hunan province.[3]

Lung meridian: distention and fullness of the lungs, pain in the supraclavicular fossa, and irritability and fullness in the chest (*), heart pain (#)

Stomach meridian: heart pain (#)

Spleen meridian: irritability in the chest, sharp pain in the epigastrium (*), irritability in the chest leading to death, heart pain and abdominal distention leading to death (#)

Heart meridian: heart pain (* & #)

Kidney meridian: irritability in the heart and heart pain (*)

---

3. Mawangdui manuscripts are recent archeological findings of texts put in the ground ~168 BCE. See p. 111-112 of *Introduction to Meridian Therapy* for details on the significance of the Mawangdui manuscripts and their symptomology.

Pericardium meridian: irritability in the heart and heart pain (*)

Gallbladder meridian: pain in the heart and flank region (* & #)

Liver meridian: distention in chest (*), irritability in the heart leading to death (#)

Thus, symptoms of the heart can be related to almost all the meridians. It is true that all the meridians connect to the heart. This is why determining the pattern is so important in rendering treatment.

1.2 Treating the Heart according to patterns

Liver deficiency: Tonify LR-8, KI-10, LV-14, and BL-18.

Liver excess: Disperse LR-2. Tonify points on the Lung or Spleen meridians.

Spleen deficiency: Tonify SP-3, PC-7, left ST-21, BL-14, and BL-20. (SP-4 and PC-6 can be tonified instead of SP-3 and PC-7.)

Lung deficiency: Tonify LU-9, SP-3, LU-1, and BL-13. Disperse LU-10 and HT-8 when the excess in the heart position does not diminish.

Kidney deficiency: Tonify KI-7, LU-5 (or LU-8), BL-23, and CV-6. Disperse SP-3 and KI-3 when the excess in the Heart position does not diminish with treatment.

1.3 Epigastric region (literally "below the heart")

CV-14 is the front alarm point of the Heart. When there is a heart problem, there is a tendency for the subcostal regions on both sides, including CV-14, to become hard. That is why there is difficulty breathing. When subjective symptoms like "epigastric fullness" and "fullness in the chest and hypochondrium" are relieved, the epigastric region also softens. The front alarm point of the Pericardium, CV-17, does not experience this effect. I find that CV-17 is more effective for diseases of the esophagus and stomach. This is why CV-17 is a useful point for cases of angina that are so-called "gastric chest pain," where pain from the stomach is felt up into the chest.

When CV-14 is hard, CV-6 under the navel is depressed. It is good to tonify CV-6. It is ideal when the epigastric region softens after the tonification of root treatment points. I also recommend using the well point associated with the pattern.[4]

1.4 Upper back region

Treating the back associated point BL-15 would serve as a local treatment for the Heart. But, as I said before, in Meridian Therapy there is a hands-off policy on the Heart, so I default to the Pericardium associated point BL-14. When there is a cardiac problem, the muscles around the upper back on the left side always become tight.

In Japan there is the phrase "to injure the heart." As noted above, traditionally the

---

4. Well points: In chapter 68 of the *Classic of Difficulties*, well points are used to treat fullness in the epigastric region.

"heart" refers to both the emotional and mental aspects of a person. It begins with being concerned, getting worried, and then becoming anxious. When such emotions go on for a long time, it becomes a "heartache." I tell my patients that even if they worry, they should not let it become a heartache. When heartaches go on for a while, only the left side of the upper back becomes tight. The right side is fine. This tightness must be relieved as soon as possible. You can give the patient one of the above root treatments that affect the Heart, depending on the pattern, along with some treatment to soften the epigastric region and treatment for the upper back. This will release the tension on the left side. Sometimes the tension doesn't go away so easily. In this case, take your time and give more treatments. Even when you are treating the patient for other symptoms, when you notice this tension on the left side, just treat it without telling the patient anything. This could prevent that patient from having to suffer in the future with a diagnosis like angina or myocardial infarction. So the upper back is a very important diagnostic and treatment area for heart problems. However, Okabe Sodo, one of the founders of Meridian Therapy, seemed to disagree.

"One must regulate the meridians. It's not going to get better by thinking like 'the heart has a problem so I'll treat BL-15 [the Heart associated point].' By regulating the meridians, the hypertrophy of the heart diminishes, the blood pressure goes down, coughing subsides, and the kidneys also get better. Nephrosis, for example, is difficult to help by treating the Kidney area. You must treat the meridians after all. Things get worse when the Kidney area is over stimulated."[5]

The above statement can also be interpreted as a warning against treating the local area too much.

1.5 Other treatment points for the heart

In addition to the above, I often use the following points for patients with heart problems.

Left axillary point: This point is level with the nipples about 5cm anterior to the vertical axillary line (see Fig. 7-1) It will be extremely tender when useful. I press both axillary regions at the same time with the tips of my middle fingers. When the point is indicated, it will stick to your fingers in addition to being very sensitive. When the left axillary point is especially tender, it is safe to assume that the heart has a problem. I like to retain an intradermal needle. You can stimulate this point with a teishin, or use a small press tack like Pyonex, but SRT and needle insertion aren't good.

PC-6: This point on the left side is especially effective for arrhythmia, palpitations, and heart pain. Simple insertion, retained needle, and direct moxibustion are all good. It is especially suited to home moxibustion treatment.

---

5. From Okabe Sodo, *Essence of Acupuncture and Moxibustion Treatment (Shinkyu chiryo no shinzui).* Tokyo: Sekibunodo, 1983.

PC-8: I use this point on the left side and locate it on the ulnar side of the index finger's flexor tendon. The point will be a hard lump on the tendon and tender.

SI-1: The one on the left is used. It is best to needle for dispersion. Small cones of direct moxa are also good. It works to alleviate shortness of breath.

Scalene point: The left side. The influence of the heart problem goes up and manifests as an induration in the supraclavicular fossa above ST-12. The more severe the cardiac problem, the more extensive and superior the indurations. They can go further up to GB-21 or even as far as GB-20. On the other side, it forms an induration around BL-14 and -15 and then goes up to GB-21 and ends at GB-20. By palpating for indurations in these places, you can deduce the patient's mental state as well as the condition of the heart.

SI-11: The one located on the left is used. There will be intense tenderness and induration. Inserting a needle and multiple cones of moxibustion is good. As you apply cone after cone of moxibustion, the palpitations and pain will diminish. Even if we don't treat the Heart or the Heart meridian, we can disperse its paired yang meridian, the Small Intestine meridian. That is why it makes sense to treat SI-1 and SI-11.

GV-10 and -11: Treat these points if there is tenderness. M-BW-25 *(jōsen/shí qī zhuī xià)* can also be used if it is tender.

2. Palpitations (arrhythmia)

Case Study 103

Patient: Female, 61 years old

Treatment Date: January 29, 2011 (she had been coming in for regular treatments)

Symptom and Situation: Palpitations which came on suddenly. I had been treating this patient for pain in the right gastrocnemius muscle, and she had previously been diagnosed with disk herniation.

Pulse Diagnosis: Spleen deficiency. Her pulse was unusually fast, but it was not irregular.

Temperature: 36.7°C. This could be a mild fever, but the rapid pulse was not due to fever.

Treatment: I performed SRT on SP-3 bilaterally, and when I checked the pulse before I went to PC-7, the pulse had slowed down. I applied SRT on left PC-6 and right SP-4 followed by five cones of direct moxibustion. I instructed the patient to press left PC-6 if the palpitations started again. I found a reaction at left ST-21 and left BL-17, so it may have been a tired Spleen, but the cause is unclear.

Progress: She had not had any palpitations or arrhythmia since the above treatment.

2.1 A case of arrhythmia (my own)

Since I reached middle age, I have occasionally experienced arrhythmias. My primary care doctor laughed and told me I had reached that age. But the EKG measurements I had taken every year showed no abnormalities. Nevertheless, since I felt short of breath a while after running, I was told that there must be some problem in my coronary artery. Early on one New Year, I drank sake at an establishment owned by one of my patients. The custom at New Years is to drink small flasks of hot sake, and I drank a bit more than usual, but it wasn't like I was drunk. Anyway, I awoke around 2 a.m. that night with palpitations. My pulse was racing. Usually when I drink too much my pulse becomes rapid, then I retain a needle in LR-1, and in a while my pulse returns to normal, and all is well after that. This time was different, however; something wasn't right. Taking my own pulse, I noticed it was irregular. The pattern was Lung deficiency so I needled LU-9 and SP-3 and checked my pulses again, but there was no change. I had some success with needling over the pulsation at CV-12, so I applied SRT for a while, but this brought no change. So I tried left PC-6, left ST-21, and CV-6, all to no avail. All this took a lot of time. I fell asleep with a needle on left LU-9. When I awoke, I checked my pulse and it was back to normal.

The next day I was busy in the clinic as usual, and about an hour into the day I felt hot and uncomfortable. I stepped outside for a minute to get a breath of cold fresh air and felt better. I went back to giving treatments, but I started to feel a bit dizzy and I started to break out in a sweat. So I went to an adjacent room, lay down, and took my own pulse. It was beating weakly at the deep level and didn't feel right. It was soft but felt sticky. I kept on sweating. Something was really wrong.

I recalled Dr. Z, an acupuncturist who had received a clean bill of health from his doctor, being told after his medical checkup that he was like a person 10 years younger than his age. Soon after that he fell ill while giving treatments and was transported to the university hospital, but he died shortly thereafter. He had had a myocardial infarction. And then there was the time I accompanied my teacher on a house call to treat his friend who suddenly took ill. It must have been a heart problem because his breathing was labored and he had reactions on his abdomen, which my teacher needled. This man died sometime soon afterward and I recall going to his funeral with my teacher. For some reason I remembered this episode that happened 50 years ago.

I retained needles in CV-22 and my left auricular vertigo point ... I checked my pulses, and they had become bigger. This was more like my normal pulse. I went back into the treatment room as if nothing had happened and resumed my work.

As long as I continue giving myself treatments with SRT, I can get over some excesses in my lifestyle. But there is a limit. There is my advancing age. I need to avoid over doing it. The former president of the Toyohari Association, Yanagishita Toshio, was the same age as me. When I was the president of the Traditional Japanese Acupuncture Society, he worked with me to improve relations between our associations. He treated an amazing number of patients every day. It was a shock when I recently heard that he had passed away, especially because he was someone I respected deeply. Even though he was 78 when he died, it is possible that his super-human work schedule had something to do with his demise.

Case Study 104

Patient: Female, 70 years old

FOC: June 2, 2008

Main Complaints: Shortness of breath. It is hard to walk up even gentle hills. Recently she seems to fall easily. She received a diagnosis of hypertrophic cardiomyopathy. Her sleep, appetite, and bowel movements are good.

Pulse Diagnosis: Sunken, slow, and deficient; Liver deficiency

Treatment: SRT on LR-8, KI-10, ST-36, LI-11, CV-12, CV-6, BL-18, BL-23, left ST-21, PC-8, GB-2, GB-21, GV-11, left SI-11, left BL-15. Direct moxibustion on LR-3, left PC-8, GV-11, left SI-11, and left BL-15. I gave the patient moxibustion points she could treat herself at home: LR-3 and left PC-8.

Progress: (2nd) Liver deficiency. Got up to urinate twice at night. For about an hour she has trouble getting back to sleep.

Comments: The shortness of breath is due to her heart condition, so I have continued to treat her. It is good to receive acupuncture treatments and do moxibustion at home, but is there anyone at home who can do it? Not that many people are able to apply moxibustion skillfully. She continues with short walks and keeps her weight down. Occasional acu-moxa treatments increase the quality of life and even extend life, but it's a process that goes on for the rest of your life.

3. Hypertension and aneurysms

Our blood pressure constantly changes. It is not stable. It is high when we become active in the morning, and we are able to move around better with higher blood pressure. People with low blood pressure feel tired and have difficulty getting going. Why does our blood pressure become high? Sending blood to every corner of the body is the function of the heart. When there is arteriosclerosis in peripheral vessels, blood pressure must go up in order to get blood through that area. When this circulatory regulation doesn't work, it can turn into occlusive arteriosclerosis, which is also known as an infarction. When this happens in the brain, it is called a cerebral infarction. If an infarction can be prevented, high blood pressure would be better for the body, but when there is hardening of the arteries, the vessels tend to rupture easier. This then causes a cerebral hemorrhage. When blood vessels have elasticity, one can avoid ruptures. All animals move toward death as their blood vessels age. How can we keep our blood vessels young and maintain their elasticity? This is the question.

When we speak of "Stomach qi" in pulse diagnosis, we are talking about this. The degree of hardening in the arteries can be clearly felt at the radial and carotid arteries, which are pulse diagnosis locations. The artery feels harder, protrudes in places, thickens or deviates. These are all signs of aging. When some hardness in the arteries is palpated in pulse diagnosis, we call this "lack of Stomach qi." When the arteries feel softer after some treatment, we say "Stomach qi has increased," which means the treatment is a success.

Can acu-moxa treatments actually soften arteries that have hardened? Early in my practice when I used to do house-calls, I treated a man close to 90 who complained of stomach pain from time to time. His abdomen at that time had distended arteries that were tender, which is the only time I have seen anything like this. They were mostly in the lower abdomen so the affected arteries must have been related to the abdominal aorta, inferior mesenteric artery, common iliac artery, and external iliac artery. They were along the Conception vessel and Stomach meridian. I reasoned that if these distended vessels were actual aneurysms, they would be hard and wouldn't be causing pain. So I did a root treatment, followed by some treatment on the back, and finished with some local treatment. I chose several points that were distended and tender on the lower abdomen and inserted needles. The arteries were distended and I couldn't insert the needles much. This was long before I had developed SRT, so I inserted the needle just a little and rotated the needle for a long time. Then I applied a few cones of moxibustion on these points after needling them.

When I paid another house call to this patient the next day, the protruding vessels were gone. His abdominal pain was also gone. I still don't really know what I was treating. In all my experience this case was the only one in which protruding vessels went away with treatment. The protruding vessels recurred along with the pain in this patient, and I repeated the same treatment several times with good effect.

3.1 Aneurysms in the abdominal aorta

There are times, on the other hand, that I discover aneurysms in the abdominal aorta. The patient doesn't notice it when the aneurysm is small since there is no discomfort. Aneurysms larger than 5cm are considered dangerous and surgery is recommended. The advances in vascular surgery are truly amazing, and I hear that there are safe surgical procedures even for elderly patients. When I find an aneurysm of the abdominal aorta, I inform the patient and the family and refer them to a vascular surgeon. I have them discuss their options. When the aneurysm is small, I do some local acu-moxa treatment. I also have the patient avoid work that may increase abdominal pressure, such as bending over to pull weeds. One 90-year-old woman in whom I found an aneurysm elected not to do surgery. She enjoyed several more years of health, but she finally died of a massive internal hemorrhage. The cause was an aneurysm in the abdominal aorta as expected, but her family told me she didn't suffer.

The consensus among Japanese scholars is that the concept of meridians or channels had its origin in arteries. If this is true, arteries that can be palpated from the surface are key points for assessing the channels. Might we get good results by treating these points? There are quite a few points over arteries that I use in my practice including LI-4, ST-4, ST-9, ST-30, BL-40, CV-7, LR-3, and KI-3. Among these, ST-9 that is directly over the carotid artery, together with GB-20 over the vertebral artery, constitute the gateway to cerebral circulation.

Unfortunately, we cannot directly palpate the vertebral artery. Anyway, when there are indurations, we can suspect arteriosclerosis. The so-called *rén yíng* pulse at ST-9, the carotid pulse, can be felt clearly. There is a pulse diagnosis method discussed in the *Vital Axis* comparing this pulse to the radial pulse at LU-8. It is said that when the carotid pulse is three times as strong as the radial pulse, it is a pulse of longevity. Yet the condition of the carotid artery is pretty much the same as that of other cerebral arteries. If this is so, it may be dangerous to press or needle the carotid artery. Nowadays the condition of the vertebral arteries can be determined by ultrasound.

There was a time when so-called "sinus-puncture" was popular among acupuncturists in Japan. Shirota Bunshi advocated needling ST-9, and my master, Miura Nagahiko, often used this method. The point was to stimulate the carotid sinus at the bifurcation of the internal and external carotid artery. When the needle tip reached the wall of the artery, the needle begins to move back and forth with the pulse. This "sinus-puncture" was held to be good for conditions like high blood pressure and asthma. I recalled this, and I also wanted to mitigate arteriosclerosis, so I started using SRT on ST-9. Deeper insertion at ST-9 can cause needle shock, so it is better to stay superficial.

There is no literature about needling arteries to reduce their hardening, but there must be some effect. I remember reading a report somewhere that needling the local area for occlusive arteriosclerosis caused angiogenesis and improved circulation. In any case, there should be no negative effect. Acu-moxa treatment on arteriosclerosis affecting the lower extremities does have a good effect in my experience. I think it should be tried more.

3.2 Treatment of hypertension

To treat hypertension, I use the standard approach of regulating the meridians with tonification and dispersion. This is the root treatment. In addition, I do the following:

1. Release tension in the neck and shoulders.
2. Tonify the deficient lower abdomen and disperse the excess in the upper abdomen.
3. Remove the coldness from the low back and legs.

These steps make the treatment complete. No other special treatment is needed for the blood pressure to settle back down to normal. If things go well, once a week treatments will resolve the problem. While undergoing treatment, warn your patient about gaining weight. They must avoid getting tense in the neck and shoulders as well as eating rich and overly salty foods. They must also get adequate exercise and receive regular medical checkups. Here are my treatment points for Liver deficiency and Kidney deficiency.

Liver deficiency: SRT—LR-8, KI-10, ST-36, LI-11, CV-12, CV-6, GB-20, GB-21, and at times disperse just GB-38. Retain needles—GV-22, auricular vertigo point, BL-18, and BL-23. Direct moxibustion—LI-11, ST-36, LR-3, BL-18, and GB-21.

Kidney deficiency: SRT—KI-7, LU-5, BL-13, BL-23, and CV-6. Retain needles—KI-7 and BL-23. Direct moxibustion—KI-7 and BL-23.

4. Hypotension

There are some people who are troubled by low blood pressure. Is hypotension really a disease? Dr. Manaka Yoshio[6] said that hypotension was like having a small nose, and that it was nothing to worry about. There is no problem when you have hypotension and no symptoms. Actually, you live longer. Your blood vessels are soft. This is why I explain to patients who complain of hypotension that there is no problem if there are no symptoms. When we make the blood pressure a problem, we can't resolve the issue. Low blood pressure does not go up so easily. If there is some disease and the blood pressure is low as a result, focus on treating the disease. When the patient doesn't have a diagnosis but still complains of symptoms, determine the pattern and treat according to the pattern and this will resolve the symptoms. Acu-moxa treatment is excellent in this regard, and can be used much more.

So I would like to summarize my standard treatments for hypertension and hypotension below.

4.1 Treatment of hypotension

Kidney deficiency: SRT—KI-7, LU-5, CV-6, CV-12, BL-13, and BL-23. Retain needles superficially in BL-23 and auricular vertigo point. Intradermal needle retained in auricular vertigo point. Direct moxibustion—KI-7, CV-6, and BL-23.

(*Note*: As much as possible, do not insert needles in deficient or weak patients. Use SRT or teishin. Direct moxibustion must also be reduced to 80% moxibustion or *chinetsu-kyu* [heat sensing moxibustion].)

Case Study 105

Patient: female, 34 years old

FOC: April 30, 1976

Symptoms and Situation: Dizziness that started four days ago. She also doesn't feel

6. Manaka Yoshio M.D. (1911-1989): A Japanese medical doctor who worked to advance and promote East Asian medicine. He served for many years as the visiting professor at the East Asian Medicine Research Center of Kitasato University.

good. Her doctor says it's because of low blood pressure, but it doesn't get any better. She also has pain at BL-2 and coughing.

Blood Pressure: 90/55

Pulse Diagnosis: Kidney deficiency

Treatment: Needles retained superficially in auricular vertigo point, CV-22, KI-7, Upper BL-10, GB-20, GB-21, and right ST-19. Simple insertion in BL-43. Intradermal needle retained in left axillary point and both auricular vertigo points.

Progress: Right after this treatment, her dizziness went away and she felt fine. She felt new and refreshed and was delighted, saying she never knew acupuncture worked this well. She recovered after just two treatments.

Q&A

QUESTION AND ANSWER NO. 5

Amount of stimulation and healing reactions (crises)

Q. After about six years of being licensed, my results have improved since first starting out, and I am feeling comfortable with my treatment style. I feel that this is a critical stage, as I am starting to develop personal preferences, but at the same time I don't wish to get caught up in my own ego or limited experience.

At this level, I have found that at the end of a treatment, many of my patients are reporting a good result, but their condition is not always completely alleviated. I do explain to them that acupuncture is a process and not a magic bullet, but I find it hard to fight the urge to end the treatment at this stage. In other words, even when I get a good result—let's say the patient reports 75-95 percent improvement—I am tempted to try to get a little more for the patient. Sometimes I do restrain myself, knowing that if I push it, I run the risk of overtreating and causing the patient to feel worse temporarily. In many American schools it is taught that this is a good thing: that the body is having a "healing crisis." It is sometimes called the "law of the cure," and the adage, "it will get worse before it gets better" is often offered to patients.

While I have had the experience of patients calling me the day after treatment in severe pain and the day after that calling to tell me they feel 100 percent better, it is a rough situation for both the patient and myself. I understand that each patient is an individual and must be considered on a case-by-case basis, but can you offer general guidelines for when to go for maximum relief and when to hold back?

A. The appropriate amount of stimulation in acupuncture is something I myself have always been concerned about. I decided to write about this because it might be a good opportunity to draw out some of my conclusions on this matter. The things written in the classics, and the things written by our predecessors, don't always work out in practice. I have tried out many things in my practice, and the following represents what I have learned and where I stand on this matter.

Conditions for mild and strong stimulation

The following are general categories and are not absolute. Please understand that these are only general guidelines.

Gender: Women tend to tolerate stimulation better, and men tend to be less tolerant.

Experience: Those who have experience with acupuncture are comparatively tolerant. When new to acupuncture, the initial anxiety and tension can cause fatigue.

Preference: Those who like acupuncture tend to be happy even if the treatment causes a little fatigue. Those who dislike acupuncture, no matter how many treatments they have, tend to tolerate stimulation less.

Season: People tend to tolerate stimulation less in the spring and summer, and better in the fall and winter.

Skin color: Those with darker skin tend to tolerate stimulation more, and those with lighter skin tend to tolerate it less.

Lips: Those with thick lips tend to tolerate stimulation more, and those with thin lips tend to tolerate it less.

Physique: When it comes to being fat or thin, the fatter person tolerates stimulation more, and the thinner person less. In the case of fat patients, there are those that have a lot of muscle mass, those that have a lot of fat, and those with water retention. Those with muscle mass tolerate stimulation well. Those with lots of fat are not intolerant, but there is a tendency to overtreat them because it's so easy to insert needles. Even if thin, muscular people tolerate stimulation well. Patients lacking muscle tone can't take a lot of stimulation.

Occupation: Those who do mental work tolerate stimulation less and those who do physical work can take more stimulation. Athletes and those who exercise tolerate stimulation well.

Urban/rural: There is a tendency for those in urban areas to tolerate stimulation less and those in rural areas to tolerate stimulation well. This is also related to their occupations.

Movements: Those who are quick in their movements tend to tolerate stimulation less, and those are slower in movement tolerate stimulation well.

Alertness: Those whose eyes move rapidly and hear everything tend to tolerate stimulation less.

Pulse quality: Those with excess, wiry, tight or sunken pulses tolerate stimulation more. Those with deficient, soft, faint or floating pulses tolerate stimulation less. *This condition is important.*

Abdomen: Those with deficient, soft, mushy and thin-skinned bellies tolerate stimulation less. Those with excess bellies that have a lot of resilience tolerate stimulation well.

Skin texture: Those with skin that is thin, soft, smooth, fine, damp or without resilience can't take much stimulation. Those who often feel pain when the needling is started, or sweat and get moist skin when there is needle sensation, can't take much stimulation. Those with fair and delicate skin are especially sensitive, and they tend to have adverse reactions to acupuncture. Those with skin that is thick, rough, bumpy or dry tolerate stimulation well. *This is the most important condition for judging tolerance to stimulation.*

Pain threshold: Those who have low pain thresholds can't tolerate much stimulation. This is a congenital tendency.

Reaction: Those who over-react to stimulation don't tolerate it well, and those who are indifferent to stimulation tolerate it well.

Depth: This is the depth of insertion. In general, superficial insertion is mild stimulation and deep insertion is strong stimulation. The classics teach that needles should be inserted deeply and retained for fat people, manual laborers, chronic diseases, and in the winter. Likewise, needles should be inserted superficially and removed right away for thin people, mental workers, acute diseases, aristocrats, and in the summer.

Size of needle: This is about the thickness of the needle. Thin needles provide mild stimulation and thick needles give strong stimulation.

Technique: The needle technique can make the stimulation weak or strong. This factor, however, varies with the practitioner. It depends on how much and how skillfully needle manipulation is done. In my case, even though I use very thin needles, I can give pretty strong stimulation. It is very important to always have a sense of how much stimulation your needling amounts to.

Response: This is about the body's response after the treatment. How does the patient feel right after the treatment, or that evening, or the next day? The amount of stimulation is appropriate if they feel refreshed, their body feels lighter, or the pain has decreased. If there is fatigue or an increase in pain, the amount of stimulation has been excessive.

State of mind: The amount of stimulation is appropriate if the patient becomes more light-hearted after a treatment. It is inappropriate when the patient's mood becomes worse.

Conclusion on Conditions for Stimulation

Putting everything together, the following can be said:

Strong stimulation is indicated when the patient is fat, muscular, does physical work, or is athletic, and movements are rough, as well as during the winter. It is also appropriate when the pulse is excessive, wiry, tight, etc., if the abdomen is tight or has resilience, when the skin is thick, rough, or dry, and in acute diseases.

Weak stimulation is indicated when the patient is thin, or has edema, their skin is soft, damp or lacking in resilience, and if they sweat easily. This is also true if they do mental work, have quick movements, and over-react to slight pain. It is also appropriate when the pulse is deficient, soft or faint, the abdomen is soft and mushy with thin skin, and the pulse at the abdominal aorta is palpated readily.

There Are Exceptions

I have classified conditions for tolerance to stimulation above, but this doesn't mean they apply in every case. These guidelines were created by human beings, and sometimes they don't work when faced with individual and unique patients.

Treating New Patients

When I see a patient for the first time I am compelled to make a judgment about the appropriate level of stimulation. The most important thing is that the stimulation not be excessive. It is said that "too much of a good thing is good for nothing," and in the case of acupuncture, going overboard is a big mistake. We must avoid overdoing it. Eighty percent of maximum tolerance is sufficient. The first thing is to identify those patients who can't tolerate much stimulation. Their movements are quick, they are not fat, their abdomen is soft, or at least not hard. Their pulse is not strong; it is soft and also floating, rootless, or hard to feel. Their skin is soft, smooth, and becomes wet with a little stress. They easily break out in a sweat. Grasping their forearm, the muscles feel soft. They also might have a depressed expression. As a rule of thumb, I treat patients with these features using super-rotation technique (SRT). Inserting needles can lead to problems. It is good to limit the number of points used as well when they are inserted. The number of points can be increased as they become accustomed to acupuncture. Eventually some needles may be inserted.

The ones that fool you are the patients who have a good physique. We acupuncturists always want to insert the needles. We insert needles in these patients believing that they can withstand stimulation because they are well built, but this can sometimes cause problems. Sometimes they have a solid body but their pulse is weak. Or their pulse is strong but their abdomen is soft and weak. Or they may talk brave, but they begin to sweat as the acupuncture is started. In all cases like this, it is better to use mild stimulation. It is important not to be fooled and to be careful even if there is only one red flag.

My Current Practice

Before I started using super-rotation technique (SRT) I used superficial insertion and sometimes inserted needles deeply. I also often made mistakes about the amount of stimulation. In most of these cases, patients complained that they felt tired afterward. This sense of fatigue goes away in a day or two. But it is a mistake in treatment. I don't make mistakes like this anymore after I started using SRT, but recently I had two or three cases that reported feeling tired the next day, or having more pain. When I paid closer attention, I found that I had inserted the needle a little bit without realizing it. After I paid more attention to my technique, these patients had no more complaints. It really takes a very small amount of stimulation in most cases. I am really concerned that the treatments of average acupuncturists amount to excessive stimulation. Unless we get it just right, patients don't appreciate it. They don't resonate with the treatment. Acupuncture and moxibustion can really be utilized much more than they are. Given the situation in Japan today, I believe at least 50% of the population could benefit from acupuncture, as it would increase their quality of life. If acupuncturists really understood this, there would be no more complaints about the declining number of patients.

When Needles are Inserted

There are many ways to do acupuncture, and it doesn't make sense to use only super-rotation technique (SRT). I myself routinely insert needle in several points, except in those cases that require extremely mild stimulation. Most places that I insert needles have strong muscle tension. You can insert a needle to a certain depth and manipulate it if you feel that a certain point on a patient is a key point for local treatment. But you may want to reduce the amount of stimulation on other points accordingly.

Healing Crisis

Now to conclude this discussion, let's think about the questions that were posed. The first was about a healing crisis. According to the questioner, many schools in America teach that it is desirable that the symptoms get temporarily worse. This is called a "healing crisis" or "healing principle," and patients are told, "Things will get worse before they get better."

In Japan also, the term *menken* is used to explain temporary aggravation of symptoms. After getting worse, the symptoms are supposed to improve, but is this really a good thing? I wonder if such an explanation is not being used as an excuse for symptoms that get worse. I believe that symptoms should gradually resolve. Even if there is a plateau in the improvement, it is best both for the patient and practitioner when recovery takes place without exacerbation. Isn't aggravation of symptoms a mistake in treatment? It does the patient no service to be told that it's a "healing principle" as a cover-up for a mistake. It is really best when there is no *menken* or healing crisis. In order to avoid this, we must strive to get the maximum effect from minimum stimulation. It is my belief that contact needling, SRT, and superficial insertion are the best means to achieve this aim.

Let's back up a little here and examine what *menken* is really about. According to the *Kampo Terminology Dictionary (Kampo yogo daijiten),* the definition of *menken* is: "Various unexpected symptoms that appear temporarily after taking an herbal formula. These include nausea, dizziness and restlessness in the chest." The text *Beginners Herbal Medicine (Nyumon kampo igaku),* published by the Japan Oriental Medicine Association, provides the origin of the term *menken*: "In the Confucian classic *Book of Documents,* it says 'Unless the medicine causes *menken* [瞑眩 *míng xuàn*—understood as dizziness and fainting spells], the disease will not heal.' Yoshimasu Todo [a leader of the Koho school of Kampo] drew on the above passage in his text *Sayings of Classics (Kosho Igen).* He wrote: 'The [classic] texts say, unless the medicine causes *menken,* the disease will not heal.' And 'When the medicine is effective, there is always *menken* and patients suffer and feel as if they are going to die.' So Todo's view was that a disease cannot be cured if one fears the *menken* [adverse] reaction of medicine."

The view of Otsuka Keisetsu, one of the leading herbalists in Japan in the 20th century and one of the founders of the Japan Oriental Medicine Association, is as follows (my summary): "*Menken* is [supposedly] a reaction that occurs in order to cure a disease. Thus believing there is no reason to fear, and taking medicines [indiscriminately] and becoming deathly ill is alarming indeed. ... We [modern herbalists] repudiate the extreme view that diseases cannot be cured without *menken* [healing reactions]."

So the Oriental medicine community in Japan is generally critical of the view of Yoshimasu Todo on this matter. What we know about this is that Yoshimasu extracted the term *menken* from the ancient Chinese classic the *Book of Documents,* which is not even a medical text, and used this to justify his aggressive approach to herbal therapy. Herbalists that followed him used this term to justify the strong reactions that occurred. I don't know the actual details of their therapy because I have never prescribed herbs, but according to the prevalent view in the Japan Oriental Medicine Association, this approach is not condoned. I really wonder about people who take this outdated idea and use it to justify healing reactions from acupuncture and moxibustion.

Ninety-five Percent Treatment

The second question that was posed was, "Even when the patient is 75–95% improved, I am tempted to try a little more treatment." Ideally we would want to give treatment until we are sure the symptoms are all gone, and they don't return even without treatment. This is also the way I feel about it. But the circumstances of patients differ. When we consider their finances, time, and effort involved in transportation, we have to think about what's best for the patient. In cases where a back strain is 90% better and the remaining pain will resolve naturally (as often happens with young people), we can explain this to the patient and discontinue treatment. What about cases like facial paralysis where the symptoms are 90% better? The results of treatment are usually good for the first few months after the onset of the paralysis, but after that the outcome is extremely poor. I would explain this to the patient and have them continue treatments (as much as possible in the first few months). In cases of chronic diseases, especially those of elderly patients, it is rare for them to get back to 100% of where they were before. You can explain this to them and have them continue treatment with their consent. In my clinic many older patients come once a week. Some keep coming for many years. Their symptoms improve gradually, if you view their condition over several years. In difficult cases (such as Parkinson's disease) the symptoms don't get any worse. This is also important. Many of those who no longer have any symptoms, or have improved 90%, come for treatment once a month. This is a mutually satisfactory arrangement.

The main thing is to decide based on individual needs. I also sense that the questioner could be thinking that since 10% of the symptoms remain, he could use strong stimulation to bring about a 100% cure. That even if it becomes worse temporarily, it could change for the better. This is a "make it or break it" gamble. If this is the idea, I do not recommend it. You are likely to lose a patient who could have become a long-term patient. Also you could foster an idea in patients that acupuncture and moxibustion are effective, but they have a dangerous edge. There is no merit to this idea no matter how we look at it. One of the sayings in Japan is, "When you are in a hurry, take the long way around." This is very aptly stated. Walking my path in life for 80 years, I am convinced that this is how life works. Patience is a virtue in large things and small. This applies to all aspects of life, and to treatment also.

CHAPTER 10

Digestive Disorders

1. Overview

There is a term "Chinese ideology." According to the Koji-en,[1] "*Chuka* (中華: *zhōng huá)* is a term used by the Han Chinese to refer to themselves, in contrast to the other, less developed races/tribes that surrounded them on all four sides. This was based on a belief that the most advanced Han culture was positioned at the center of the world." In other words, the idea was that China, the Middle Kingdom, was the most valuable and important. Considering the national politics of the world at the time, China wanted to boast. This is only to be expected. In recent years, China seems to be making a comeback. Does that mean that Japan will become the Eastern Barbarians again?

This idea that there is something important at the center can also be seen in East Asian medicine. Among the five yin organs, the Heart has a special place, but aside from that organ, the Spleen is the most important. So they positioned it in the middle. In abdominal diagnosis, the area around the navel is the Spleen diagnostic area. On the face, the nose is the place to look for the state of digestion. Both of these are found at the center.

When a patient has an appetite, the disease resolves quickly. Recovery takes longer when they can't appreciate the flavors in their food or are not interested in eating. That is why we must always ask about a patient's appetite along with their sleep and elimination. When a patient looks a couple of pounds (1kg) overweight, we can assume that their physical condition is good. But of course it's a problem if the appetite is too good, and there are many patients these days who are upset over too big of an appetite. This trend toward overeating could be related to having lived through lean times. It may be time to reconsider our tendency for lack of exercise, overeating, and the preference

1. *Koji-en*: Authoritative Japanese dictionary, published by Iwanami Shoten, Tokyo, 1991.

for rich foods in light of Chinese ideology of two-thousand years ago.

1.1 Stomatitis (canker sores)

In my practice I see stomatitis quite often, even though few patients come in with that as their main complaint. I ask patients if they have sores in their mouth. If they say yes, I ask them to let me look in their mouth. The mucous membranes on the inside of the cheek or on the tongue turn red or white, known as aphthous ulcers. In bad cases they ulcerate into open sores. It is painful when certain things come into contact with the sores. The root treatment for stomatitis is to treat the Stomach, and the branch treatment is the shoulders. It is good to treat the Spleen and Stomach meridians as well as the neck and shoulders.

When the pattern is Spleen deficiency, I use points like SP-3, CV-12, left ST-21, left BL-17, and left BL-20. Moxibustion is also effective on reactive Stomach meridian points on the abdomen and tight points on the shoulder and upper back. The effect is even better when the patient is able to do moxibustion at home.

As for the local area, you can place the tip of the needle gently on the sores themselves, and this can have an immediate effect. It hurts to prick the sores, so just brush the sores gently with the needle tip. When you examine the submandibular lymph nodes (see Fig. 7-2 on p. 193) on such patients, you sometimes find they are swollen. It also works to needle the swollen lymph nodes. I recommend using SRT or superficial insertion of just a couple of millimeters on these lymph nodes. These days there are cases of stomatitis due to various viruses and severe cases may require referral to a specialist.

1.2 The Spleen

So what exactly is the Spleen, as spoken of in the classics? As one of the five yin organs, the functions of the Spleen are as follows:

1. Digestion
2. Water metabolism (moves excess fluids out of the body)
3. Creation of qi and blood
4. Houses the mental function of intention (意 yì)

Among these functions, digestion is one that is found in Western medicine. Comparing the Spleen with the other four yin organs, however, there is something different about it. Whether it is the Lung or the Kidney, their functions are almost the same as in Western medicine, but the Spleen is not the same at all. The spleen in Western medicine has no digestive function. Perhaps they got it wrong then in the ancient dissections. The pancreas is the one involved in digestion. The Spleen mentioned in the classics must be the pancreas. That is what the classical scholar Dr. Iemoto[2] says in his text,

2. Iemoto Sei-ichi M.D. (家本誠一): A renowned classical scholar and president of the Chinese Classical

Suwen Commentaries.[3] This makes things much easier to understand.

The treatment of the Spleen as a digestive organ is done via the Spleen meridian. We use the five-phase points SP-2 or -3 and PC-8 or -7. In addition, we use the back associated point BL-20 and the front alarm point LR-13, along with points on the paired yang meridian. This is the standard practice in Meridian Therapy, but there is one more point that needs to be mentioned. It is ST-21 on the left side. It becomes reactive when there are digestive disorders or diabetes, and acu-moxa treatment yields good results. This could actually be the front alarm point, and it is close to LR-13. Maybe the alarm point has moved. As a drinker, I get good use out of this point. When there is sensitivity to pinching, if the patient is a man, he loves to drink alcohol in general. When there is an induration at ST-21 on the left, he tends to love the Japanese distilled beverage called shōchū. Sometimes I even guess the local brand of the shōchū they are drinking when I find this reaction, and patients are surprised. This reaction probably indicates stress or fatigue in the pancreas.

A reaction at left ST-21 is related to pathology of the pancreas, stomach, or descending colon, with pancreatic issues being the most likely. Recently I have seen more women with pancreatic diseases, including pancreatic cancer. With this reaction I also have to consider diabetes. If the patient gets regular checkups, I will get their records and pay particular attention to the A1c and amylase numbers. The symptoms of pancreatic disease include excessive appetite or diarrhea and loss of appetite. If the patient doesn't have any data, I have them go get a medical check-up.

Case Study 106

PATIENT: Female, 61 years old

FOC: July 4, 2008

MAIN COMPLAINT: Pain in tongue

SYMPTOMS AND SITUATION: She has had continuous pain in the right occipital region and stinging pain in the left half of her tongue for 7-8 years. The pain in the tongue becomes bad at least once a month. The painful spot in the occiput is between Upper BL-10 and Yanagiya's GB-20, right on the inferior margin of the occiput. She has neck and shoulder tension. She has always been a light sleeper and recently she has started taking medication to get to sleep. Her appetite is not so good. She has two bowel movements a day, and urination is normal. She weighs 39kg (86lbs) and her height is 152cm (5ft).

HISTORY: Meniere's disease and uterine cancer

PULSE DIAGNOSIS: Liver deficiency

Medicine Research Society (中国古典医学研究会) in Japan.

3. *Suwen Commentaries* (素問訳注 *Somon Yakuchu),* Tokyo: Ido-no-Nippon Sha, 2009.

Treatment: Root treatment – SRT on LR-8, KI-10, ST-36, LI-11, BL-18, and BL-23.

Local treatment – Needles retained superficially in left TB-16 and reactive points on right occiput. Other treatment – SRT on GV-22, CV-12, BL-43, auricular vertigo point, GB-21, and BL-58. Direct moxibustion on CV-12, LI-11, ST-36, GB-21, left TB-16, right occiput point, left BL-18 (depressed), left BL-20 (depressed), and LR-1.

Progress:

(3rd) July 22 – No pain for one day, but pain returned thereafter.

(4th) Aug 1 – Pain persists, so I inserted a needle about 5mm in left TB-16 and asked about the pain, and she said the tongue pain was gone. So I retained another needle in the reactive area on the right occiput to see how things went, and the pain disappeared.

(5th) Aug 6 – The tongue pain is better but there is still some pain in the right occiput.

1.3 Esophagitis

In recent years the diagnosis of reflux esophagitis has become more common. Patients complain of heartburn, regurgitation of some contents in the stomach, and pain under the sternum. I find points like CV-12, left ST-21, upper ST-19, and left BL-17 to be effective. If there is a reaction at CV-17, this point can be used as well. It should definitely be used if the patient tends toward psychological or mental issues.

Also, drinkers who consume whiskey and shōchū without dilution tend to injure their esophagus and get esophagitis. We should know better, but ...

2. Gastric diseases

Now I will discuss diseases of the upper digestive tract including gastritis, gastric ulcers, as well as duodenal ulcers. The symptoms that come up clinically for the stomach include stomach pain, loss of appetite, heartburn, nausea, and occasionally vomiting. If the symptoms before a meal are worse than after a meal, suspect an ulcer or a pre-ulcerous condition. If the symptoms are worse after the meal, suspect gastritis. For an accurate diagnosis, we need to rely on the imaging studies. When patients show no improvement with acu-moxa treatments, suggest to those who have yet to get a biomedical diagnosis to get a medical exam. It often happens, however, that no abnormalities are found even when a patient has symptoms such as discomfort in the gastric region. They call this "functional dyspepsia," but it is what we call "incipient diseases" in East Asian medicine. We can work with this, and it will improve.

2.1 Examination

When the tongue has a thick coating, suspect some abnormality in the digestive system. A thin white coating is fine, but following changes to a coating that is thick and white, or yellow or dark, is an indicator for how the treatments are working.

Among the methods of abdominal diagnosis is sensitivity to pinching and indurations. Points that are sensitive to light pinching or that reveal a soy-bean sized nodule with light pressure are targets for treatment. Points that are tender with pressure can also be treated, but there is a concern that we might end up just depending on what the patient says and treat too many points.

Sensitivity to pinching tends to appear in the upper abdomen above the level of the umbilicus. It usually indicates a mild pathology in the underlying internal organ. These are changes that don't come up in imaging, so it serves as detection of incipient diseases and for prevention. When the pathology progresses, the point becomes indurated. In Meridian Therapy this is called a change in the qi level progressing to the blood level. I have found a general correspondence between sensitive or indurated points and organ pathologies, as follows:

CV-14: **heart**[4] and stomach

CV-12: stomach

LEFT ST-21: **pancreas**, stomach, and colon

RIGHT ST-21: duodenum and gallbladder

LEFT ST-19: **heart** and stomach

RIGHT ST-19: **gallbladder** and liver

RIGHT ST-24: **duodenum**

RIGHT LR-14: **liver**

So the points are selected based on their reaction, but the point with the most pronounced reaction must be palpated. This will yield unexpected results. It is better not to use too many points.

2.2 Acupuncture

For simple cases I retain needles superficially in three points and use SRT on everything else. When I find one good point, such as left ST-21, I rotate the needle superficially, inserted for 30 seconds to a minute. When patients have gastric diseases, they tell me this feels very good. The five-phase points are very effective for diseases of the internal organs, so the treatment of abdominal points and five-phase points are bookends of the treatment. I suggest you practice superficial rotation on your own abdomen until you can do it in a way that feels good to patients.

Actually, another set of points along with those on the abdomen is the back associated points. Given the viscero-cutaneous reflexes, I see the back associated points as a branch treatment (local treatment) for diseases of the internal organs. So I would also

4. The organs in **bold** are those more likely to be associated with reactivity at these points.

recommend treating reactive back associated points. For example, when a patient has stomach symptoms and isn't feeling well, palpate left BL-20 if he has Spleen deficiency. You usually find a depression or an induration. Insert a needle carefully in the middle of the reaction—very slowly. When you reach a depth of about 5mm, continue rotating the needle and apply a few minute up-and-down movements. Both you and the patient will feel a pleasant sensation. When there is an internal organ disease, you get good results when you use this technique on one point. Otherwise, you can retain needles superficially: three points on the abdomen and four on the back associated points. Also retain one intradermal needle in the most reactive point.

As far as the root treatment, Spleen deficiency is the most common, but other patterns also occur, such as Liver deficiency. The thing is to follow the pulse diagnosis and not be pushed around by the symptoms. Among the five-phase points, I often use the tonification points, source points, and well points.

2.3 Moxibustion

I generally apply five half-rice-grain sized cones on the points where I retained needles on the abdomen and back. On the arms and legs, I choose from among points like ST-36, SP-4, SP-6, KI-3, LR-3, and LI-11. The outcome is much better when patients are able to do moxibustion at home. People are different. Some make up their mind and do the moxibustion at home, some only allow moxibustion to be done on them in my clinic, and others don't tolerate moxibustion at all. The case below is an example of the latter.

Case Study 107

Patient: Female, 66 years old

FOC: February 14, 2011

Main Complaints: Reflux esophagitis and gastritis. Her sleep, appetite, and bowel movements are normal.

Pulse Diagnosis: Lung deficiency

Treatment: SRT on LU-9, SP-3, CV-12, left ST-21, left upper ST-19 (Fig. 10-1), ST-36, LI-11, BL-20, left BL-18, BL-13, GB-21, Yanagiya's GB-20, and BL-58.

Progress:

(2nd) Lung deficiency. She's a little better, but is experiencing hay fever.

(3rd) Spleen deficiency. She is burping, but without reflux.

(7th) Liver deficiency. She's doing fine. No more symptoms. We conclude treatments.

Comments: Reflux and contents of stomach coming up into the mouth turned into simple burping before resolving. When she was finally better, her pattern had become Liver deficiency.

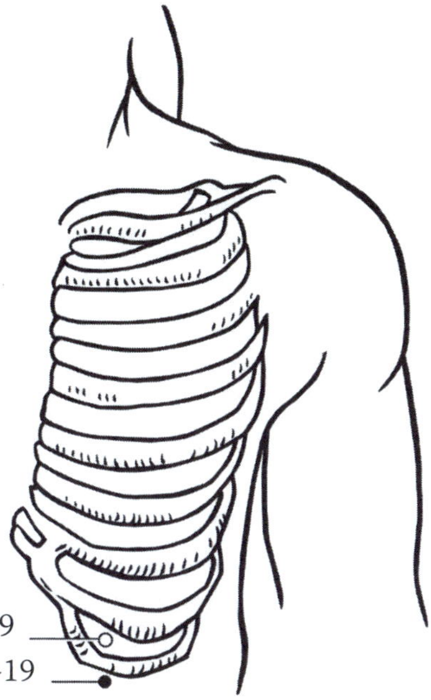

Fig 10-1 Upper ST-19

3. Asthenic constitution

I see quite a few patients who just don't have energy. Simply stated, they have a weak constitution. If we exaggerate, we can say they have problems all over. They feel weak, their head feels heavy, their appetite is poor, their stomach hurts, their abdomen and bowels ache, they have diarrhea or soft stools, they tend to catch colds, can't tolerate cold or heat, and sweat easily. They also get chilled in their hips and lower extremities, they have low blood pressure and they have no stamina or will power, so they always want to lie down.

This is more than a chronic condition, but something from birth. The patient just doesn't know what to do about it. Examinations at the hospital show no abnormalities, but these patients suffer a lot. Can acu-moxa treatments do something for them? My conclusion is acu-moxa is very good. They will become stronger. Their symptoms will go away, or at least diminish, and they won't be as bothered by them. This is a long-term condition, however, and it takes prolonged treatment, a year or at least several months. Can the patient persist with the treatments? If you don't have much experience, it's hard to declare, "It's OK, you'll get better." On the other hand, if you don't respond confidently, it's possible that the patient will terminate treatments before they get better. It would be good if you could skillfully explain, encourage, sympathize, and nurture these patients so they continue treatments. When the results start to show, they become very pleased and behave as if you are some kind of guru.

The key to treatment is to improve the appetite. Use abdominal diagnosis, tongue diagnosis, pulse diagnosis, and meridian palpation to assess the condition of the Spleen and Stomach. If you are not sure about the pulse diagnosis, you can provisionally treat them for Spleen deficiency. Going by the rationale in East Asian medicine that both the blood which nourishes the body and the qi that protects the body are created by the Spleen and Stomach, restoring health to the gastrointestinal system is their path to health. Truly, the Spleen is the master of the five yin organs.

The thing to be careful about in treatment is not to insert needles deeply. You might even say that insertion will make them worse. I recommend SRT. Even if you only use SRT, you need to limit the number of points used. Moxibustion is also necessary for treatment, but use techniques that are comfortable and pleasant, like 80% moxibustion. These patients don't have stamina, so they can't tolerate the heat that normal patients can. They tend to drop out if the treatments are too strong. Moxibustion at home is also useful, but teach them to make small cones (or use stick-on moxa) so they stay with it.

3.1 Treatment of asthenic patients

For the abdominal treatment, I use CV-12 and CV-6. These are important points: the former increases postnatal qi and the latter increases prenatal qi. Especially on CV-12, I continue the SRT for a relatively long time. It is good to do it for as long as the root treatment tonification points (about 10 seconds). When there is a reaction (sensitivity to pinching or induration) at left ST-21, this becomes an important treatment point. There is a correlation between the amount of reaction at ST-21 and the physical condition of the patient.

On the back, check points below BL-17. Often back associated points on the left side are especially depressed. If there are tender or indurated points, these become good treatment points, but these patients don't have sufficient strength to deal with a lot of treatment. It is better to treat points that are depressed and feel good to be pressed. I tend to use points like BL-17 and BL-20 (or BL-21). If you find a depression among GV-9, -10 and -11, you can treat it, but often there is no reaction. Don't use it if there is no reaction or tenderness in the depressed point. While you're at it, sometimes it is good to use Onodera's point on the left. When the right Onodera's point is also depressed, it's okay to treat both. I apply both SRT and moxibustion on this point. I also like to treat BL-36 when there is a reaction.

Among the five-phase points, I use SP-3 (or SP-4, the network vessel point) and PC-7 (or PC-6, the network vessel point) along with ST-36. I look for indurations at SP-4; otherwise I look for depressions. It goes without saying that correct point selection depends on pulse diagnosis.

Finally, if there is insomnia, treat M-LE-5 *(shitsumin/shī mián)* with direct moxibustion. Keep applying more cones until the heat is felt strongly in the heel. If the heat is felt right away, apply five small cones.

When the above treatment is continued once a week, the patient will gradually begin to change. Ask about their appetite every time. It will go up and down, but gradually will improve over time. I recommend a traditional Japanese diet to my patients. The main course is semi-brown rice that is refined 30 to 50%. It has to be chewed well—50 to 100 times. The key is to eat the side dishes after eating the rice slowly. When other flavored food is eaten together with the rice, people tend to swallow it too quickly. When patients follow this diet for several months to a year, first their abdomen become bigger. They put on some weight. Later on they become bigger in their back and hips, and it is obvious when you look at them or touch them. You know they've gained a couple of pounds. When they have more energy, their movements become more dynamic and their muscle mass also increases. All they need to be careful of at that point is overeating and gaining too much weight. If they had low blood pressure, it can start to turn into hypertension and they could become susceptible to diseases of excess.

Case Study 108

Patient: Male, 65 years old

FOC: July 11, 2006

Main Complaint: Fatigue

Symptoms and Condition: This man has a history of sciatica. He gets tired very easily. His left leg has burning pain. His appetite and sleep are okay with medications. He has received acu-moxa treatments before, but each time he gets so tired, he thinks maybe he is not cut out for acupuncture.

Pulse Diagnosis: Kidney deficiency

Treatment: Root Treatment – SRT on KI-7, LU-5, BL-23, BL-13, ST-36, and LI-11.

Direct moxibustion on BL-23, BL-13, ST-36, and LI-11. Branch Treatment – SRT on CV-12, CV-6, GB-20, and GB-21. This was followed by direct moxibustion on CV-12 and CV-6.

I instructed him to apply direct moxibustion at home on points he could do himself: ST-36, LI-11, CV-12, and CV-6.

Progress:

(2nd) July 18 – Lung deficiency. He told me that unlike previous acupuncture treatments in other clinics, he didn't become fatigued after my treatment. His exhaustion was gone so he was able to trim his bonsai plants. He still has pain in his left hip.

(3rd) Lung deficiency. Thick yellow tongue coating.

(7th) Tongue coating thin and yellow.

He had 22 treatments in 2006 and 2007. In June of 2008 he reported that he no longer felt chilled. By December his energy had become ample and his pulse had become a bit hard. He had 11 treatments in 2008. He was feeling strong. I told him acu-moxa treatments were only needed when he has some symptom but that it was desirable to continue moxibustion at home. Reviewing the frequency of treatments, I notice that a year after starting treatments, the number of treatments per month began to decrease.

By a year or two later when he was down to about one treatment a month, he was quite a bit stronger. So this shows that regular treatment for one year is important. When they start feeling better, these patients get more enthusiastic about moxibustion treatments at home. They also get motivated to persist with acu-moxa treatments. This is a positive feedback loop. The pattern was often Lung deficiency, but sometimes it was Liver deficiency.

Case Study 109

Patient: Female, 48 years old

FOC: October 2, 2006

Main Complaint: Stomach pain and lower abdominal pain

Symptoms and Condition: She has chronic gastrointestinal problems with constant stomach pain and lower abdominal pain. It varies with stress and what she eats. She is in a bad mood when her stomach is not feeling good. She tends to vent on whomever is around. Her appetite and sleep are normal.

Pulse Diagnosis: Sunken and thin; Lung deficiency

Treatment: Root Treatment – SRT on LU-9, SP-3, ST-36, LI-11, BL-13, BL-20, and left BL-21. Branch Treatment – SRT on left Onodera's point, CV-12, CV-6, and left ST-21.

Direct moxibustion on all of the above points except LU-9 and SP-3.

Progress:

(2nd) Liver deficiency. Pain is mild.

(3rd) Liver deficiency. Her amylase values increased and her doctor commented that she may have chronic pancreatitis. Three treatments given in October.

(6th) Liver deficiency. She feels dizzy when she moves her head. Three treatments given in November.

(11th) Appetite is a little better.

(15th) Appetite is good. Five treatments given in January 2007.

(16th) She had some abdominal pain.

(17th) She doesn't feel good at times. Four treatments given in February.

(May 2007) She is gaining a little weight. Four treatments given in May.

(September 2007) Two treatments given. She wrote me: "It is an especially hot summer this year, but I am doing well. This summer is really different. I'm sure it is the effect of your treatments. My stomach doesn't hurt anymore. Every time I have a meal, I think of you and am thankful. I am able to stay in air conditioning from morning to night without any deep fatigue or discomfort. I awake thinking that if this is a dream, I don't want to wake up from it. It is because of you that I don't have any stomach pain or need to lie down during the day, so I am able to fulfill my duties at home such as preparing meals without any problem."

(**October 2007**) Four treatments given. She wrote me while traveling in Japan: "I am in Tokyo. I am so happy because I can eat without worrying. It was so hard when I had to keep going without eating! I remember how difficult it was. I move around much more than usual. I have been able to keep up with my schedule. But I wonder sometimes, whose legs are these? Please treat my legs also in my next treatment."

—Total number of treatments in 2007: 41.

—Three treatments given in January 2008. She wrote me saying, "I had insomnia around the New Year and was very busy, but my body is feeling fine. I am grateful for what you've done for me."

—Three treatments given in March 2008. She wrote me while traveling abroad: "I went to Germany, Hungary, and the Czech Republic. This is my last night on the trip, and I've been able to enjoy the meals. Today, the last day, I tried ice cream and some special sweet wine. I think that, thanks to you, I'll be able to arrive home in good shape. March 23 from Budapest." She also took a trip to Great Britain the same year.

—Three treatments given in January 2009. She had a mild fever of 37.1°C. Five treatments given in March 2009. She ran a high fever for two days.

I got another letter from her on March 2, 2010: "I am on a train from St. Petersburg to Moscow. I am having a great trip. There is lots of snow and it's cold, but I am feeling good and very happy."

Comments: This patient had frequent stomach and abdominal pain, which made her irritable and trouble for those around her. She was exceedingly careful about what she ate because the wrong food caused stomachaches and diarrhea. Her love of classical music went beyond a hobby, and she lived to attend concerts. She managed somehow to travel to concerts around Japan, but after a year of treatments she went to Europe. Everything went smoothly and it seems she gained confidence. Her lower abdomen filled in and became stronger. She got a little more fat on her waist and hips. She no longer became annoyed at people around her and was always in a good mood. I have had her apply stick-on moxa to points on her abdomen and low back every day. We are trying bi-weekly treatments instead of the almost weekly treatments of the first couple of years. The ideal is monthly treatments. Recently I haven't seen her for a while. In other words, she is doing well. Her pattern differed with each treatment, but Spleen deficiency was primary. The secret to her success is getting regular treatments for a long time. It is surprising that this patient was able to go to Russia in the extreme cold of winter. She writes often and I have been able to keep track of her physical condition.

3.2 Summary on treating asthenic patients

Acu-moxa treatments are ideal for those with weak constitutions who complain of a generalized weakness, especially a weak gastro-intestinal system with poor appetite and having low blood pressure and a tendency to get cold. If possible, persist with weekly treatments. Also have the patient apply moxibustion at home that is not too strong. When they continue this regimen for a year, they will become robust. The main thing is to persevere.

Pulse diagnosis: Spleen and Lung deficiency are common. Treat for Spleen deficiency if you are not sure.

Needle technique: Use SRT, do not insert needles.

Acupuncture points: Include SP-3, PC-7, CV-12, left ST-21, BL-17, BL-20, and left Onodera's point as indicated.

Moxibustion points: Include CV-12, left ST-21, ST-36 (or PC-6 & SP-4) BL-17, and BL-20 as indicated.

4. Gallbladder diseases

4.1 Gallstones (cholecystolithiasis)

In traditional plays by traveling troupes that made the rounds of villages in Japan, when a beautiful woman crumples in pain, the cause is usually Shaku (abdominal accumulations). This is usually a trick to draw the attention of a man, but if it were real, it would probably be a gallstone attack. The pain of a gallstone attack is said to be quite something. Once a man in his 60s waiting his turn in my waiting room got a sudden pain in his abdomen. The pain and sensitivity was in his right subcostal region. Before the ambulance arrived, I tried needling SP-3, but there was no effect. The outcome was that he had an infection in his gallbladder, it was critical, and he had surgery right away. Yet it was surprising that the pain would come on so suddenly. I was told that he was fine before that.

I don't have any experience treating gallstones, but it seems quite possible based on my success with treating kidney stones. The pattern would probably be Liver or Spleen deficiency. The well points, cleft points, and tonification points would be good candidates. If it were Liver deficiency, I would choose among points like LR-1, LR-6, LR-8, GB-34, LR-14, GB-24 (these two points are in intercostal spaces), BL-18, BL-19, and right GB-41. If it were Spleen deficiency, I would choose among points like SP-1, SP-3, SP-8, LR-13, upper ST-19, BL-20, and BL-49.

4.2 Cholecystitis (gallbladder inflammation)

For this condition also, I have no established treatment protocol because of lack of experience, but I've treated many cases that I suspect were cholecystitis. The symptoms include stomach pain, heaviness, and discomfort in pit of stomach, and tension in the right midback. Few complain of pain directly in the right subcostal region. Below are a few findings that may indicate cholecystitis.

❶ Tenderness and or induration at right upper ST-19

Position yourself on the right side of the patient. Press reactive points on the right subcostal region around upper ST-19 and LR-13 toward the ribs with fingers of your right hand. You will feel resistance in the point and the patient will feel pain. It's very clear when you compare it to the reaction on the left side.

❷ Sensitivity to pinching at right upper ST-19

❸ Tenderness next to spine at level of BL-19, the Hua Tuo *jiá jǐ* (M-BW-35) point below T10.

❹ Tenderness and/or induration at right GB-34. Compare with the point on left.

The more of the above findings there are, the more likely it is that the patient has gallbladder inflammation. According to the text recommended by Dr. Manaka Yoshio, *Acupuncture Point Diagnosis,*[5] when there is a reaction at right GB-41, it indicates gallstones.

To treat cholecystitis, in addition to the points listed in the last section for the treatment of gallstones, needle CV-12, CV-6, ST-21, and ST-36. Also retain an intradermal needle in ST-19 or upper ST-19 on the right. Apply direct moxibustion at right GB-34 (or GB-41) and right BL-19, or its Hua Tuo *jiá jǐ* (M-BW-35) point. Further instruct the patient to avoid oily foods and to eat more sour (acidic) foods.

5. Diseases of the colon

My fight with tuberculosis began with trying to recover from intestinal tuberculosis. The diarrhea day after day was really a strain. I thought I would take constipation over diarrhea, but now that I'm old and have experienced it, I find it not much better. It is best to have normal bowel movements, of course. Anyway, the main symptoms of colon disease is diarrhea or constipation and abdominal pain. Nowadays I hear a lot about irritable bowel syndrome. This seems to have a connection with psychological issues, and we need to keep this in mind as we treat it. Of course, this means that SRT and superficial needling is effective. It seems that the intestines function independently of the brain. In the current thinking in Japan about physiological regulation, the intestines and autonomic nervous system are called the "second brain," and the skin and peripheral nervous system is called the "third brain."

5.1 Acu-moxa treatment of constipation and diarrhea

Many patients these days are constipated, and many use laxatives. Ask them about their bowel movements, and if they are constipated, give them acupuncture for it. My

5. *Acupuncture Point Diagnosis (Xué wèi zhěn duàn fǎ)* by Gai Guo-Cai, translated into Japanese by Sugi Mitsutane. *Tsubo Shindanho* Yokosuka, Ido-no-Nippon Sha, 1984.

treatment is superficial insertion in CV-12, left ST-21, and left BL-17. Then I insert a needle about 1cm in either ST-27 or SP-14 on the left. I apply small sparrow-pecking motions and withdraw the needle. This usually clears up the bowel problems. But often patients say their bowel movements improved for three days or a week, but then they became constipated again. This means they need more regular treatments. I have also tried using dispersion on SP-4 and direct moxibustion on Sawada's HT-7 (see Fig. 6-3, p. 183), but the results are not that clear. There are some stubborn cases of constipation that do not respond to acu-moxa treatment.

In contrast, diarrhea responds well to acu-moxa treatment. But we must remember that diarrhea is a reaction of the body to expel undesirable things from the body, so we don't always want to stop it. Diarrhea in the early stages of a cold is a good example. It clears things up. I read an article that said many patients died when E. coli was rampant, when their diarrhea was forced to stop. They died because they couldn't expel their toxins. Acu-moxa treatments let the body determine how best to respond, diarrhea ends naturally, and the patient recovers.

The pattern is usually Spleen deficiency. Sometimes it is Lung deficiency. This makes sense when we think about the Large Intestine meridian, the yang meridian paired with the Lung meridian. So treat the Large Intestine meridian along with the Lung meridian. Of course, use the front alarm point ST-25, but also try distal points like LI-11, LI-10, LI-7, and LI-4. The closer the point is to the wrist, the deeper the relationship to the abdomen. Then there is Kidney deficiency. The Kidney meridian goes around the anus, so it works well for diarrhea and hemorrhoids. The diarrhea associated with the Kidney meridian will be marked by tenesmus. Diarrhea with frequent urge to defecate, but ineffective evacuation, is usually a case of Kidney deficiency. In cases of Spleen deficiency, one feels relief after defecation. This kind of diarrhea can be left alone, but the Kidney deficiency type requires attention.

The front alarm and back associated points associated with the pattern (GB-25 and BL-23 in cases of Kidney deficiency) can also be effective. The sea points (KI-10) are also useful for diarrhea. You can also use points around the navel (CV-9, CV-7, and CV-4) and the lumbo-sacral region (BL-52, BL-25, and BL-32). Those points that are good for diarrhea should be avoided when the patient is constipated.

Sometimes when the diarrhea is really bad, undigested food comes out. One can suspect confusion in the brain when the diarrhea is really bad, so look for reactive points on the head (GV-20), upper spine (GV-10 & -11) and between the lumbar vertebrae (GV-4 and M-BW-25 *[jōsen / shí qī zhuī xià])*. If any of these points are tender, they become good treatment points.

5.2 Polyps

The detection and removal of polyps in the gastrointestinal tract has become simple in recent years with the use of endoscopes. I once had an elderly female patient who was told every year that she had polyps in her colon. She came to me saying the number was especially high this year, so she wanted to do moxibustion treatments at home to get rid of them. She did the moxibustion, and her physician noticed the marks on her abdomen and asked what they were. She told him she had been doing moxibustion to eliminate the polyps, and the doctor criticized her. Undeterred, she continued with the home moxibustion for an entire year. In the examination the following year, the many polyps she had (according to the patient) were all gone. Her doctor didn't say anything.

The patient I am seeing now is a 69-year-old woman. She comes for treatment every other week. She also does moxibustion on herself at home. In past years, intestinal polyps were found in her medical exam, but she told me there were none this year. Her doctor asked about the moxa scars on her abdomen, and when she told him, he said it must really hurt. Actually, I am treating this patient for joint disease, but the moxibustion points on her abdomen are CV-6, CV-12, ST-27, and GB-29. This is clear evidence that regular moxibustion treatments can cure polyps.

5.3 Ileocecal pain

Pain in the ileocecal region is usually appendicitis. When antibiotics don't work, it requires surgery. Actually, multiple cones of direct moxibustion on the induration at CV-6 can be effective for appendicitis. When my mother was 80 years old, she had abdominal pain in the ileocecal region with an induration at CV-6. I applied cone after cone of direct moxibustion for three hours, and she was able to avoid surgery.

Also the Fukaya moxibustion point *kaiyu* (快俞)on the right can be effective if there is a reaction. This point is about 3 units lateral to spinous process of L4, or lateral to BL-25 wherever there is tenderness or induration.

Sometimes people experience pain around the surgical scar for appendicitis. It tends to occur when people are under a lot of stress. When you insert a needle superficially into the tight point around CV-6, a needle sensation is felt in the ileocecal region and the pain goes away. It also feels good to needle tight points in the ileocecal region itself, but in my experience the pain gets worse later. Direct treatment is safer when you use a teishin. I like to reduce the stimulation even more by placing the teishin at a 20-30 degree angle. I also treat right BL-25 and SP-3.

5.4 A case of irritable bowel syndrome

When it comes to the suffering of one's own family, people seem to really lose their composure. This is understandable, but one woman kept calling me about a grandchild who lived in Yokohama (about a thousand kilometers from my office). I started to wonder if she had mental issues. Her story was that her granddaughter had been having diarrhea and abdominal pain for one month. The girl was a sophomore in high school (17 years old). She had stomach and abdominal pain when she woke up, when she ate and after she ate, and also had diarrhea. She didn't feel much relief after these bowel movements, and still had the urge to defecate. She couldn't go to school because of the pain. At the hospital she was given the diagnosis of irritable bowel syndrome. She was taking medications, but they had no effect. When she got hungry and ate, she had more abdominal pain and diarrhea. Her parents were at a loss about what to do.

Her grandmother, this woman who kept calling me, asked me if I could help this girl if she came south and stayed with her while she received treatments from me. So this girl came to see me all the way from Yokohama. Her first treatment was November 27, 2009. Her pulse was sunken, slow, and deficient. The Liver and Kidney positions were weak. Her abdomen was deficient overall with some depressions and protrusions, but nothing out of the ordinary. I treated her for Kidney deficiency. I used SRT on KI-7, LU-5, BL-23, BL-25, and LI-7. I also treated CV-12, CV-6, SP-6, GB-21, and BL-32. If I wasn't careful, over treatment might cause blood in the stools, so it was a bit nerve wracking.

She came for treatment again the next day (2nd treatment: Nov. 28) and told me that she had an appetite in the evening so she had a normal meal. She went to the toilet to defecate in the morning, but nothing came out. She had had no pain. I gave her similar treatments that day and the following day. She came for another treatment a week later (4th treatment: Dec. 5). She told me she was just fine for three days. After that she had soft stools every morning. I asked how she was spending her time, and she told me she was reading constantly.

This reminded me of when I was young. After reading without a break for a year, I found myself at the threshold of tuberculosis. I advised her to take a break from reading now and then to do some thinking on her own. Her pulses on the left side were weaker, but I treated her for Spleen deficiency. Her pulses balanced after I tonified SP-3.

(7TH) Dec. 28. Her abdominal pain and diarrhea returned. I treated her for Kidney deficiency.

(8TH) Dec. 29. Her symptoms went away.

(9TH) Dec. 30. Her pattern was Liver deficiency, but her pulses were fairly balanced even before the treatment. Her pulses had resiliency and it felt like an example of good Stomach qi. I wondered if this time the effect of treatment would last.

Back in Yokohama she got a referral to an acupuncturist to continue treatments, but these treatments didn't work as well. When she returned to Ohita to get more treatments from me, her mother asked me why she was still refusing to attend school when she had no more abdominal pain. I thought she could be having difficulty at school with a certain subject or a teacher. When I asked the girl myself, she told me that her homeroom teacher and her club activities supervisor was the same person, and that she had a disagreement with this teacher over her club activities. Probably this teacher had a strong personality. Then the question was, could I give her an SRT treatment (for the mind) that would give her the mental resilience to deal with this situation. I was curious to see if acupuncture could change her attitude. Anyway, she overcame this challenge and a few years later she was accepted into a college of her choice.

Nowadays we hear a lot about irritable bowel syndrome (IBS). Diarrhea is common with IBS, but when you receive a diagnosis with a big name like this, it seems really serious. IBS is a disease that affects the colon, of course, but we can get good results when we think about it as a psychological issue rather than just a yin and yang organ issue and treat it accordingly. It is a good thing to use our brain, but when there is stress added to mental exertion, symptoms manifest in the body. We can get good results when we disregard the physical issues and treat IBS as a psychosomatic disease. Since this is a disease that is on the rise, we need to be mindful and address it correctly.

5.5 A case of food poisoning

Case Study 110

Patient: Male, 77 years old

FOC: April 23, 2012

Main Complaint: Diarrhea

Symptoms and Condition: He had had diarrhea 20 times over the three previous days, and it hasn't stopped. He thinks it was caused by some raw fish he ate. He has been eating only rice porridge ever since.

Pulse Diagnosis: Kidney deficiency

Treatment: SRT on KI-7, KI-10, LU-5, BL-23, BL-52, CV-12, CV-6, BL-32, and ST-36.

Direct moxibustion on M-LE-1 *(uranaitei/lǐ nèi tíng)*[6] (heat felt after two cones, five cones applied), 10 cones on BL-52 and five cones on BL-23 and BL-32.

Advice: Stop eating rice porridge, and instead eat rice and chew well. Eat anything else except for greasy foods. Do not try to stop the diarrhea with other remedies.

Progress: (2nd) April 24 – Diarrhea stopped. Passing gas, feels good.

Summary

1. Judge whether the diarrhea is due to food poisoning.
2. Diarrhea will continue until the toxin is fully expelled.
3. It is risky to force diarrhea to stop.
4. Diarrhea can be stopped naturally and comfortably with acu-moxa.

5.6 A case of pain in lower left abdomen

In some cases, abdominal pain does not originate in the internal organs. A 62-year-old man came in on March 8, 2010 complaining of pain in lower left abdomen. His appetite and elimination were normal, and his sleep was also okay. He had a history of kidney stones, and had a medical exam, but no abnormality was found. He was told that the CT scan showed that he had a history of a fracture in his left femur. He is scheduled soon for a stomach and colon exam.

The pain extends from the lower left quadrant to the side around to the Girdle vessel *(tai-myaku/dài mài)*. It hurts primarily during movement, but sometimes at rest.

6. M-LE-1 *(uranaitei/lǐ nèi tíng)*: The primary indications for M-LE-1 in Japan are food poisoning and abdominal pain.

Orthopedic exam showed a positive Patrick's test on left. Shudo's GB-29 was tender, and there is inguinal pain at rest. Examining the patient in the left side up position, I found tenderness and induration at the Iliac point, ischial point, a point over the greater trochanter, as well as Onodera's point. It seemed to me that this patient was feeling pain from his lateral hip in his abdomen. Did he have any intestinal problem? His pulse presented with Lung deficiency, so it was conceivable that his Large Intestines were weak. But the pain didn't seem to be coming from the Large Intestines. I applied SRT on both LU-9 and SP-3. Then I applied SRT and direct moxibustion on the left side only on the following points: ST-21, Iliac point, Ischial point, a point posterior to the greater trochanter, Onodera's point. The pain at rest was gone after this treatment. There was no pain with movement either. The patient started saying that maybe he should cancel the medical exam if the pain went away. I still wasn't certain, so I told him to get the exam just to be sure.

6. Diseases of the anus

The disease of the anus that we encounter in our practice is hemorrhoids. Acu-moxa treatments can have some effect on hemorrhoids. When I was young, I had five fistulas around my anus, but they all healed thanks to acu-moxa treatments. I wrote about this in *Finding Effective Acupuncture Points.*[7]

The first thing about hemorrhoids is to eliminate the causes. These are constipation, diarrhea, liver disease and things that increase intra-abdominal pressure. A patient must do things to improve his physical condition such as being mindful about drinking and eating to regulate his gastrointestinal system, quit smoking and reduce alcohol intake to reasonable amounts, as well as getting regular acu-moxa treatments. The symptoms associated with hemorrhoids are bleeding, pain, and anal prolapse. The pain in the anus is especially hard to live with.

The treatment of hemorrhoids is along the lines of that detailed above for diseases of the colon. The most common pattern from the pulses is Kidney deficiency. When you insert a needle in KI-7, a sensation can be felt in the abdomen. Lung deficiency and Spleen deficiency are also possible. Use the back associated points in addition to the five-phases tonification points. BL-13, BL-15, BL-17, BL-20, BL-23, BL-25, and BL-26 are all good, but BL-23 and BL-26 are at the top of the list.

When it comes to local treatment, BL-32 is the best. If you can get the needle into the second sacral foramen, the needle sensation will reach the lesion in the anus. The sacral foramina are not so large, so it's not that easy to hit the mark. Angle the needle downward. BL-32 shows the strongest reaction among the points on the sacrum, but BL-33 and -34 could also work. Trust your fingertips and locate the point where your finger comes to a stop.

The second best local point is BL-35. It's half a unit lateral and slightly superior

7. See discussion of BL-32 in *Finding Effective Acupuncture Points*, p. 93.

to the tip of the coccyx. I insert the needle in the side-lying position with the top leg flexed, and the sensation reaches the anus. The effect is good when the needle sensation reaches inside the anus. The effect is less when the sensation just goes to outside the anus. Insertion of two units is required for patients of normal build. The thinner needles feel more comfortable, but in order to get the sensation to go right where you want it, you might need to use a thicker needle if your skills are not advanced. I recommend starting out by using a No. 5 gauge (0.24mm) needle. When the sensation reaches the anus, it feels very strong, and patients cry out. These days I mostly use a 40mm No. 3 gauge (0.20mm) needle and get good results with less depth and needle sensation.

Once a middle-aged man came in for treatment of back pain. He had hemorrhoids and was going to have surgery the next day. I needled BL-35 on both sides while I was at it. The next day at the hospital he was told his hemorrhoids had healed and he didn't need an operation. This patient was a farmer in the busy season and was very grateful for my treatment. He came back later and gave us a 30kg sack of rice and my wife and I were very appreciative.

6.1 Treatment of anal prolapse

Early stages of anal prolapse also respond well to acu-moxa treatments. It's difficult to recover when it becomes chronic and the sphincter muscles become slack. In such cases, I recommend surgery. These days, it is day surgery so it's a lot easier.

Anal fistulas, on the other hand, are a complicated condition. I suffered quite a while with anal fistulas, which were from tuberculosis, but these days I hear this is rare. I believe acu-moxa treatments will be effective if you look at it from the standpoint of regulating the whole body.

Case Study 111

Patient: Female, 49 years old

FOC: April 4, 1998

Main Complaints: Hemorrhoids with occasional anal prolapse, headaches and cold feet, constipation

Pulse Diagnosis: Kidney deficiency

Treatment: SRT on KI-7, KI-10, LU-5, LU-4, CV-12, left ST-21, CV-6, left ST-27, LI-11, GB-20, GB-21, GV-12, BL-11, SI-11, BL-23, BL-25, BL-32, and BL-58.

Direct moxibustion on GV-20, LU-5, BL-32, and left BL-52.

Progress:

(2nd) April 10 – Lung deficiency. The anus went back in after the treatment, but it began to come out a bit yesterday.

(3rd) May 30 – Lung deficiency. Her symptoms are gone.

Comments: This treatment was over a decade ago, and there are many unnecessary needles. Since that time, this patient doesn't have symptoms associated with hemorrhoids, but has had constipation from time to time. Making her bowel movements comfortable prevents recurrence of hemorrhoids and also improves the general effect of the treatment.

Case Study 112

Patient: Male, 30 years old

FOC: August 30, 1989

Main Complaint: Anal prolapse that is very painful

Pulse Diagnosis: Kidney deficiency

Treatment: SRT on KI-7, BL-13, BL-23, BL-32. Simple insertion on LU-8, KI-10, BL-58, and left BL-35. Direct moxibustion on GV-20 and BL-25.

Progress:

(3rd) Sept. 2 – He is feeling much better.

(4th) Sept. 4 – Lung deficiency. Pain is better.

This patient had a recurrence in 2000 and 2006, but in both instances he recovered after several more treatments. This case history includes needle techniques other than SRT, especially the point next to the sacrum, BL-35. There is an immediate effect when a 2-inch insertion into this point causes a sensation to radiate into the anus. The question is whether you can get the sensation to reach the painful point inside. This case resolved in four treatments the first time, but now this patient reminisces that the pain went away in just one treatment. He must have been deeply impressed by the mystery of how pain like this can be resolved completely, not at a hospital, but with just acupuncture.

7. Diseases of the esophagus

In many years of clinical practice, you run into unexpected situations. You need to be prepared for anything, but it's hard to know what to do if you don't have much experience. Especially when it's an acute condition. Is it an emergency requiring a trip to the hospital, or can acu-moxa take care of it? We are required to make a snap judgment. In acute cases we tend to want to send patients to the emergency room, especially considering the safety issue, but this is not a good default strategy.

7.1 Case of esophageal spasm (esophageal achalasia)

Case Study 113

Patient: Female, 16 years old

FOC: July 7, 2007

Main Complaint: Recurrent vomiting

Situation: This young woman came in carried by her two parents. When I tried to take her pulse, she broke out in tears, and reached for her mother who was standing next to us. After managing to calm her down, I figured out that she had a Lung deficiency pulse, which was also floating and rapid. Her temperature was 37.5°C. Anyway, I couldn't get over how immature this girl was. In the Edo period, 16 years was a marriageable age. In the Shogun's harem, young women like her were getting involved in power struggles. Right ... this is the 21st century. But this doesn't make it any easier to deal with her. Did she have a psychological issue like depression?

I asked her parents and they told me she's been going to the hospital of the University of Osaka for the last two years. She even had an operation on her esophagus, but it was unclear if it had been of any benefit. Once she began vomiting, she couldn't stop. She felt nauseous when tired or had a fever. She had reflux esophagitis and had received the diagnosis of esophageal achalasia.

How to treat such a delicate patient? From the symptoms, SRT was indicated, but judging from her emotional state, she might move suddenly. If the needle went in at all and she felt any pain, I wouldn't be able to treat her anymore. The patient was sitting up and bent forward.

Treatment: I used a teishin and applied some rapid rotations, even though they were not as smooth as with normal needles: LU-9, SP-3, CV-12, ST-21, BL-13, BL-20, GB-20, and GB-21. I placed a Pyonex press tack on GV-14 because I decided that she was in the early stages of a cold. Normally, I would apply multiple cones of moxa, but this patient wouldn't tolerate it. The press tack was just a substitute. The patient left being carried on her father's back.

Observations: What was I to make of this disease? It was a problem in the esophagus, and because she'd already had surgery, there was organic or structural pathology. But my intuition told me that this was a psychosomatic condition. How would this patient do? More than that, would she be willing to come again for a treatment? I was concerned and curious at the same time. Let's take a closer look here at the rare disease of esophageal achaleasia.

> **Esophageal achaleasia** (synonym: esophageal spasm). A motor dysfunction of the esophagus in which the lower 1-4cm of the esophagus constricts, while the upper end becomes abnormally large. The cause is unknown. The primary symptom is problems swallowing. Also, there is retention of food within the esophagus and reflux, and sometimes pain behind the sternum. These symptoms come on relatively acutely with changes in the environment and mental stress. The progress of this disease is chronic and the symptoms repeatedly improve and then get worse. Exacerbation tends to happen especially with emotional disturbances. X-rays reveal a smooth and symmetrical occlusion of

> the esophagus on the bottom end, and expansion on the upper end. The size of the expansion is often between 3-4cm, but it gets as large as 6-10cm in extreme cases. Endoscopes reveal esophagitis, and cancer must be ruled out. Often the bottom end of the esophagus remains closed. Treatment protocols for psychosomatic medicine are used. ... Otherwise, advice on diet and life-style, expansion of lower esophagus with balloon dilation, and in extreme cases surgery can be considered.[8]

So the lower end of the esophagus constricts while the upper end becomes abnormally large. In extreme cases it gets as wide as 10cm. It comes on suddenly with mental stress. Since the cause is unknown, it is probably a psychosomatic disease. SRT is indicated for psychosomatic conditions, but I had no choice but to use teishin on this patient. Would she let me give her a real treatment?

Progress:

(2nd) July 21 – It had been two weeks since she first came in and this time she was all smiles. She had had no symptoms since the last treatment. She had Liver deficiency. I was able to treat her with SRT lying on the table in the normal way.

(3rd) Aug 4 – Another two weeks has passed. Her pattern remained Liver deficiency after this.

(10th) Nov. 10 – Four weeks since last treatment. Reaction at GV-9 and -10. SRT and moxibustion applied.

(11th) Dec. 22 – Six weeks since last treatment. She gets nauseous before her period. SRT and five small cones of moxibustion applied on SP-6 and BL-52.

—15 treatments in 2008. 11 treatments in 2009. 14 treatments in 2010.

Comments: She almost had a recurrence of her symptoms in 2010 due to studying so hard for her nursing exams. She weathered it with acu-moxa treatments and she safely passed the nursing board exam, and she went to work at a local hospital. Her parents who had been worried that she might be going crazy at one time were overjoyed. In June of 2011 this young woman sent me a box of candy from her first paycheck. It had been four long years. I believed that, as long as she could receive periodic acupuncture and take care not to catch colds, get stressed out or overworked, she could prevent the recurrence of the esophageal spasm. It's been five years now, and I'm sure she will be a good nurse.

It is hard to draw any conclusion without treating many cases, but it seems that esophageal spasms can be treated with acu-moxa. It's a strange phenomenon where the lower end constricts and the upper end expands, which can probably be viewed as a manifestation of a psychological disorder. If this is true, operations and balloon dilation should be left to the very end as last resorts. This is a case that points to the untapped potential of acu-moxa treatments.

---

8. Nanzando Medical Dictionary CD-ROM, Pro Medica Ver. 3, 2007.

7.2 Mandibular torus

I encountered a strange phenomenon called mandibular torus (protuberance) while I was treating the above patient. What is this, I was asked one time about 10 months after she had first begun treatments? She had gotten a fever from a cold and had recurrence of vomiting. Then a hard protuberance formed behind her lower incisors. It looked like she had two rows of teeth. Her physician as well as my own dentist who I referred her to had no idea what it was. Checking resources on dentistry and oral surgery I found the term mandibular torus, which is a bone growth known as external hyperostosis that occurs on the inside of the mandible. What was amazing was that, when she came in for another treatment a week later, this protuberance was gone without a trace (photos 10-1 & 10-2). What happened? I would like to claim that the acu-moxa treatment is what cured it, but it was a fascinating phenomenon.

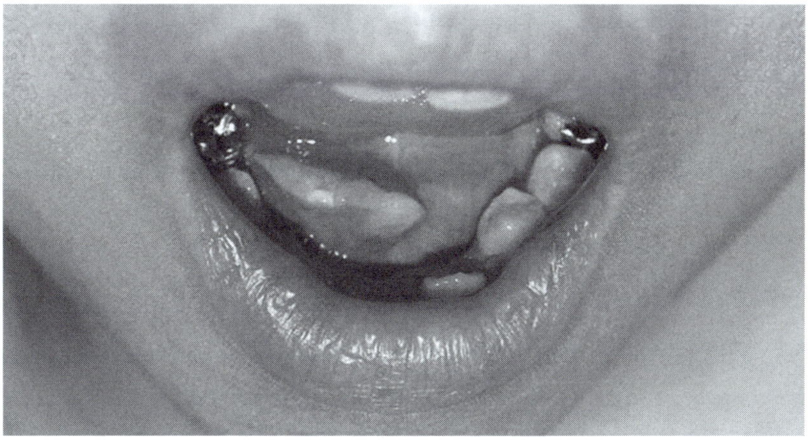

Photo 10-1 Mandibular torus

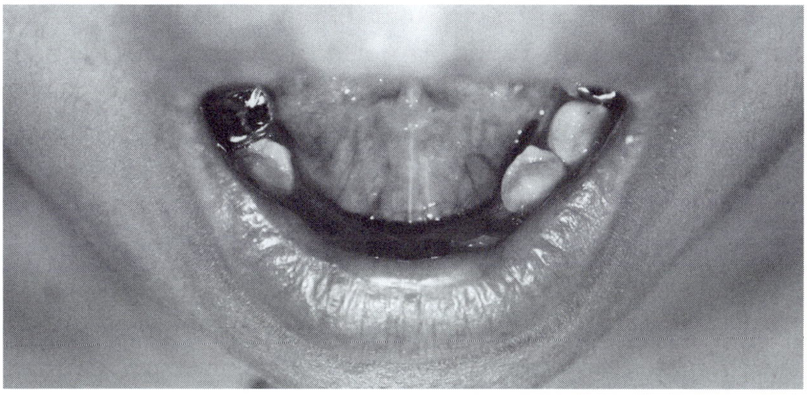

Photo 10-2 No more mandibular torus

Summary

- Esophageal spasms are often a psychosomatic disease. Such diseases are best treated with SRT or teishin.

7.3 Case of esophageal dysfunction

Case Study 114

Patient: Male, 56 years old

FOC: April 7, 2012

Symptoms and Condition: He has trouble getting food down since January 2011. He is an English professor at the university, and his burping was getting worse and worse so he went to the Kampo herbal out-patient clinic in the university hospital in September. The herbal treatments haven't helped much. Food gets stuck in his esophagus, and sometimes it takes a long time to go down. He has esophageal spasms during a meal and regurgitates copious amounts of saliva. His stools are hard and sometimes rabbit-like, and he has a hard time passing them.

History: Type C Hepatitis, renal tumor, bladder tumor, and hiatal hernia

Pulse Diagnosis: Kidney deficiency

Treatment: SRT on KI-7, LU-5, CV-12, CV-6, ST-36, LI-11, Upper BL-10, Yanagiya's GB-20, GB-21, BL-58, BL-2, and left ST-12. Direct moxibustion on CV-12, CV-6, KI-7, BL-13, left BL-17, BL-23, and Yanagiya's GB-20.

Progress:

(2nd) Apr 14 – He is no better. Spleen deficiency. Add an intradermal needle retained in left auricular vertigo point.

(3rd) Apr 21 – Occasionally there are days he feels better.

(4th) Apr 28 – Liver deficiency. Intradermal needle retained in induration at left ST-21.

(5th) May 12 – Sometimes he feels better for three days in a row. Liver deficiency. His right upper back between BL-15 and -17 is hard and there are tender points.

(6th) May 26 – Perhaps the herbs from a different hospital are working, but he feels quite good recently. Liver deficiency. Intradermal needle retained in induration at CV-14. Also needles retained superficially in LR-1. SRT applied on left LR-8 for one minute.

(8th) Jun 30 – Lung deficiency. Tenderness and sensitivity to pinching at ST-19, -21 and -27 on the left. SRT on reactive abdominal points.

(9th) July 28 – He is doing very good. Liver deficiency. No reactive points on the abdomen. Indurations at BL-13.

Comments: This patient is an Australian and is also very sensitive. When I asked him how he was doing each time, he would occasionally reply, "Better." He traveled from outside my prefecture to see me, so I told him I would recommend a good acupuncturist closer to him, but he said he liked me. When you look at his history, it is clear that it isn't just caused by stress or psychological issues. I am still treating him, and hope that he will one day reply that he's the best he can be. Then we can toast to our success with champagne!

CHAPTER 11

Liver Diseases

1. Overview

When it comes to diseases of the internal organs, I have both hope and uncertainty. Can we really treat internal organs with acu-moxa? It seems to me that the acupuncture profession in Japan has heretofore concentrated on the treatment of musculoskeletal problems. This trend continued within acupuncture associations, and it influenced even the Japan Traditional Acupuncture and Moxibustion Society. The reason could be the perception that acu-moxa doesn't work that well for internal organs and there is still no scientific rationale for the treatment of internal organs. In other words, our profession has been hesitant to take on the challenge.

Personally, I have taken on all kinds of diseases in the pursuit of the potential of acupuncture. I still continue to take on new diseases. Sometimes it doesn't go so well, just as many in our profession believe, but on the other hand I sometimes get unexpectedly good results. The thing is to give it a try if possible.

It seems that our profession is starting to open up a bit and I see reports on treatment of internal organ diseases. But there is a bottleneck in this pursuit.

We cannot get a correct diagnosis of internal organ diseases or determine if we are getting a result without medical technology. This is inconvenient for an acupuncturist because most of the time we must seek the help of hospitals and universities. The cooperation and instruction of doctors is indispensable. What is an acupuncturist in private practice to do? One must be creative and make connections.

When I look back to acupuncture in an earlier era, my predecessors successfully treated internal organ diseases. My own teacher also treated quite a few internal organ diseases, but he didn't write reports about it. When I think of all my predecessors who didn't report on this, I think there were quite a few unreported case histories. It takes a lot of resolve to publish such a case history.

1.1 Medical treatments plus acu-moxa

When a patient has tests at a hospital, as often as possible have them show you the results. Take a copy and save this with their charts. It is even better when you get the comments of the primary physician. If the patient hasn't been to a clinic or hospital and you suspect liver disease, refer them to a specialist. Use the diagnosis of this physician as your reference to proceed with acu-moxa treatments. Have the patient get a check-up from time to time. Once a month is enough. Medical treatment along with regular acu-moxa treatments is the best approach for a patient. I doubt that there are any acupuncturists who would say don't take drugs or get injections, but our attitude in giving acu-moxa treatments must be to complement medical treatments. This is a posture that applies across the board in the treatment of internal organ diseases.

1.2 Examination for liver disease cases

■ Abdominal palpation

Palpate around the right subcostal region with light stroking, pinching, light pressure, and sometimes heavy pressure. In general, if there are any reactions, I check the whole abdomen in layers. First, when there is sensitivity to pinching, I press the point gently, then I press a bit stronger. Where there is no sensitivity to pinching, I press the point gently, then I press a bit stronger. It's up to the practitioner but I progress from superficial to deeper palpation. If there is an induration, it can be used as a treatment point. Common points are ST-19, ST-21, and ST-24 on the right; CV-12 and CV-14; ST-19 and ST-21 on the right upper ST-19 (see Fig. 10-1). As for the alarm point of the Liver, LR-14, sometimes I find it at the bottom end of the ribs, at other times the reaction is stronger in the intercostal space, and sometimes in-between these two locations. The point is wherever the reaction is most pronounced in this area. In the lower abdomen it is common for there to be a deficiency around CV-6.

■ Back associated point palpation

Look for reactions between BL-17 and BL-23. It is especially common to find indurations around BL-18 on the right. Sometimes there is a bulge in the muscles in this area. Also look for deficient associated points. You can save time if you palpate deficient points as follows: Liver deficiency BL-18 and BL-23, Spleen deficiency BL-15 and BL-20.

■ Pulse diagnosis

The pattern must be determined from the pulse. Just because there is liver disease doesn't mean it is Liver deficiency, but there is that tendency. The majority of cases end up being Liver deficiency. Cases of Liver excess are hard to treat. Those who don't have an appetite are often Spleen deficient. Those who tend to catch colds, or tend to get depressed, could have Lung deficiency.

In terms of pulse qualities, the pulses balance out with treatment for those with soft pulses, but those who tend to have hard or rapid pulses are difficult to treat.

1.3 Treatment of liver disease

- Root treatment: For Liver deficiency, apply SRT on LR-8, KI-10, and LR-3.
- Retain needles and apply direct moxibustion afterwards on the back associated points, BL-18 and BL-23. Also apply direct moxibustion on ST-36 and LR-3.
- Treat abdominal reactive points, typically ST-19 and LR-14 on the right, CV-12 and ST-21 on the left.
- Apply SRT on GB-20 and GB-21.

❶ Retain intradermal needles in abdominal reactive point, choosing one point among ST-19, LR-14, and CV-12.

❷ Treatment frequency: Once a week. Two or three times a week is even better, but considering that treatment takes a long time, make sure that the patient can keep it up and doesn't drop out. Ask the patient if they felt tired after the last treatment. If they feel fatigued afterward, the stimulation was too strong.

❸ Suggest moxibustion at home. Patients can do moxa on themselves if the points are on the abdomen or legs. The minimum point prescription would be ST-36, LR-3, CV-12, and right ST-19. If someone can do moxibustion for them, BL-18 can be added. The vast majority cannot get any help with moxibustion, but there is not much difference in results as long as one is diligent.

The above is the treatment for Liver deficiency, but for other patterns, just change the root treatment tonification points and the back associated points. The treatment points on the abdomen depend on which points are reactive, but just look for the same ones that show up with Liver deficiency if you are not sure. For the direct moxibustion in cases of Spleen deficiency, use PC-6 and SP-4 along with the associated back associated points.

Another thing to be careful about is the patient's psychological state. Find out by inference if they are depressed by asking about their sleep, appetite, and elimination. Depressive patients require lighter treatments with less insertion.

When treatments like this are continued once a week, in cases that respond quickly, improvement can be seen in one month. Even in those that are not so responsive, the liver enzyme values will go down in three months. Pay attention to the GGT, among the liver enzyme values. It is said that a person is more likely to get cancer when the GGT remains high. When the liver enzyme values improve, the patients become excited and they are motivated to continue treatments.

In many cases the liver enzyme values go down after just one acu-moxa treatment. If you were to ask me for which non-musculoskeletal conditions acu-moxa is most effective, I would say internal organ diseases and then mental disorders. Among internal organ diseases, liver diseases are the easiest to cure and kidney diseases are the hardest. Of course, it also depends on how many cases you treat. It can be tricky but is well worth the effort.

Summary

1. To treat liver diseases pay attention to pulse pattern and abdominal findings.
2. Retain needles superficially in abdomen and then retain one intradermal needle.
3. Also use the related source and back associated points.
4. Keep your eyes on the GGT values, they are the hardest to change.

2. Liver function abnormalities

Case Study 115

Patient: Female, 66 years old

FOC: November 17, 2009

Main Complaint: Liver function abnormality due to chemotherapy

History: malignant lymphoma

Pulse Diagnosis: Transposed radial artery on right. Treated as Liver deficiency.

Treatment: SRT on LR-8 KI-10, CV-12, right ST-19, left ST-21, CV-6, ST-36, LR-3, LI-11, BL-18, BL-23, and GB-21. The needles were retained superficially in abdominal points and back points after SRT. Direct moxibustion on CV-12, left ST-21, ST-36, LR-3, and BL-18. Moxibustion at home recommended.

Progress:

(2nd) Nov 25 – Her husband recently retired, is home every day now, and she is depressed. The blood test values seem to be improving. AST 58 → 51, ALT 47 → 39, creatinine 0.71 → 0.59 (normal), blood sugar 112 → 115.

(6th) Dec 29 – Blood test values improved: AST 43, ALT 36, creatinine 0.68, blood sugar 115.

(9th) Jan 26, 2010 – Blood test the day before showed normal values for liver enzymes and blood sugar, but creatinine was high (AST 26, ALT 23, creatinine 0.74).

(13th) Mar 2 – Creatinine 0.74, blood sugar 114

(17th) Apr 2 – AST 20, ALT 15, creatinine 0.71, blood sugar 112

(20th) Apr 27 – Creatinine 0.69 (normal), blood sugar 109 (normal)

(22nd) May 31 – Creatinine 0.71, blood sugar 112

(24th) June 25 – Creatinine 0.72, blood sugar 108 (normal)

(28TH) July 27 – All values normal: AST 24, ALT 19, creatinine 0.68, blood sugar 109

(32ND) Sept 3 – Blood sugar 120

(35TH) Sept 28 – Tested negative for breast cancer.

(36TH) Oct 5 – Creatinine 0.73

(39TH) Nov 9 – Creatinine 0.75, blood sugar 114

(43RD) Dec 12 – Creatinine 0.78, blood sugar 106

(50TH) Feb 25, 2011 – Creatinine 0.73, blood sugar 112

(54TH) Mar 29 – Creatinine 0.70, blood sugar 108 (both in normal range)

(59TH) May 6 – Creatinine 0.68, blood sugar 106 (both normal)

(61ST) May 24 – Creatinine 0.66, blood sugar 95 (both normal)

(63RD) June 7 – Creatinine 71, blood sugar 110

(67TH) July 15 – Creatinine 0.71, blood sugar 108

(70TH) Aug 16 – Creatinine 0.69, blood sugar 105 (both normal)

COMMENTS: In this case the liver function abnormality was due to chemotherapy, but she also had abnormalities in the function of the kidneys and pancreas. The GGT value was close to normal to begin with, so I tracked the changes with acu-moxa treatments in the AST and ALT for the liver function, and creatinine for the kidney function and the blood sugar lever for the pancreas.

The liver function improved early on, but the kidney and pancreas didn't improve so easily. Her indicators for these organs continue to be marginal now, but her primary physician says the values are barely above the normal range so it isn't really that bad. In the beginning this patient was diligent in doing moxibustion at home, but she stopped because her values improved and sometimes the moxa points itched. Of course, the risk of infection at wounds increases with diabetes, so it was just as well. Her doctor did not prescribe any medications so the above results were obtained solely from weekly acu-moxa treatments with me.

While the results were due to this patient coming regularly for a long time, there is a story behind this. Her brother is an acupuncturist and was the student of Jyo Ikkaku (1879-1945), one of the disciples of the legendary moxibustion master Ken Sawada.[1] He advised her saying, "Go get treatments from Shudo sensei. Don't let up on treatments because Western medicine can't do what acu-moxa can do."

Anyway, the general tendency is for fairly rapid improvement in liver function, but kidney function isn't easy to improve. I will discuss this in a later case in the section on kidney diseases in the next chapter on urogenital diseases. Blood sugar levels also require

1. Ken Sawada (1877-1938): One of the leading figures in acu-moxa in Japan in the early 20th century who created the treatment system *Taikyoku (Taiji)* Therapy. He primarily practiced moxibustion but he influenced the acupuncture profession through his students.

dietary therapy and appropriate exercise and is not something that can be changed with acu-moxa alone. Nevertheless, acu-moxa treatments do aid in the reduction in blood sugar. I will discuss this further in the section on diabetes in Chapter 14.

Case Study 116

Patient: Female, 75 years old

FOC: April 1, 2011

Main Complaint: Insomnia and liver function abnormality

Blood Test Values: Mar 19 – AST 40, ALT 49, LDL 150

Pulse Diagnosis: Liver deficiency

Treatment: SRT on LR-8 KI-10, LR-3, ST-36, LI-11, GB-20, and GB-21.

Needles were retained superficially in CV-12, right ST-19, left ST-21, BL-18, and BL-23.

Direct moxibustion on BL-18 and BL-23. Moxibustion recommended at home at CV-12, right ST-19, left ST-21, ST-36, LR-3, and M-LE-5 (shitsumin/*shī mián*).

Progress:

(4th) June 17 – Test results from June 2 – AST 21, ALT 19, LDL 115. Her physician is surprised. Her insomnia continues.

(7th) Sept 6 – AST 23, ALT 20, GGT 36 (all within normal range)

Comments: This patient is among a group of women that comes for treatment once a month. After she was told she had liver function abnormality, she kept up moxibustion treatments at home for a while. Now, it seems like she is lazy and uses excuses like itchiness and being busy. If the liver function becomes bad again, however, I'm sure she will become serious again. She is taking care of her husband handicapped by a stroke, so she thinks it's the stress. She has been getting treatments with me for four years now, so I'm sure that if necessary, she will comply if I give her the word.

Case Study 117

Patient: Female, 72 years old

FOC: March 23, 2011

Main Complaint: She had a medical exam and was told she had liver function abnormalities.

Blood Test: (H denotes high, L low) April 8 – total bilirubin: 1.3 (H), AST: 296 (H), ALT: 437 (H), LDH: 342 (H), ALP 813 (H), GGT: 366

Lymphocytes: 0.81 (L), eosinophils: 0.90 (H)

Pulse Diagnosis: Liver deficiency

Treatment: SRT on LR-8, KI-10, ST-36, LR-3, LI-11, GB-20, GB-21, right BL-43, BL-17, CV-6. Needles retained superficially in CV-12, right ST-19, left ST-21, BL-18, and BL-23.

Direct moxibustion on right ST-19, ST-36, LR-3, BL-18, and BL-23.

Moxibustion recommended at home at CV-12, ST-36, and LR-3 (points she could do herself). In addition to instruction for daily moxibustion at home, she as advised to come in once a week for treatments.

Progress:

(4th) Apr 23 – Some high values went down. ALP: 813 → 624, GGT: 366 → 266.

(25th) Oct 26 – ALP: 342 → 301, GGT: 45 → 17.

Comments: The values became normal in the August exam, after about five months of treatment. The GGT value settled within the normal range. She told me that her mother-in-law, who lived with her, was over 90 and had dementia. As her mother-in-law had strong legs and walked around, this exhausted her mentally and physically. Her liver function abnormalities could be because of this stress. Recently she has been coming for treatment once or twice a month, which is ideal for maintenance.

2.1 Story of treating incipient liver disease

Sometimes strange symptoms make one suspect liver disease. For example, a 47-year-old woman, a dental hygienist, came in recently. She had chronic constipation, and one day she strained to pass stools, and this caused a splitting headache in her right occipital region. She had an exam at a neurologist including a CT scan and MRI, but there was no abnormality. She was told she had excess neck and shoulder tension (*katakori*). The pain continued unabated, so she had a nerve block injection in the occipital region. This relieved the pain a little, but she continued to have pain in her right shoulder, neck, and temple.

When she came to me, the center of the pain was Upper BL-10, and I suspected occipital neuralgia. When I examined her abdomen, I found something funny about the right subcostal region. I went around to the right side of the table to palpate carefully and found a hard area about 5cm in diameter around ST-20. Pressing gently with my middle finger, it was tender and hard to the touch. I also found a tender induration at GB-34 on the right. This made me suspect liver and or gallbladder disease. When I asked her about it, she told me that her liver had some problems. She had been told that her gamma GPT was a bit high. She also liked to drink. But it wasn't until recently that she was told about a possible liver problem. Her pulse pattern was Liver deficiency, but it wasn't a wiry pulse. She is taking drugs to reduce blood pressure. From the above, I deduced that she had a liver function abnormality, and this influence moved up her right side and brought on the neck and shoulder stiffness. I believe that treating the liver will have a positive affect overall, so I am treating her incipient liver problem. More than her shoulders, I am focusing on improving her liver. I am paying careful attention to see how she does.

2.2 Other liver problems

Liver cancer (see Chapter 14: Cancer and Acu-moxa Treatment).

Q&A

QUESTION AND ANSWER NO. 6

For which diseases is acu-moxa effective?

Q. For which diseases is acu-moxa effective? Does it work for all diseases?

A. Acu-moxa is effective for many diseases, but it works well in some cases and not so much in others. I have listed those conditions that have proven to respond well to acupuncture in my own practice. They are from a pamphlet that I created for my patients.

CONDITIONS THAT RESPOND WELL TO ACUPUNCTURE

dizziness	facial paralysis	facial nerve spasms
colds/coughs	tonsillitis	asthma
hiccoughs	stomach pain	headaches
neck spasms	cervical syndrome	neck/shoulder tension
frozen shoulder	tennis elbow	baseball elbow
reflux esophagitis	liver dysfunction	spinal stenosis
low back pain	disc herniation	kidney stones
sciatica	femoral neuritis	osteoarthritis in knee
chilblains	neuralgia of all kinds	depression
poor appetite	fatigue/low energy	carpal tunnel syndrome

continued >

pancreas dysfunction	diarrhea/constipation	irritable bowel syndrome
trigger finger	menstrual pain	fetal malposition
bladder infection	leg cramps	growth pains
sprains	arthritis	insomnia
loss of motivation	post-herpetic neuralgia	

CHAPTER 12

Urogenital Diseases

1. Overview

I am not feeling too good about writing this chapter. This is a category of diseases that constitutes a small minority of cases in my clinic, and furthermore the results are not that good. It is one of the limits of acu-moxa treatments. The ideal would be for a person to gain the skills and knowledge of a medical doctor as well as the skills and knowledge of a good acupuncturist. Such a person would be able to deal with patients with complicated diseases that are seen in hospitals.

What kind of results can be obtained with patients with urogenital diseases? We can't come to a general conclusion until many cases have been treated. There is an issue with an acupuncturist's access to such patients in Japan, and this is one thing our whole profession has to seriously consider. As I have said, acu-moxa has unlimited potential, and it is effective for a wide range of internal organ diseases. Our collective future becomes brighter when each acupuncturist records good results. We might even say this will contribute to the welfare of mankind. Acupuncturists have a long way to go.

When I think of urogenital diseases, I recall an incident in my early childhood. It was just before I entered grade school, so I must have been five or six. I had some discomfort with urination. It hurt. So I would quit urinating, but then the urge to urinate would arise again. I would urinate again, and it hurt, so I would stop again. I recall how uncomfortable this was. In those days we didn't see the doctor much at all. It was probably a urethral infection, so without the antibiotics that are available these days, it is doubtful that medications would have solved my problem. I think my parents must have tried all sorts of home remedies, but I clearly recall how putting a hot water bottle on my lower abdomen stopped the pain with urination, and I was able to urinate comfortably again. I must have been suffering a lot, and the relief must have really made an impression. In my old age I sometimes get this symptom from my childhood. Is it my prostate? When I remember to warm my lower abdomen, things go quite nicely.

2. Bladder infections (cystitis) & related symptoms

I have seen this condition quite often in my practice. When the symptoms are severe, I send the patients to the university hospital. Antibiotics work very well. If the germs causing the problem can be identified, using the drugs that are effective against those germs will cure the problem. But sometimes the patient doesn't get any better. Also, sometimes no germs are found at all. This is known as non-microbial cystitis (allergic cystitis[1]). Acu-moxa treatments are indicated here. Acu-moxa treatments are especially suited for non-microbial cystitis.

The keys to treatment are as follows:

1. Determine the pattern and give a root treatment.
2. Treat the lower abdomen – branch treatment.
3. Treat the lumbo-sacral region.
4. Treat the cranium. Calm mental confusion.

The most common pattern is Liver deficiency. Kidney and Lung deficiency also occur. The meridians that need attention are the Liver, Kidney, Lung, and Bladder. The Triple Burner also needs attention.

Liver deficiency – LR-8, KI-10, and KI-3.

Kidney deficiency – KI-7, KI-10, and LU-5.

Lung deficiency – LU-9, SP-3, and SP-9.

The Lungs have the function of "regulating the water passages," and they help expel water. This is very much connected with the function of the Bladder. Sometimes people forget this, but it must be borne in mind.

2.1 Relationship between the lower abdomen and the bladder and urethra

Reactions often appear in the lower abdomen when there are urogenital diseases. Here's yet another personal experience. Once after recovering from a cold, I had some trouble passing urine. The more I worried about it, the worse it became. I had an exam at the hospital and was told that my prostate was slightly enlarged, as might be expected of someone my age. I was still concerned so I got a referral to a urogenital specialist and I was told the same thing—that my prostate was enlarged to an extent expected for my age. Otherwise there were no abnormalities.

I took my own pulses and treated myself for Lung deficiency. I did contact nee-

1. Allergic cystitis: Also known as interstitial cystitis or bladder pain syndrome (BPS).

dling on LU-9, and wonder of wonders, I was able to pass my urine without difficulty. Thinking it over, I decided that the function of my Lungs had declined and the function of "regulating the water passages" had been impaired. Tonifying the Lung meridian resolved the problem.

Anyway, before I made this discovery, in order to do the prostate exam, they had inserted a catheter in my urethra. The next day I found urinating very painful. Since there was some blood in my urine, they must have injured my urethra. I palpated my own lower abdomen and found an induration the size of a soybean at CV-4, and it was tender. When I inserted a needle into this induration, I felt a sensation radiate to my urethra where it had been injured. This is evidence that the bladder and urethra (and the urogenital system in general) are intimately connected to the lower abdomen. The pain with urination stopped with just this one needle in CV-4. So I confirmed this relationship by treating myself. This is why I know treatment of the lower abdomen is effective for urogenital diseases.

2.2 Acu-moxa treatment of urogenital diseases

So what points are effective for urogenital diseases? This depends on which points are manifesting localized changes. The related meridians, in addition to the above-mentioned Lung meridian and Conception vessel, are the Kidney, Stomach, Spleen, and Bladder meridians. When you palpate the Conception vessel from CV-2 up to CV-7, often you find that there is deficiency (depression) somewhere between CV-4 and CV-6. Sometimes you find a tight band instead. In either case it is an indication of Kidney deficiency. When you insert a needle in the tight band or induration, often there is a radiating sensation to the urethra. You can insert a needle when the point is depressed, but you must insert the needle more skillfully.

On the Kidney meridian, reactions tend to appear below the midpoint between the navel and the pubic bone (KI-12, -13 & -14). I insert needles between 5-10mm in the lower abdomen. The classics mention deeper needling, but I find that shallow insertion works better. Deep insertion is risky. When the patient is really deficient, I only use SRT.

I also like to palpate laterally just above the pubic bone in both directions from CV-2. Sometimes I find a tender point, and it serves as a good treatment point. In acute cases with frequent urination or pain with urination, the needles can be briefly retained in the reactive points on the lower abdomen. One must be careful, however, not to let go of the needle because the depth changes when the supporting hand on the abdomen is released. Keeping the hands on the needle allows one to gauge the response.

Direct moxibustion on reactive points on the lower abdomen is also good. Sometimes I do multiple cones of moxibustion (20-30) on the most reactive point.[2]

In the sacral area, look for reactive points among BL-28, BL-32, BL-33, and BL-53. I find that BL-32 shows up most often. I also look for a reaction just above the sacrum,

2. Moxibustion on abdomen: Some patients cannot tolerate direct moxibustion on their abdomen. Other ways to add more stimulation are to insert a needle about 5mm and retain for about 5 minutes, retain an intradermal needle, and heat the point with a moxa pole or warming device.

the extra point M-BW-25 *(jōsen / shí qī zhuī xià)*. Otherwise, I palpate BL-23 and BL-52.

On the legs I often find reactions in points like SP-6, LR-8, and BL-59. These points can be treated with acupuncture, moxibustion, or both.

One more thing. Patients who have a bad bladder infection, or have it repeatedly, tend to become irritable and upset. Probably the condition is affecting their mind and causing some confusion. To calm them down, it is good to give some treatment on the cranium, occipital region, and neck/shoulders.

Sample Treatment (Liver deficiency)

- SRT on LR-8 and KI-10.
- Insert needles in CV-3, CV-6, and BL-32.
- SRT on BL-59, GV-22, GB-20, and GB-21.
- Superficial retained needles in BL-18 and BL-23.
- Direct moxibustion on CV-3, CV-6, SP-6 (or LR-8), BL-23, and BL-32.

For acute cases, give treatments every day until it improves. For chronic cases, give a treatment every 5-7 days. Female patients especially tend to get recurrent bladder infections at the change of seasons, exposure to heat or cold, or from fatigue. They need to be careful not to let their feet get too cold or hot (not to walk barefoot on hot surfaces). They also need to increase their fluid intake. I ask patients with recurrent bladder infections to do moxibustion at home on points like SP-6, CV-7, and CV-6 (or CV-3).

Case Study 118

Patient: Female, 77 years old

FOC: March 6, 2012

Main Complaint: Difficulty urinating starting 20 days ago. She had no idea what is causing it. A urological exam showed no abnormalities. She was told it was because of her age, but she just isn't satisfied. She has a sore throat and occasional coughing. Her feet are cold.

Pulse Diagnosis: Kidney deficiency

Treatment: SRT on KI-7, LU-8, LU-5, CV-12, CV-6, BL-13, BL-23, BL-58, GB-20, and GB-21. Direct moxibustion on KI-7, CV-6 BL-23, and BL-32. Also on M-LE-5 *(shitsumin/shī mián)* until she felt the heat after three cones.

Progress: (2nd) Mar 13 – It has become easy to urinate, except at 4 a.m.

(3rd) Mar 26 – Lung deficiency. She is completely better. She is mystified. She mentioned this to the doctor at the hospital and was told to facilitate urination by making a sound as if she were a child (?). I told her that in East Asian medicine, urination can become difficult not just with urogenital problems, but by the weakening in the function of the lungs. She seemed perplexed, naturally.

(4TH) Apr 2 – Lung deficiency. No coughing. She is better all around. We decide to extend the interval between treatments.

Comments: This seems to have been a functional disorder rather than a bladder infection. There is no way a doctor can understand that this is related to the Kidney and Lung function unless he knows about the yin and yang organs of East Asian medicine. It is mysterious to the patient, and even though there is no major problem, it must be unsatisfying not to understand my explanation.

Case Study 119

Patient: Male, 62 years old

FOC: June, 2012

Main Complaints: His legs are paralyzed since his surgery for a herniated lumbar disk two years ago. He doesn't have any hopes for the paralysis, but there are two symptoms he just can't live with: sharp pain in his urethra when urinating, and strong pain from the knees down to the ankles.

Examination: He can move his right leg a little, but he can't move his left leg much at all. His sensory nerves are damaged as well. He can walk a little by wearing leg braces, but he has difficulty in my clinic which has steps and isn't entirely free of obstructions. I doubt if there will be any effect on the motor paralysis, but there might be some effect on the pain with urination. We decide to give it a try.

Pulse Diagnosis: Kidney deficiency

Treatment: SRT on KI-7, LU-5, BL-10, BL-13, BL-23, BL-59, CV-12, CV-4, CV-2, BL-32, and Ischial points. Direct moxibustion on CV-4, KI-7, BL-23, BL-32, and BL-59.

Progress: For personal reasons, this patient stopped coming after four months and 11 treatments. I had started inserting needles at some points after the second treatment. About 5mm at the Ischial points and about 1cm at CV-2. I also applied 5-10 sparrow-pecking movements. I also tried SRT on points like KI-1. Near the end the pain with urination was bad in the morning, but it wasn't that bad during the day. The greatest pain on a scale of 1 to 10 was 8. So he got some relief although not complete. There was no effect at all on the motor paralysis, but there was a significant reduction of pain in his lower legs.

3. Prostatic hypertrophy

Parts of our body that worked well while we were young don't perform the way we want them to in old age. In the end they are even considered to be ancient relics that get in our way. It is really a shame. It is one thing to treat machines in this way, but I am talking about the prostate.

After a certain age the prostate begins to enlarge and this is treated as a disease. It is really a great shame! The first symptom is frequent urination at night. You wake up with the desire to urinate (phase 1: stimulation stage). Then you have difficulty urinating and incomplete urination (phase 2: residual urine stage). Finally, urine retention becomes greater and there is incontinence (phase 3: chronic urine retention stage).

Acu-moxa treatments are effective in the first stage. It works especially when moxibustion is practiced at home. I have a case that had been considering surgery because the PSA[3] value became high, but was able to avoid surgery when the value came down after a few months of moxibustion. These days patients tend to dislike direct moxibustion, but in the case of prostate problems there is less resistance because the patient is male and usually quite old. In the final stage there is urinary retention, or the inability to fully empty the bladder. Actually, sometimes acu-moxa treatments can be effective even at this stage. After my standard Meridian Therapy treatment, I insert a needle in BL-53. I reported on my use of this point in the *Journal of Japanese Acupuncture and Moxibustion* (May 1960 issue, No. 381):

> How to locate BL-53: measure three finger widths up from the tip of the coccyx and then measure laterally four or five finger widths. Press this area with the tip of your thumb and locate the depression. This is BL-53.
>
> Insertion technique: Use a four inch #6 or #7 needle (0.26 or 0.28mm). Aim the needle slightly medially and insert gently. In obese patients, the supporting hand *(oshide)* must press firmly to insert the needle. With thinner patients, the pudendal nerve, which is the target, can be reached when the needle is inserted about 9/10s of the way. When you hit the nerve that is the target, the needle sensation reaches the lower abdomen, genitals, or anal region. There is an effect no matter where the sensation is felt. Even if no sensation is felt the first time, the patient will begin to feel it after the second day of treatment.
>
> Until you are practiced at this technique, the needle runs into the pelvic bone or touches the sciatic nerve and doesn't feel good. If this happens, withdraw the needle part way and change the direction of the needle and reinsert.

The above passage comes from an article I wrote on behalf of one of my mentors in Ohita, Nakamura Yaeko. The first two of the following case studies are from this article, and they date back to the 1950s.

Case Study 120

Patient: Male, 75 years old

Main Complaints: Urinary retention; at present he is unable to urinate at all. He was about to go to the hospital when his wife suggested acupuncture and he decided to try it first.

Pulse Diagnosis: Kidney deficiency

3. PSA (prostate-specific antigen): One of the proteins specific to the prostate. Normal value is under 4.0ng/ml.

Treatment: Needles inserted in KI-7, KI-9, KI-11, BL-52, GB-25, and BL-32. Direct moxibustion on CV-3 (tender point). Deep insertion in BL-53 bilaterally. The left side did not produce a sensation in the lower abdomen at first, so the needle was inserted twice and the second time produced the sensation.

Progress: The evening of the treatment the patient urinated large quantities. The next day he felt a little urine retention. After five treatments the uncomfortable feeling of retention also disappeared.

Case Study 121

Patient: male, 70 years old

Main Complaints: Urinary retention which started a few days ago. He went to the hospital today. He was told there was nothing wrong with his prostate or bladder, but that it was neurological. He received urethral catheterization.

Pulse Diagnosis: Liver deficiency

Treatment: Acupuncture for Liver deficiency (LR-8, KI-10, and CV-6) along with insertion in KI-11. Deep insertion in BL-53. The patient was thin so he felt a strong sensation at the tip of his penis at a depth of about 3 units.

Progress: The feeling of retention went away after a few treatments and did not recur.

3.1 Summary on treating prostatic hypertrophy

To treat prostatic hypertrophy, follow the same protocol as bladder infections given in the previous section. In cases of Kidney deficiency, the treatment would look as follows:

1. SRT on KI-7, KI-10, and LU-5.
2. Insert needles in CV-4 and KI-11.
3. Retain needles superficially after SRT on BL-13, BL-23, and BL-32.
4. Direct moxibustion on CV-6, KI-7 (or KI-3), BL-23, and BL-32.

Case Study 122

Patient: Male, 70 years old

FOC: November 30, 2009

Main Complaints: He is receiving medical treatment, but his PSA value is unusually high. It started at around 2.7 and gradually went up to 10.5. This took about five years. Surgery has been recommended but he wants to try moxibustion.

Pulse Diagnosis: Kidney deficiency

Treatment: After standard acupuncture treatment for Kidney deficiency (first three items above), direct moxibustion applied on KI-7, right KI-3, CV-4, BL-23, and BL-32.

Progress and Comments: This patient was the picture of health, and loves acu-moxa, but he especially likes moxibustion. His PSA value became normal after seven months of my treatments and regular moxibustion at home. Of course, he didn't need surgery. Two and a half years later he is having no trouble. He is one of the senior members of our Prefectural Council and is active far beyond expected for his age.

4. Prostatitis

When a man gets a sudden fever, frequent urination, and pain with urination, he consults a urologist in a hurry. He receives a diagnosis of prostatitis or pyelonephritis. In the former case, often the cause is *Escherichia coli.* It is resolved by judicious use of antibiotics. But sometimes it transitions to a chronic infection. There are also cases of aseptic prostatitis.

The symptoms of prostatitis include frequent urination, feeling of retention, pain with urination, pain after ejaculation, discomfort after urination, and dull pain or discomfort in the perineal and lower abdominal regions. They say there is an indescribable discomfort in the lower abdomen which is present even when not urinating. Just as with bladder infections, it causes mental agitation. Chronic prostatitis seems to be hard to deal with even at hospitals. Then patients start making the rounds of different urologists, which is called "doctor shopping" in Japan. There is the medical term prostatodynia. It refers to cases of prostate pain and symptoms that mimic prostatitis when there is no infection or inflammation. When things get to this level, it starts to look like a psychological issue as well. I think that SRT would be applicable to such patients.

4.1 An interesting case of prostatitis

A 30-year-old man suffering from prostatitis for several years came for treatment. He had many of the symptoms listed above. I treated him for Kidney deficiency in the beginning, but more recently I have been treating him for Liver deficiency.

His first treatment was on March 1, 2011. Palpation revealed nothing outstanding. There was some tenderness at BL-32 and the Conception vessel was soft in his lower abdomen. The Kidney meridian on his abdomen seemed tense. I gave him the standard treatment for prostate problems.

SRT on LV-8, KI-10, KI-3, ST-36, LI-11, CV-12, CV-3, SP-6, GB-20, GB-21, BL-43, BL-18, BL-52, and BL-59. Needle inserted 5mm in CV-6 pointed diagonally downward; five sparrow-pecking motions were applied. Needles retained superficially in BL-23. Needles also retained in BL-32 after five sparrow-pecking motions at 5mm. Direct moxibustion on BL-23, KI-7, CV-6, BL-32, and M-LE-5 *(shitsumin/shī mián).*

This patient was diligent about coming for treatment. When his symptoms were bad, he would become irritable and also had pain in his epigastric region. At times like this, I found a reaction at left ST-21, retained an intradermal needle there, and his epigastric pain would go away. These days he doesn't have any pain in his prostate. He has discomfort from a prickling pain down his medial thigh. It appears to be more like neuralgia of the obturator nerve. I used a teishin to treat this, and the pain went away. Recently he is complaining of decreased libido. This is a big deal for a young man!

Summary

1. Acupuncture and moxibustion are effective for prostatitis.
2. Treat KI-7 or LR-8 along with CV-6, BL-23, BL-32, and SP-6.

5. Kidney diseases

Soon after the conclusion of the Second World War, a middle-aged woman took some medicine that was in her cabinet. She didn't know what the medicine was for, but she just took it because she didn't want to waste it. Something like this would be unthinkable these days, but those were desperate times. This is a true story.

Right away her skin broke out in a rash. She had a doctor nearby take a look at it, but he didn't know what to make of it. He wouldn't even touch her. He may have thought that it was some contagious skin disease. Eventually she started to get edema, and her urination became scanty.

She came to get treatment from my master, Miura Nagahiko. Right after the treatment she urinated copiously and then her problems resolved. Probably the old medications had caused kidney dysfunction and skin rashes. It was really amazing. Of course, it was about my teacher's skill, but also it demonstrated what acu-moxa treatments can do.

Although acu-moxa treatment works well for diseases of the internal organs, it doesn't seem to work as well when it comes to kidney diseases. This is on the opposite pole as how well acu-moxa treatments work for liver diseases. Of course, there are always exceptions.

5.1 A case in which dialysis was avoided

This was over 20 years ago, but a 53-year-old woman was delivering milk to each of the departments of the prefectural government. Her complexion was bad. One of the government workers asked her what was wrong. She told him the doctor ordered her to start kidney dialysis tomorrow. He said to her, "Go see doctor Shudo. You can do dialysis if he tells you to go see the doctor."

I misplaced the precious chart recording the treatments, but the following is what happened based on this patient's and my own recollection:

When she was 40, she had had a hysterectomy in which her uterus and ovaries were removed. She had fatigue after the surgery and was examined by a doctor nearby. The results showed that the urine sugar levels were normal after 30 minutes but became abnormal after one hour. She had her urine tested every month, but the results were always the same. She continued getting exams at the hospital for three years, but eventually she stopped going. If she had continued getting the exams, she may have prevented it from getting worse. Anyway, 10 years went by and by the time she started having symptoms, her condition was already serious.

Once after she came home from a trip to Nagasaki, she became so fatigued that she didn't want to do anything. She had no appetite and didn't even want to drink. She could no longer urinate. Two days later, by which time her weight had decreased 7kg, she went to a urologist for an exam. She was told to come back with her family and that they were going to start her on dialysis the next day. She just happened to run into one of my patients who recommended she should see me first.

So I decided to at least try acu-moxa, and near the end of the treatment, I applied 10 cones of moxa on M-LE-5 *(shitsumin/shī mián)*. She did not feel any heat on these points. This was back when it was just my wife and I working in my clinic, and I had a lot of patients so we were really busy. So I asked her to go home and apply moxibustion on M-LE-5 *(shitsumin/shī mián)* herself until she could feel the heat. She went home and it took 57 cones before she was able to feel any burning sensation on this point on her heels. About five minutes after that she had the urge to urinate, and she released a small amount urine. She was amazed because until then she had been unable to urinate at all. She came for acu-moxa treatments every other day for two or three weeks, and then she came once a week for about a month. After that she continued treatments about every other week, and during this time I recommended she eat brown rice and watermelon sugar (which is said to have diuretic properties).

After she started feeling better, she went to a different urologist for an examination. She was told that her urine was too clear for someone with kidney problems, and she should come again in one week for another exam just to be sure. But the results a week later were just the same. They could not detect any kidney dysfunction. It's been over 20 years since then and this patient has been able to lead a normal life without dialysis.

Even when she explains to the urologist that acu-moxa treatment cured her, he doesn't accept her story. He said if just acu-moxa could cure such diseases, there would be no need for doctors. The patient was stunned, but it can't be helped. For a doctor, such a thing seems impossible. The patient wants the doctor to be happy that they have recovered, but doctors can't deal with it. This happens often.

Once when the ocular pressure of a patient with glaucoma went down to normal, an ophthalmologist shook his head. When told that this was accomplished through acu-moxa, he didn't believe it. He laughed as if it were a joke. This actually isn't a bad response. Some doctors get angry. They say, "There's no way acu-moxa could work." They hold the assumption that acu-moxa doesn't work; they don't want to believe it works. It is their professional pride. But the reception of acupuncture around the world is not so narrow. In China, Korea, and the United States, governments and doctors are passionately involved in acupuncture research. What about Japan? I just hope that we don't find ourselves far behind, like falling behind in the race to develop information technology.

The doctors that I associate with have had the experience of patients who didn't get any better at hospitals recovering quite simply with acu-moxa, so they are used to it. Since that time, they studied up on acupuncture and utilize it in their practices. Of course, their patients really trust them too. Too bad this is a rare breed of doctor in Japan.

5.2 Observations about this successful case

So, once she learned it worked, the above patient was very diligent about doing moxibustion at home. She did moxibustion not only on M-LE-5 *(shitsumin/shī mián)* but on points on her abdomen, low back, and legs. Her urine output became normal and 20 years thereafter her exams show no abnormalities. This is the only case where the patient was told she needed dialysis and got away without doing dialysis, but it shows the unlimited potential of acu-moxa. Let us consider why acu-moxa was effective in this particular case.

Patient could have had a constitution for which acu-moxa was especially effective: In later years, this patient got liver disease as well as diabetes, but she overcome them both with acu-moxa. She did, however, require a bypass operation for her heart.

Diligence in home moxibustion treatments paid off: The patient doing regular moxibustion at home is huge. Unlike acupuncture, moxibustion is not about subtle stimulation, so bigger cones seem to work better. The results are not so good for patients who can't do moxibustion at home.

5.3 Acu-moxa treatment for kidney diseases

Follow the same protocol as for prostate disease. The pattern is often Kidney deficiency.

Kidney deficiency: SRT on KI-7 (or KI-3), KI-10, LU-5, and BL-23. Direct moxibustion on KI-7 and BL-23.

Spleen deficiency: SRT on SP-3, SP-6, PC-7, and BL-20. Direct moxibustion on SP-6 and BL-20.

Liver deficiency: SRT on LR-8 (or LR-3), KI-10, and BL-18. Direct moxibustion on LR-3 and BL-18.

Branch treatment points for all cases: ST-36, LI-11, CV-6, CV-7, CV-9, and BL-32. Direct moxibustion on M-LE-5 *(shitsumin/shī mián)* until the heat is felt. One additional special point I use is the auricular kidney/bladder point (Fig. 12-1). When the point is indicated, there will be tenderness if this part of the ear is pressed. There is a strong response when using an electric point locator. Retain a needle or an intradermal needle.

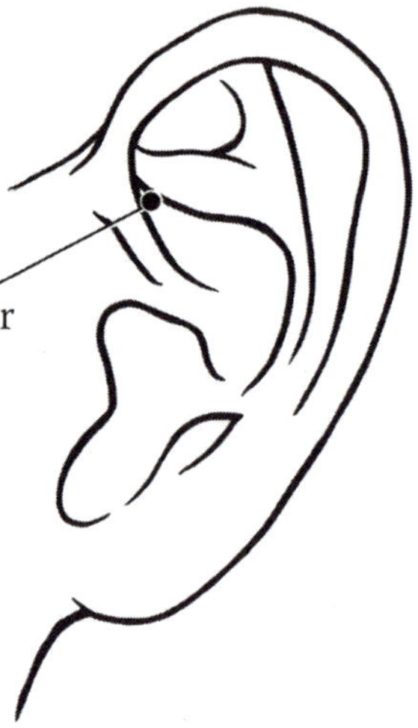

Fig 12-1 Auricular Kidney/Bladder point

Summary

- The key is regular moxibustion at home: M-LE-5 *(shitsumin/shī mián)*, KI-7, CV-6, and BL-23.

Case Study 123

Patient: Male, 61 years old

FOC: June 25, 2011

Main Complaint: Left kidney was removed because of a tumor on June 12. The function of the right kidney is not good.

Pulse Diagnosis: Kidney deficiency

Treatment: SRT on KI-7, LU-5, ST-36, CV-6, CV-12, BL-52, and BL-39. Needles inserted 5mm in BL-23 and sparrow pecking applied for 30 seconds and then needles retained. Direct moxibustion on KI-3, ST-36, BL-23, and M-LE-5 *(shitsumin/shī mián)*, which was tender.

Progress:

(2nd) July 30 – Creatinine 2.5mg/dl in blood test on July 25.

(3rd) Aug 10 – Her doctor asks, "Shall we begin dialysis?" She begins moxibustion at home instead.

(4th) Sept 16 – Results of blood test were good enough that her doctor said they could put off dialysis.

(6th) March 10 – Creatinine 2.2mg/dl in blood test on Jan 26.

Observations: The normal level for serum creatinine is 1.0mg/dl for adult males, so it is still too high. In this case the patient is not diligent about treatments, so it's difficult to do much more, but it is clear that the acu-moxa is having an effect.

CHAPTER

13

Gynecological Diseases

1. Overview

Over half the population of the human race is female and women receive acupuncture in greater numbers than men. I wonder why this is. Perhaps it is because women are more complex and delicate. Nevertheless it seems that women, more than men, are innately capable of enduring pain. This must be God's dispensation for their giving birth to babies. The main physiological feature of women (in contrast to men) is menstruation. Since this is the case, for women between middle school and their mid-50s, we must consider the menstrual cycle and regulate it if necessary.

How do we find out about abnormalities in menses? One can read the intake questionnaire or ask the patient directly, but I use the following method. Standing at the feet of the patient lying supine on the table, I press SP-6 on both sides with the base of the anterior surface of my thumbs.[1] I move my thumbs over the point, not in a vertical direction (along or against the meridian), but horizontally (across the meridian). When it feels like I'm up against bone, this is normal. When it is puffy or feels like there is some meat stuck to the bone, this indicates menstrual problems. Usually women with menstrual issues wince even when I work over SP-6 lightly this way. It is very painful. Even when there is no menstrual pain or irregularity, this sensitivity at SP-6 shows up when there is a gynecological problem. Of course, SP-6 becomes reactive with leg problems and internal organ problems as well, so it's not definitive, but there is a high probability. Aside from SP-6, reactive points for gynecological diseases include CV-4 and ST-28 on the lower abdomen, BL-27, BL-32, and M-BW-25 *(josen/shí qī zhuī xià)* in the sacral area, and BL-17 and BL-52 on the back. Aside from what the patient tells me, I can surmise the degree of gynecological problem from the reactivity of these points.

---

1. See Fig. 1-4 in *Finding Effective Acupuncture Points* for palpation with distal thumb joint.

2. Menopausal syndrome

Menopause is generally understood as the cessation of menses in women aged between 45 and 55. Menopausal syndrome is used to denote situations in which women in this age group complain of various symptoms, but medical exams show no abnormality. For a time, autonomic dysregulation was a popular term in Japan, but menopausal syndrome seems to be close to this. People understand that it's the aging process, but still they wonder if something can't be done about it. This is also like frozen shoulders or adhesive capsulitis, which is called "50-year-old shoulder" in Japan. Menopausal syndrome is related to the decrease in reproductive hormones. It is something every woman goes through, but some seem to get by without any symptoms. They seem to slip past this particular barrier.

According to the view of Dr. Atoyama, a professor at Osaka Medical University, menopausal syndrome has three primary causes: First is a deficiency of estrogen with the decrease in reproductive hormones (endogenous factor). Second is a socio-cultural reason as a woman's role changes (environmental factor). Third is suffering alone because one's character is innately serious, fastidious, and inflexible such that interpersonal pressure is felt from all sides (psychological factor).

The symptoms of menopausal syndrome vary, but the most common one is known as a "hot flash," where one suddenly breaks out in a sweat and then feels chilled afterward. Otherwise, there is cold hands, feet, and low back area, stiffness in the neck and shoulders (*katakori*), and flushing. Hormone replacement therapy is the main method of Western medical treatment. Doctors in Japan also prescribe antidepressants or Kampo herbal formulas.[2] Psychological counseling or psychiatry is the other side of the coin in Western medical approaches. In the most recent thinking, the approach in medicine is whole person treatment that aims to improve the quality of life for middle aged and elderly women. This is close to what we try to do in East Asian medicine.

2.1 View of menopause in East Asian medicine

In the first chapter of *Basic Questions* is the following passage:

> At the age of seven the Kidney qi in girls become ample and they get a new set of teeth and their hair grows long. They begin to menstruate at 14 and menstruation becomes regular when the Conception vessel opens up and the Penetrating vessel becomes abundant. Thus, they are able to bear children. At 49 they have menopause when the Conception vessel becomes deficient and the Penetrating vessel goes empty.

There is not much difference between what is recorded in ancient China and the life cycle of women around menstruation today. When the function of the right Kidney

---

2. Kampo formulas: Japanese herbal medicine that developed from Chinese medicine is called Kampo. Many medical doctors in Japan prescribe Kampo formulas (usually in granular form) which are reimbursed by the national insurance system.

(uterus) becomes abundant, the Conception and Penetrating vessels become functional in women to cause menstruation every month.

Not much is said about blood in acu-moxa therapy in Japan, but Kampo herbal therapy places emphasis on blood stasis (*oketsu*) in the treatment of women. Blood stasis occurs when old blood stagnates in some part of the body (usually the lower abdomen). This is a circulatory disorder, but the blood itself becomes thick and viscous. There is a dark color in the lips, tongue, under the eyes, and in the skin. It is a dark red or purplish color. Also, there is tenderness or induration in the lower abdomen, especially on the right side. There is tenderness with light pressure, but there may or may not be tenderness with heavy pressure.

If we view this as a circulatory obstruction unique to women, then the above abdominal finding becomes a tool of assessment along with tenderness at SP-6. In herbal therapy, blood-moving herbs are used to clear blood stasis. In traditional acupuncture, people like myself believe that it is enough to regulate qi and blood. So, along with the root treatment, we focus on treating SP-6, the lower abdomen, and the lumbo-sacral region. Among the organs, the Liver is known to store blood. Women regularly lose blood every month, so they are susceptible to anemia, or Liver (blood) deficiency. Congestion or stagnation of blood is Liver excess. There is also a strong connection with the Kidney (the function of the adrenals).

2.2 Treatment of menopause

Patterns and symptoms

Liver deficiency: gets very hot and then cools down right afterward

Liver excess:

- Spleen deficiency, Liver excess— chilling/flushing and constipation
- Lung deficiency, Liver excess—strong appetite, overweight

Kidney deficiency: chilling and heaviness in lower back and legs, tension in lower abdomen, easily fatigued, tinnitus and loss of hearing.

Root treatment

Liver deficiency: Tonify LR-8 and KI-10. Disperse only GB-38.

Spleen deficiency: Tonify SP-3. Disperse LR-2 if Liver excess.

Lung deficiency: Tonify LU-9. Disperse LR-2 if Liver excess.

Kidney deficiency: Tonify KI-7, LU-5, and CV-6.

Branch treatment

Five cones of direct moxibustion on SP-6; if possible, have the patient continue at home. Retain intradermal needle in SP-6 if moxibustion is not possible at home. Acupuncture followed by direct moxibustion on induration around ST-27. Also treat BL-17, BL-18, BL-23, BL-27, BL-32, and GB-21.

Use the above as a guide and treat to regulate the condition of the whole body. Don't insert needles in patients with a tendency toward depression; use only SRT. Look for tenderness between the spinous processes between GV-9 and -11. Apply direct moxibustion to any area that is tender or retain an intradermal needle if moxibustion is not possible. Also do moxibustion on M-LE-5 *(shitsumin/shī mián)* if the patient has insomnia. The above approach is useful for all gynecological issues.

Case Study 124

Patient: Female, 52 years old

FOC: January 24, 2011

Main Complaints: Headaches, neck/shoulder tension, nausea and stomach issues

Examination: I found considerable tenderness at SP-6. There is an induration in the abdomen at ST-27 on the right. This is a sign of blood stasis. The lower abdomen is deficient. I also found an induration at GB-20 on the right.

Pulse Diagnosis: Sunken and thin; Liver deficiency

I told the patient, "The abnormality I found at SP-6 indicates that your reproductive hormones are out of balance. Your symptoms will improve if you apply moxibustion on this point every day. Considering your age, it could be related to your menopause. You don't have your period, do you?"

She responded, "I am being treated for menopausal syndrome now. I do have my period. My symptoms are almost impossible to bear. It's about to make me crazy."

So all of her symptoms had a deep connection to her menopause. I don't usually ask in detail about menstrual problems, so I almost missed this important point.

Treatment: SRT on LR-8, KI-10, CV-6, CV-12, LI-11, BL-2. Needles retained superficially in SP-6 and auricular vertigo point. Needles inserted but not retained in right ST-27, right GB-20, GB-21, and Yanagiya's GB-20.

Direct moxibustion on LR-3, SP-6, right ST-27, BL-18, BL-23, GB-21, and right GB-20.

Progress: Her symptoms, including her stomach issues, resolved in three treatments over about two weeks. I advised her to return twice a month to maintain her health.

Observations: Once the symptoms are resolved, treatments can be terminated, but the problem is that the symptoms tend to recur. The ideal would be to continue weekly treatments for three months. If the symptoms do not recur, back off to once every 10 days and then twice a month, and finally to once a month. The stage of menopause is cleared this way, but occasional acu-moxa treatments can be recommended for health maintenance.

3. Fetal malpresentation (breech position)

It was Dr. Ishino Nobuyasu, an obstetrician who used a lot of acu-moxa in his work, who first reported that moxibustion on SP-6 was effective in correcting fetal malpresentation. This was surprising because it was traditionally said that inserting needles at SP-6, LI-4, and GB-21 would cause a miscarriage. He turned the concept around. This relates to the idea that you can actually get a great effect if you can skillfully insert a needle in points that are forbidden to needle. It is all a matter of degree. (See the excerpt from Dr. Ishino's writings at the end of this section.)

Having tried moxibustion on SP-6, I found that it did indeed work this way. Perhaps it is the function of the point, a concept that is becoming popular in Japan. Perhaps SP-6 is a point that is directly connected to the uterus.

The practitioner places the pad of his thumbs on the margin of the tibia and moves the distal joint over the bone to find something that feels odd. It is hard to describe, but it feels "gummy." I apply SRT and then do 10 cones of direct moxibustion. This is the main point for patients with fetal malpresentation, so I apply more cones to add emphasis. If possible, I have the patient apply five cones at home once a day.

3.1 My treatment for fetal malpresentation

The treatment to prevent fetal malpresentation is called for after the fifth month of pregnancy, so it is uncomfortable for the patient to lie on her back. Even if she can, it is better to treat her in the side-lying position. I take the pulse with the patient sitting on the treatment table. After that the patient lies on her side, but I have them flex the hip and knee of the top leg so the legs are not together. This way I can palpate the medial aspect of the bottom leg. In cases of Liver deficiency, I apply SRT on LR-8, KI-10, KI-3, and SP-6 on the bottom leg. Then I apply moxibustion on SP-6.

Then I go around to the back of the patient and perform SRT on BL-58, BL-32, BL-27, BL-23, and BL-52 as well as GB-20. If the patient also has sciatica or low back pain, I add treatment to the Ischial point and the Iliac point. Then I have the patient lie on her other side and repeat the above treatment on that side. I finish up the treatment with the patient seated on the table and superficially needle GB-21 and LI-11. If you want to be extra careful, these last two points can also be done with the patient side-lying.

Miura Yoshio, a member of my local study group, says, "Kidney deficiency is most common [with breech position]. Abdominal sounds can be heard after a teishin is manipulated over KI-7, and you can tell the fetus is beginning to move." This is understandable when you consider the function of the right Kidney.[3] If the pulse indicates Kidney deficiency, the points at the beginning of the treatment can be changed to KI-7 and LU-5.

When it works well, just one treatment is enough to return the fetus to the normal position. If this is not the case, it is best to continue treatments about twice a week until it does. The treatments can be concluded when an examination at the gynecologist shows that the fetal position is normal. It is ideal if the moxibustion on SP-6 is contin-

---

3. The right Kidney: In chapter 36 of the *Classic of Difficulties (Nanjing)*, it is stated as follows: "The two kidneys are not both kidneys. The one on the left is the kidney; the one on the right is the gate of life *(mìng mén)*. The gate of life is where the spirit essence resides and it's tied to source qi. In males it stores essence, in females it connects to the womb."

ued until birth. Mothers are convinced when you tell them that moxibustion not only corrects the position of the fetus, but eases labor and delivery so that the baby becomes a bright child. This will convince them to stick with the moxibustion at home.

I had two cases where the fetal position did not correct after a few treatments. In both cases, the umbilical cord was wrapped around the neck of the fetus. This is known as nuchal cord. Even when a gynecologist or a midwife manually corrects the fetal position, it is said that the position reverses again.

Anyway, acu-moxa treatments are an ideal way to treat fetal malpresentation. I would like to see this application become more widespread.

The benefits of this approach are as follows:

1. The treatment is simple, and no complicated techniques are required.
2. It doesn't take many treatments so the cost of treatment is inexpensive.
3. It reduces the mental and physical pressure on the expectant mother.

Ideally, one could determine the pattern as done in Meridian Therapy and give a root treatment with SRT. Then the mother's mood improves and she feels motivated. This could reduce the stress around labor and delivery to prevent postpartum depression.

Case Study 125

Patient: Female, 31 years old

FOC: July 3, 2010

Main Complaints: Low back pain and fetal malpresentation (5 months pregnant)

Pulse Diagnosis: Liver deficiency

Treatment: SRT on LR-8, KI-10, ST-36, LI-11, BL-58, BL-59, BL-18, BL-23, BL-52, Iliac point, SP-6, BL-27, and GB-21. Direct moxibustion on SP-6.

Progress: (2nd) July 17 – Kidney deficiency. She was told that the baby was now sideways, not breech. (4th) Sept 18 – The baby's position is normal. She has some sacral pain and a sense of obstruction in her throat, but she was told everything was normal at the hospital.

Case Study 126

Patient: Female, 32 years old

FOC: January 17, 2011

Main Complaints: Low back pain and fetal malpresentation (33rd week or 8 months pregnant). The baby has been breech since the 25th week of pregnancy. She was told that there was not enough amniotic fluid. She also has stiffness in neck and shoulders.

Pulse Diagnosis: Liver deficiency

Treatment: Teishin used on LR-8, KI-10, ST-36, SP-6, LI-11, GB-20, GB-21, BL-18, BL-23, BL-58, BL-59, BL-52, BL-27, and Ischial point. Direct moxibustion on SP-6.

Progress: (2d) Jan 21 – Kidney deficiency. She felt the baby moving around a lot on her way home from the last treatment. She was told at the hospital that the baby was sideways.

The delivery was normal, as was the baby.

Case Study 127

Patient: Female, 36 years old (dentist)

FOC: August 18, 2001

Main Complaints: Fetal malpresentation (9 months pregnant). Also hemorrhoids, frequent urination, incontinence, rhinitis, and stiffness in neck and shoulders.

Pulse Diagnosis: Liver deficiency

Treatment: SRT used on LR-8, KI-10, ST-36, SP-6, GB-20, GB-21, BL-52, Ischial point, BL-58, BL-59, and M-HN-3 (*yìn táng*). Five cones each direct moxibustion on SP-6 and BL-67.

Progress: (2d) Aug 21 – Lung deficiency. Temperature 37 °C. Insomnia. Also did direct moxibustion on GV-20 and GV-12. She felt some fetal movement during the treatment.

(4th) Aug 28 – Lung deficiency. Some fetal movement felt after the moxibustion. An exam on Aug 30 showed the fetal position had become normal. In the exam on Sept 7, it was found that the baby turned around completely once, so now it was facing in the opposite direction.

(7th) Sept 14 – Fetus 2000g. She had labor pains on Sept 28, but the baby was delivered by Caesarian section because it was small.

Comments: It is said that it is difficult for the position of the fetus to correct in the 9th month. The fact that the position corrected in this period, and that the fetus was able to continue turning, is evidence of the effect of acu-moxa treatments.

Case Study 128

Patient: Female, 29 years old

FOC: October 5, 2011

Main Complaints: Fetal malpresentation (6 months pregnant). She also has constipation and stiffness in neck and shoulders.

Pulse Diagnosis: Liver deficiency

Treatment: SRT on LR-8, KI-10, SP-6, KI-3, GB-20, GB-21, BL-23, BL-25, BL-32, BL-58, and BL-59. Five cones each direct moxibustion on SP-6, GB-21, and BL-59.

Progress and Comments: In an exam one month later, the fetus was in the normal position. This effect was probably due to performing the treatment in the earlier stage of pregnancy at six months.

3.2 Dr. Ishino on SP-6 moxibustion for pregnancy[4]

SP-6: the point for easy birth

I started using the point SP-6 right after the war (late 1940s) since I applied moxibustion on this point and corrected a baby in breech position. Later on, I learned that moxibustion on this point made the labor and delivery easy, and furthermore, the baby that was born grew strong and healthy.

Moxibustion for easy birth and its effects

A pregnant mother doing moxibustion on SP-6 is not just for the mother's body, but it also has a pronounced effect on the baby as well. What is clear is that the digestive system of such a baby is strong and they develop a sense of rhythm and they move nimbly. When you compare mothers who have done moxibustion to those who haven't, there will probably be a difference in the health of their children.

How to apply moxibustion

Based on old texts and my accumulated experience, the time to begin applying moxibustion on SP-6 is around the fifth month of pregnancy. By that time, it is thought that any morning sickness is usually finished and the placenta is stable and the growth (of the fetus) is on track. The number of cones of moxa to apply on SP-6 increases from 7 to 14 to 21 based on the number of months pregnant as follows: 5-6 months 7 cones, 7-8 months 14 cones, 9-10 months 21 cones.

Morning sickness

Overeating has the reverse effect, so reducing food intake becomes the treatment method. Keep the daily intake under 1500 calories. The mother must rest in the later stages. Otherwise, she must be careful to get enough exercise.

Breech position

In 1950 I reported in an Oriental Medical Association [meeting] on a case in which I corrected a baby in breech position with moxibustion on SP-6. The fetus moves around inside the mother for about five months, so breech position must be corrected after the second half of the sixth month, and the seventh and eighth month of pregnancy. In the final stages of pregnancy, the baby's head descends into the pelvis, and it becomes difficult to correct the position.

---

4. From Ishino Nobuyasu, *A Woman's Life and Oriental Medicine* (*Jyosei-no-Issho-to-Kanpo*). Tokyo: Midori Shobo, 1983.

4. Morning sickness and disorders during pregnancy

Common disorders that occur during pregnancy include morning sickness, low back pain, sciatica, and fetal malpresentation (discussed in the previous section). Doctors have trouble treating pregnant patients with colds and neuralgia because they can't use drugs or injections. In contrast to this, acu-moxa treatment applied judiciously can have a positive effect not only for the mother, but also the fetus. So acu-moxa is highly recommended, but one must be careful in giving treatment to pregnant patients. My rule of thumb is to not insert needles and to primarily use SRT.

Serious cases of morning sickness are very distressing. Sometimes there is nothing left to throw up and expectant mothers vomit blood. Morning sickness is not easy to treat, but results can be obtained. As far as the pattern, Spleen deficiency is common. So SP-3 and PC-7 are the main points for the root treatment, but the Extraordinary vessel point combination SP-4 and PC-6 also works well. As long as the pulse is not rapid, needles can also be retained superficially in these points.

Murata Morihiro, a member of my study group, reported in NAJOM[5] that applying SRT on SP-1 for one minute resolved morning sickness.

Case Study 129

Patient: Female, 32 years old

FOC: August 12, 2008

Main Complaint: Morning sickness. She is five months pregnant and has bad nausea.

Pulse Diagnosis: Spleen deficiency

Treatment: SRT on SP-3, PC-7, PC-8, LI-11, ST-36, GB-20, GB-21, BL-20, BL-15, and BL-23. Needles inserted superficially and retained in auricular vertigo points.

Five cones of direct moxibustion on SP-6.

Progress: The morning sickness resolved in one treatment.

Subsequently: She came in again on September 29, 2011, five months pregnant, with morning sickness. Again, the presentation was Spleen deficiency. The difference in this treatment was that I also used left PC-6 and right SP-4, applying SRT followed by direct moxibustion. I also retained an intradermal needle at left PC-6. This treatment resolved her morning sickness.

Case Study 130

Patient: Female, 35 years old

5. *North American Journal of Oriental Medicine*, Vol 19, No. 55, July 2012, "Treatment of Morning Sickness" by Murata Morihiro.

FOC: February 25, 2011

Main Complaints: She is eight months pregnant and has inguinal pain (at the origin of the pectineus muscle). The pain is mostly on the right side, but the left side also hurts a little. She gets cramps in her calves (gastrocnemius muscles). She has stiffness in her neck and shoulders.

Pulse Diagnosis: Liver deficiency

Treatment: (She is able to lie supine!) I did some SRT on the local area since she was pregnant. Usually I would insert needle 5-10mm and apply sparrow pecking three times. Then I retained intradermal needles in tender points in the inguinal region. Next I applied SRT on Yanagiya's GB-20. Then I had the patient sit on the table and repeated SRT on GB-30. After that I did the standard Liver deficiency treatment: SRT on LR-8, KI-10, ST-36, LI-11, BL-58, BL-59, GB-20, GB-21, BL-18, BL-23, BL-27, and BL-32. I concluded with five cones of direct moxibustion on SP-6.

Progress: (2nd) Mar 9 – Her pain has diminished. I did some more local treatment on the inguinal region, but this time I inserted the needles a little.

Case Study 131

Patient: Female, 38 years old

FOC: April 5, 2011

Main Complaints: She is seven months pregnant and has low back pain and stiffness in the neck and shoulders. She also has palpitations and fatigue.

Pulse Diagnosis: Lung deficiency, Liver excess

Treatment: SRT on LU-9, LR-2, and SP-6 in supine position. Next, in the side-lying position, I performed SRT on BL-52, Iliac points, BL-27, BL-59, Scalene points, and GB-20. I concluded with direct moxibustion on SP-6, BL-52, the Iliac points, and BL-27.

Progress: Her morning sickness resolved with just one treatment.

5. Menstrual pain and dysmenorrhea

Menstrual pain seems to cause a lot of suffering. Women miss work, and in extreme cases they are hospitalized every time. Other symptoms of dysmenorrhea include distention of the abdomen, headaches, nausea, vomiting, feeling weak, diarrhea, loss of appetite, and irritability. Those cases that are caused by endometriosis, adenomyosis, uterine fibroids, or pelvic inflammatory disease are known as organic or secondary dysmenorrhea. Those cases without such pathology are known as functional or primary dysmenorrhea. Functional dysmenorrhea is thought to be caused by excess production of prostaglandin or otherwise vasopressin.

5.1 Acu-moxa treatment for menstrual pain

Unusual amounts of menstrual bleeding: Kidney deficiency is primary. The Liver meridian has a special connection to all secretions (including menstrual blood and vaginal discharge). When you treat the Liver meridian, there is a tendency for very scanty secretions to actually become copious. This is very useful for scanty menstruation. For menorrhagia, we treat the Liver meridian through the Kidney meridian to reduce the amount of bleeding.

Dysmenorrhea: This is Liver and Kidney deficiency, with Gallbladder imbalance. (Okabe Sodo[6])

My sense is that acu-moxa treatments are quite effective for menstrual pain. For branch treatment I recommend three successive cones of "stick-on moxa"[7] on BL-52. It's not painful, so young people especially like it. It works even better when patients can do this moxa treatment every day at home.

Next is moxibustion on SP-6. This too works better when done regularly at home. Direct moxibustion is the most effective way. Even if a patient creates a small scar on this point, it isn't a problem because it's not in a visible location.

In terms of meridians, the Liver and Kidney are most closely related to menstrual problems. Usually I treat for Liver deficiency. When the menstrual flow is excessive, however, I like to make the treatment of the Kidney meridian primary, as Okabe suggests. I of course use standard points like KI-7 and KI-10, but I like to use LR-3 for the Liver meridian.

One patient who was being hospitalized every month with extreme menstrual pain was very pleased and told me that she no longer needed to be hospitalized thanks to acu-moxa treatments.

I had a young woman who had married a man in Tokyo show up with her mother who lives here. She wanted to get pregnant. She conceived after just one treatment. Three years later she showed up again saying she wanted another child. This time it also took just one treatment to get a child. It almost seems too good to be true, but I have many cases where women conceived in the course of receiving treatments for menstrual pain or if Liver deficiency is treated.

Case Study 132

Patient: Female, 25 years old

6. From Okabe Sodo, *Essence of Acupuncture and Moxibustion Treatment (Shinkyu Chiryo no Shinzui).* Tokyo: Sekibunodo, 1983.

7. Stick-on Moxa: An indirect moxa product that uses a cardboard with adhesive on the bottom to buffer the heat from the moxa material on top. Introduced as *Ibuki* moxa in Birch and Ida, *Japanese Acupuncture: A Clinical Guide.* Brookline: Paradigm Press, 1998.

FOC: June 6, 2001

Main Complaints: Menstrual irregularity. She also has low back pain, neck and shoulder stiffness, eye strain from computer use, weak digestive system, and lack of appetite. She has sores on her lips and in her mouth, constipation, and frequent urination. She wants to get pregnant.

History: Asthma and lumbar disk herniation

Pulse Diagnosis: Liver deficiency

Treatment: SRT used on LR-8, KI-10, CV-12, CV-6, ST-27, BL-2, Upper BL-10, GB-21, BL-43, SI-11, BL-18, BL-23, BL-27, BL-32, and BL-59. Direct moxibustion on SP-6 and BL-52.

Progress: In the course of treatments (bi-weekly) over a year she complained of asthma, delayed menses, and menstrual pain. Her pattern shifted from Liver to Kidney, to Lung and Spleen deficiency. She gave birth to a healthy child in September 2002. The next year she gave birth to her second child. She no longer complains of menstrual irregularity or pain.

6. Ovarian tumor

For an acupuncturist it is difficult to differentiate the condition of the ovaries, so we must rely on examinations by specialists. I have treated several cases with ovarian tumors, and the tumors disappeared according to the patients.

Case Study 133

Patient: Female, 64 years old

FOC: April 22, 2011

Main Complaint: She has pain in her left low back with movement since a month ago. She was told she had an ovarian tumor after an examination at a gynecologist.

Pulse Diagnosis: Liver deficiency

Treatment: SRT used on LR-8, KI-10, ST-36, LI-11, CV-12, CV-6, ST-27, GB-20, GB-21, BL-17, BL-18. Also on the right side only BL-20, BL-23, BL-27, and BL-59. Direct moxibustion on SP-6, BL-23, BL-27, and GB-21.

Progress: She received 40 treatments by the end of that year. Her pattern was usually Liver deficiency. I instructed her to apply direct moxibustion on SP-6 every day, and she was faithful in this home treatment. Her physical condition became very good, and the tumor that was 5cm from a CT scan disappeared. She is in the best physical shape that she can remember.

7. Other gynecological conditions

7.1 Coughing and gynecological issues

Here is a case where the patient made the round of hospitals in our area trying to get help for her persistent cough, and it finally stopped after acu-moxa treatments with me. Her pulse indicated Liver deficiency, but I found an abnormality in her lower abdomen. It was a large lump that could be palpated so it must have been a fairly large uterine fibroid tumor. Since she had the chronic symptom of coughing, she needed a different medical examination than what she had already been receiving. Up until then she had been seeing internal medicine doctors, like respiratory specialists, so I referred her to a gynecologist. After a while, she came back to thank me and reported that she had been discharged from the hospital. She had an operation and it turned out that her abdomen had contained a bucketful of fluids!?! Her cough went away completely after the operation. Why? It could be understood that the symptom was a result of the ascitic fluid putting pressure on her lungs. This is related to patients with edema from kidney disease coughing when lying in the supine position, but the cough subsiding when they sit up.

Anyway, this patient must have been delighted because word got out and many women came to see me for a check-up (?). I did find two women with fibroids, but it didn't turn out so well. One of them turned out to have uterine cancer instead of fibroids and she passed away in two years. Anyway, coughing is not always due to problems in the respiratory system.

7.2 Migraines and menstruation

In my experience, there is a strong relationship between migraines and the menstrual cycle. Patients with migraines need to regulate their menses.

7.3 Compensatory menstruation

This case was back in the days when I did house calls. A woman in her late 40s complained of neck and shoulder stiffness and low back pain—typical symptoms of menopause. I asked about her menses and she told me she had stopped menstruating 10 years ago. She seemed to think this was normal. What was going on?!? Come to find out, she experienced copious nosebleeds once a year. Then went back to normal as if nothing had happened. I figured that this bleeding was taking the place of menstruation.

Sure enough, as she continued to receive weekly acu-moxa treatments from me, her menstruation started again, and she no longer had massive nosebleeds. So this could be called "compensatory menstruation."

This story has a sequel. The grandchild of this patient, a girl in upper grade of elementary school, had a nosebleed that wouldn't stop. She came to me for acu-moxa treatments. The moxibustion, especially at BL-12, was effective in stopping the bleeding. Nose bleeding must have been an inherited constitutional tendency.

7.4 Uterine tumors and low back pain

This story continues. I was treating the 70-some-year-old mother-in-law of the above middle-aged patient. I was giving whole body treatments for her complaints of neck and shoulder stiffness, low back pain, and leg pain. One day I was treating points on her abdomen and I just happened to palpate her inguinal region. There were large lumps in her lymph nodes. Oh no! I referred her to a gynecologist but it was too late. Her uterine cancer was in an advanced stage.

I also treated a woman in her 40s whose mother-in-law told me that her low back pain was probably due to cancer because she had undergone surgery for breast cancer. I gave her a series of treatments, but we found out later that she had uterine cancer. It must have metastasized to her spine.

Some patients know they have uterine cancer but absolutely refuse surgery. As long as they are fully informed, we can give acu-moxa treatments as palliative care. There is a definite benefit. The key is not to insert too many needles. It will exhaust the patient if you do. I recommend using SRT or contact needling, or teishin treatments. We can expect a strengthening of their immune function. The depression lifts and they feel happier. The pain also diminishes and their appetite improves. Just be mindful about keeping the stimulation light.

7.5 Uterine fibroid tumors

We can treat fibroids as long as they are egg-sized. Those that are fist-sized or bigger, however, require surgery. Okaba Sodo, one of the founders of Meridian Therapy, said this. I have no experience of complete cures for uterine fibroid tumors. Even though they are benign tumors, and there is no danger, it is inconvenient when they become really large. And they could turn out to be uterine cancer. I have known women who suffered and died from uterine cancer, so I think that it's better to surgically remove them at an appropriate time when they are still small. At least this is what I have come to believe from my experience.

7.6 Uterine ptosis

I understand it really doesn't feel good when the uterus sags. They say it is felt especially when walking around. Extreme cases turn into uterine prolapse, but it is better to have surgery if things go that far. Acu-moxa treatments can be effective in mild cases of ptosis. The discomfort ceases. On the abdomen, treat points around CV-4. Find the tightest or most depressed points above or below CV-4 and insert a needle. When a needle is inserted shallowly, a light comfortable sensation extends to the urethra (or the vagina or the cervix). On the low back, treat BL-23, BL-27, and BL-32 with SRT. Also on the legs, treat SP-6 with SRT. As far as meridians, the Spleen, Kidney, Liver, and Bladder are involved. Among these, the Spleen and Liver meridians are most important.

7.7 Acu-moxa for postpartum issues

Women who have just given birth tend to flush. The lower burner becomes deficient so the upper burner becomes excessive and this causes flushing. This is known as "upper excess lower deficiency." It can cause dizziness known as blood vertigo. In the Mubun school of acupuncture[8] there is a famous technique called "Fire Drawing Needle." According to *Compilations of the Secrets of Acupuncture*, the Mubun school text, "This needle technique [is applied] in the middle between the two kidneys [zones] 3 units below the navel. It is a technique in which [the point] 3 units below the navel is needled to pull down the qi that is rising when there is dizziness that is blood vertigo after giving birth. Even when there is no dizziness after giving birth, it is good to needle about three times within 31 days. After all, pathology in general when one is upper excess and lower deficiency, the qi always rises [flushes]. Use the Fire Drawing Needle for people like this."

When there is postpartum dizziness, it is good to do this Fire Drawing Needle technique on points on the lower abdomen like CV-6 and CV-4. Deficiency in the lower abdomen inevitably causes excess or tension and hardness between the bottom of the xiphoid process and CV-12. The excess in the upper abdomen disappears by performing the Fire Drawing Needle technique. The above passage says "when there is dizziness," but there doesn't have to be any dizziness to use this technique. Just tell your postpartum patients, "I'm going to do the 'Fire Drawing Needle' to direct the qi downward and prevent postpartum flushing." Then carefully tonify points in the lower abdomen using SRT. And this technique is not just for postpartum mothers; there are many people whose lower abdomen is deficient (and prone to flushing). So the application of this technique is limitless.

7.8 Discriminating the sex of the fetus

❶ Compare the strength of the pulse on the right and left sides. When the left side is stronger, it is a boy. When the right side is stronger, it is a girl.

❷ Have the pregnant mother stand facing away from you. Ask her to turn around and look at you. When she turns around to the left it is a boy; when she turns around to the right it is a girl. The above two methods come from the yin-yang principle where the left is yang and male, the right is yin and female.

❸ When the face of the pregnant mother is severe, it is a boy. When the face of the pregnant mother is gentle, it is a girl.

The first two of these sayings are from the classics and the third is a traditional belief in Japan. In my experience, the first two are correct most of the time. These days, ultrasound and imaging makes it possible to determine the sex very accurately, but sometimes it is unclear. When you can guess the sex of the baby correctly, patients trust you more. You can just tell them that this is how they determined the sex in the old days. There are two more methods mentioned in the *Pulse Classic.*[9]

---

8. Mubun school: This traditional Japanese style of acupuncture has been discussed in detail in *Introduction to Meridian Therapy*, p. 89-90.

9. *Pulse Classic (Mai jing)* by Wang Shu-He, c. 280.

❶ If the pulse is floating it is a girl, if the pulse is sunken it is a boy.

❷ When there is a hard knot in the mother's left breast it is a boy. When the right breast is hard it is a girl.

Q&A

QUESTION AND ANSWER NO. 7

How to prevent illness

Q. Please tell me how to prevent illness.

A. I summarized the following points about preventing illness. Please use it for the benefit of yourself and your patients.

The principles of disease prevention

(1) No smoking

When you can't quit by yourself, consult a doctor or a smoking-cessation clinic to get nicotine patches.

(2) Diet

Always eat breakfast, but eat only to 60% of being full. Eating until you are full or over eating becomes a cause of dementia. Chew each mouthful over 50 times. When you chew well, this stimulates the cerebrum and prevents dementia. Don't eat side dishes together with rice. The secret is to eat rice by itself. Japanese food is the ideal diet. Japanese cuisine is sought after and incorporated all over the world. In the modern era Japanese have been adopting an American diet and shortening their lifespan. Eat more vegetables. Eat less meat. It's good to remove the fat. Brush your teeth well after a meal. It has been found that periodontal diseases can cause many diseases.

(3) Alcohol consumption

Drink about ¾ cup of sake (or wine) daily. The World Health Organization discourages alcohol consumption, but in Japan, sake is known as the king of medicines. They say drinking moderately nurtures the digestive system, so a little alcohol improves digestion and brightens the spirit. Recently it has been found that those who drink a little have a lower chance of getting myocardial infarctions and cerebral embolisms. Drinking to excess, however, is not good for you. The substance acetaldehyde, which is created when breaking down alcohol, can cause cancer and various diseases.

(4) Exercise

Be sure to get some exercise. The ideal is said to be one hour a day or 10,000 steps. It is enough, however, just to walk at a fast pace for 20 minutes three days a week. Also, be sure to use your fingers. Moving the thumbs especially is said to stimulate the brain. Typing, piano, and the abacus can be done for the fun of it, without worrying about proficiency, as a way of preventing senility. Massaging the fingertips is also very good. Gently massage the fingertips with your thumb and index fingers. While you are at it, massage your toes the same way. The fingers and toes are connected to the internal organs and brain, so this massage is very beneficial. It is also good to make a habit of calisthenics, yoga, qigong, Taiji, abdominal breathing, skin brushing and other health regimens. Standing on one leg is also good for balance and preventing falling. Be sure, however, not to overdo anything.

(7) Sleep

Around 7 hours of sleep is good. People who oversleep tend to get dementia.

(8) Stress

Do your best to reduce your stress levels. If you are going through difficult times, try to change your attitude. When there is no stress at all, however, a person is more likely to get dementia. It is fine to be concerned, but don't let yourself become anxious.

(7) Vocalization

Use your voice. Singing, reciting sutras, doing karaoke, reciting poetry, and reading out loud are all good. Remember, however, to breathe abdominally and to keep your attention at your abdomen. The effect is not as good when just the throat is used.

(8) Conversation

Having a social life is very beneficial to one's health. People who live alone become like animals. You can talk to your television if you live alone. Women especially have a clear head when they have people to talk to.

(9) Hobbies

It is good to take an interest in things. Computers, e-mails, and learning foreign languages is recommended. Rather than trying to improve your overall ability, which can be stressful, just work on learning more vocabulary. Even if you learn to speak just a little, that's a great accomplishment.

(10) Neck and shoulder tension

Katakori, or neck and shoulder tension, can cause cerebral embolisms and dementia. Nobody dies of back pain, but many people die because of chronic neck and shoulder tension. It is important to release tension in the neck and shoulders to improve cerebral circulation.

(11) Acupuncture and moxibustion

Acu-moxa is a medicine that treats disease before it appears. By taking the pulse we can determine which organs and meridians will have a problem, and then give treatment to correct it. This is known as "treating disease before it starts." Moxibustion that can be done on oneself is also effective. The power of moxibustion should not be underestimated. There are countless cases of difficult diseases that have resolved by regularly doing moxibustion for a long time. It is a simple method that anyone can practice to prevent disease and promote health.

CHAPTER 14

Other Diseases

1. Cancer and acu-moxa treatment

In this day and age it is said that one out of two people in Japan will get cancer, and one out of three will die of it. So the issue of treating these patients with acu-moxa is inescapable. This is why I am devoting a section to this topic. In years past, it was forbidden to say that acu-moxa was effective for treating cancer. I recall the heated debate over whether to feature an article on cancer treatment by Ohta Rinsai in the newsletter of my local Ohita Acupuncture Association. It was because this article claimed that acu-moxa was effective for cancer. Recently, the All-Japan Acupuncture and Moxibustion Association has taken up the theme of acu-moxa treatment for cancer. It is known that acu-moxa is effective for a wide range of diseases, and it is necessary to clinically evaluate how much acu-moxa works for cancer. In this section, I will consider this question from the cases of cancer that I have come across.

The three primary methods of treatment for cancer are surgery, chemo-therapy, and radiation. It is held that once the patient gets past the acute phase, any treatment that strengthens immunity is good. This is where complementary medicine comes into play and acu-moxa treatment is one option.

1.1 My past experiences treating cancer patients

Hepatic cancer: He was a priest of a Buddhist temple. This was early in my practice when I did house calls. I mostly treated tender points. There was a mass in his abdomen that I palpated. He had a bad case of constipation, and he was happy that my acupuncture treatment gave him a good bowel movement. I inserted needles and it was deep needling compared to what I do today. I probably needled into the abdominal mass, even though it is said that tumors are aggravated when you stimulate them directly.

In one more case, I palpated hardness in the right subcostal region in a male patient with liver disease. He loved to drink, and he was happy because acu-moxa treatments always made him feel better. He eventually passed away with hepatic cancer. Perhaps I should have been more strict and told him he needed to quit drinking even if he wouldn't have liked me. Or perhaps it is okay to have a shorter life in which you do as you please. This question also applies to the issue of smoking.

Uterine cancer: She was an elderly woman. I made house calls once a week to treat her low back pain. One day, I happened to palpate her inguinal region and found swollen lymph nodes. I referred her to a gynecologist and it was found that she had uterine cancer.

In another instance, I treated a middle-aged woman who had a history of breast cancer. Her main complaint was low back pain, but it turned out that her cancer had metastasized to her spine. (The above two cases are mentioned in Chapter 13 in section 7.4 "Uterine tumors and low back pain.")

Uterine cancer and coughing: An elderly patient had persistent coughing for two years. I found a tumor in her lower abdomen when I did abdominal diagnosis. I referred her to a gynecologist, suspecting a uterine fibroid. Her cough went away after she had surgery, but it turned out that she actually had cancer. (This case is mentioned in Chapter 13 in section 7.1 "Coughing and gynecological issues.")

Stomach cancer: She was a middle-aged woman with stomach pain. This patient came from a neighboring prefecture. Her stomach pain resolved with just one treatment, her appetite returned, and her expression became bright. There was a lump about 5cm across around CV-12. She was aware that this was cancer. She did well for a while, and she even talked about moving closer (so it would be easier to get treatments), but gradually she started to become very fatigued and terminated treatments.

Lung cancer: A middle-aged man with terminal lung cancer. I gave him several treatments, but there was no effect. The treatments did not alleviate his pain.

Metastasized spinal cancer: I saw this patient 40 years ago. Her main complaint was low back pain. X-rays showed no abnormalities, and several acu-moxa treatments had no effect. Her tendon reflexes were exaggerated and she had pain with percussion at M-BW-25 *(jōsen/shí qī zhuī xià)*. It was extremely painful. I recommended another medical exam and she was admitted into a national hospital. Shortly after that her legs became paralyzed. One month later it was finally determined that she had spinal cancer that had metastasized from her pancreas.

Malignant lymphoma: I saw an elderly woman in her 70s. She had swollen submaxillary lymph nodes. The medical exam revealed that she had cancer. She was hospitalized for a time, but as she became terminal, she insisted that she just had to receive acu-moxa treatments. So she got special permission from her doctor and came to my clinic a few times for treatment. Unfortunately, the treatments had no effect.

1.2 Case histories of cancer treatment

Case Study 134

Patient: Female, 80 years old

FOC: June 20, 2008

Symptoms and Condition: There is a shadow in her right lung. Six years ago she had a medical check-up and was told that the CT scan revealed a shadow in her right lung. They have been monitoring this every year, and surgery is being recommended because the shadow is growing. She doesn't want to have surgery. She has pain in her knees and right shoulder. Sleep, appetite, urination, and bowel movements are all normal.

History: Pneumonia and hypertension

Pulse Diagnosis: Liver deficiency

Treatment: SRT applied on LR-8, KI-10, CV-6, CV-12, right LU-1, GB-20, GB-21, GV-10, SI-11, BL-17, BL-18, BL-23, right M-UE-48 *(mae kengū/jiān qián)*, and medial M-LE-16 *(shitsugan/xī yǎn)*. Direct moxibustion on LI-11, ST-36, CV-12, right LU-1, GV-10, right SI-11, right BL-17, PC-8. Additional direct moxibustion points on subsequent treatments were BL-18, BL-23, ST-35, M-LE-16 *(shitsugan/xī yǎn)*, and right M-UE-48 *(mae kengū/jiān qián)*. She continued with moxibustion at home.

Progress: (3rd) Jul 18 – Her lymphocytes increased suddenly.

(13th) Dec. 9 – The shadow in the CT scan became lighter. Lymphocytes continue to increase. She received 14 treatments in 2008.

(25th) Aug. 25, 2009 – The tumor in the chest is holding steady. It is not growing. She feels a bit dizzy. A subarachnoid hemorrhage has been discovered. She was told that the MRI shows that she had a cerebral embolism in the past. She received 22 treatments in 2009.

(43rd) Jun. 8, 2010 – X-rays show that the shadow in her chest has shrunk from 4.7cm to 2.2cm. Her doctor asked, "What happened?" She received 23 treatments in 2010.

(62nd) Jul. 5, 2011 – She is not getting any exams this year.

Comments: Her daughter entered acupuncture school even though she was middle-aged. She wanted her mother to choose acupuncture and moxibustion over surgery also because she was advanced in age, so she sent her to my clinic. The patient also did not want surgery. She lived two hours away by car, however, and couldn't come for treatment that often so she did moxibustion at home. Her husband was over 80 years old, but he was still working as a teacher in an acupuncture school. He did the moxibustion on his wife, and he applied many cones on his wife without giving up. After three years, however, he started to complain that he was getting tired of it. Her cancer didn't get any worse and her condition was good, so he was being optimistic that things would continue to go well. There is what is called "pseudo-cancer" with a lung tumor, so it could actually be benign. Yet I would like more time with this patient to witness the event of the tumor completely disappearing.

Case Study 135

Patient: Female, 70 years old

FOC: December 5, 2003

Symptoms and Condition: She fatigues very easily. She had an operation for stomach cancer 10 months ago (Feb 8). The cancer had spread all over her abdomen, so the incision was closed without excision. She is on medications. She has no appetite. Her weight is 37kg. She has cold feet. There is no strength in her voice. She has not been told that she has terminal cancer.[1]

History: Thyroid disease and ovarian tumor in her youth (both resolved), glaucoma, cataracts (surgery scheduled)

Pulse Diagnosis: Sunken, rapid, and deficient; Spleen deficiency

Treatment: SRT applied on SP-3, PC-7, ST-36, CV-6, CV-12, KI-27, BL-2, GB-20, GB-21, GV-14 (very tender), left SI-11, BL-18, BL-20, and BL-23. Direct moxibustion on ST-36, BL-18, BL-20, and BL-23. She was instructed to apply moxibustion at home on the above eight points.

Progress:

(2nd) early Jan 2004 – She had no pain.

(7th) She has no energy.

(9th) She has an appetite.

(12th) Her complexion is better and her appetite is good. She received 11 treatments in 2004. Aug. 24, 2005 – She is going to have surgery for cataracts. Direct moxibustion on LI-11. She received 6 treatments in 2005.

(18th) Jan. 31, 2006 – Lung deficiency. Her appetite is good. She received three treatments in 2006, and three treatments in 2007 (Jan, Feb & Sep).

(24th) Feb 2, 2008 – Liver deficiency. Her appetite is good. Tinnitus in right ear.

(26th) Liver deficiency. She got pain in her tongue eating pickles. Her weight is 41kg, so she has gained 4kg. She received four treatments in 2008.

(28th) Liver deficiency. She has become a bit plump. She received two treatments in 2009.

(30th) Apr 14, 2010 – Liver deficiency. She has not done any moxibustion since New

---

1. Disclosure of terminal diagnosis: It is not uncommon in Japan for the patient to remain uninformed about a terminal diagnosis. Disclosure is dependent on the family's wishes and the patient's mental status.

Years. Problem with liver function. She received just one treatment in 2010.

(31ST) Mar 28, 2011 – Liver deficiency. Right knee pain. Extra moxibustion points treated on the knee. Her liver function is fine. She is doing fine in 2012.

COMMENTS: What is noteworthy about this case is home moxibustion treatment over eight years. The patient told me she is going to retire from her work as a nurse to take care of her own mother. Food began to taste good again after nine months of acu-moxa treatments. Initially her pulse indicated Spleen or Lung deficiency, sometimes Kidney deficiency. By the end of 2006 it became hard to distinguish between Lung and Liver deficiency, and by 2007 her pattern changed to Liver deficiency. Currently she does gardening, including weeding, and she is the picture of health. It has already been eight years since she had cancer, and there is little doubt that the remission was due to acu-moxa treatments, especially moxibustion. This case reveals the potential of acu-moxa treatments.

Case Study 136

PATIENT: Female, 76 years old

FOC: August 22, 2005

MAIN COMPLAINTS: Sciatica in left leg, ankle pain, knee pain, Ménière's syndrome, tumor in right lung

PULSE DIAGNOSIS: Liver deficiency

TREATMENT: SRT applied on LR-8, KI-10, LI-11, CV-6, CV-12, GB-20, GB-21, BL-18, BL-23, left Gluteal point, right SI-11, right LU-1, ST-35, M-LE-16 *(shitsugan/xī yǎn)*, and GB-40. Direct moxibustion on LI-11, ST-36, ST-35, M-LE-16 *(shitsugan/xī yǎn)*, left Gluteal point, BL-25, right SI-11, right BL-13, and right LU-1. She was instructed to do moxibustion at home.

PROGRESS: This patient did moxibustion faithfully at home and came for treatments almost every week in 2005 (18 times). She received 36 treatments in 2006. She received 20 more treatments up until March 2007. She resumed treatments in October 2008 and received 9 treatments. She received 16 more treatments up through September 2009. She received 11 treatments in 2010. The size of the tumor was unchanged in July 2010. She received 19 treatments in 2011. Most recently she has been coming in about twice a month.

COMMENTS: In the six-year course of treatment, I treated this patient for a tumor in her lung along with joint pain. Having said that, I used just a couple of extra points like LU-1 and SI-11 for the tumor. It hasn't diminished or disappeared, but the patient is doing fine. Ménière's syndrome was alleviated along with her sciatica, while the knee pain has come and gone. These treatments could be preventing the progress of her tumor.

Summary

1. Always keep in mind the possibility of a tumor.
2. Direct moxibustion is especially effective for the treatment of cancer.
3. Acu-moxa treatments support patients going through conventional cancer treatment.

1.3 Things to bear in mind when treating cancer patients

The following things need to be kept in mind as one takes on the treatment of patients with cancer.

❶ It is imperative to have the patient undergo a medical exam to confirm the nature of the cancer, if they haven't already. If there is any doubt about cancer, advise the patient to get a thorough exam, and refer them to a medical facility capable of doing this. It is risky to undertake acu-moxa treatments without a diagnosis.

There are some patients who believe in acu-moxa so much that they say, "I only want to be seen by you." Don't indulge such patients. When there is a definitive diagnosis of cancer and the patient wants acu-moxa treatment, we need the informed consent of both the patient and their partners or responsible family member. If the cancer is advanced, the patient will gradually deteriorate. There can be hard feelings when a patient does not fully understand the role of acu-moxa and hopes for too much. It is very important to fully inform the patient and family members.

❷ Don't forget to clearly explain the benefits of acu-moxa treatments to the patient and family members. Explain in a simple way how acu-moxa treatment strengthens immunity, lifts the mood, and alleviates pain. When depression associated with a life-threatening illness lifts, this also helps slow down the progress of the disease.

❸ Determine the pattern (yin and yang organ pattern).

❹ Focus on the root treatment and keep the branch treatment to a minimum. Select effective points that have a broad effect.

❺ Use mostly SRT (super-rotation technique). When the patient is emaciated or in a great deal of pain, use SRT or teishin only for treatment. Teishin is best for terminal patients. It can reduce the pain. A few needles can be inserted when the patient is in good condition.

❻ Moxibustion also must be kept light. Use smaller cones of direct moxibustion or remove the cone before it burns all the way down.

1.4 Post-surgical treatment for cancer patients

Acu-moxa treatments are highly recommended for post-surgical patients. Treatments before surgery are also good. Western medical treatments at a hospital and acu-moxa treatments can have a combined effect. This is borne out in the case study below, and I'm sure many acupuncturists have encountered this in their own practices. The satisfaction of the patient, the doctor, and the acupuncturist can be expected. It is a real opportunity for acupuncturists, and we must study more about how to be helpful in these situations.

Case Study 137

Patient: Male, 65 years old

FOC: October 16, 2006

Situation and Symptoms: He had surgery to remove a tumor in his left femur on July 10, 2006. I treated him for pain related to this surgery starting in October of 2006. He had a second operation in April of 2007. After the operation, there was pain with moving and walking. He also has low back pain.

History: Cerbral embolism, angina pectoris, and hypertension

Pulse Diagnosis: Liver deficiency/Lung deficiency ··· Liver excess/Lung deficiency ··· Lung deficiency/Heart excess

Palpation: Heat felt at left M-LE-16 *(shitsugan/xī yǎn)*. The surgical scar on the medial thigh extends about 20cm above SP-10. It feels like the muscles have been shaved off, and the tissue is hard. There is tenderness at the lower margin of the scar (SP-10) and this matches exactly with where the patient has pain. He experiences pain and fatigue from his low back and hips down to his lower leg during movement and when walking. He says that treatment alleviates the pain and eases the movement of his body.

Treatment: Only the details of more recent treatments will be given here. With Liver deficiency, SRT is applied on LR-8, KI-10, CV-6, CV-12, LI-11, right ST-36, GB-20, and GB-21. Needles retained superficially in BL-18, BL-23, and BL-25. Needle inserted 3mm in left SP-10 and sparrow pecking applied. Needle inserted 5mm in left side and sparrow pecking applied at ST-36, GB-33, ST-32, and Onodera's point.

Direct moxibustion on leg points on the left including ST-36, SP-10, GB-31, BL-59. Moxibustion on back associated points on the left side, especially BL-25.

Comments: In six years, this patient has received 490 treatments. There has been a clear effect in preventing recurrence and alleviation of his symptoms. I am continuing to see this patient twice a week (as of June 2011).

Case Study 138

Patient: Male, 18 years old

FOC: June 18, 2011

Main Complaints: He had surgery in February 2011 for synovial sarcoma[2] that started

---

2. A relatively rare form of malignant synovioma, which occurs mostly between that ages of 10 and 40 and affects males and females equally. It tends to occur often in the lower extremities, especially the hip and knee joints adjacent to joint capsules, synovial sacs, and tendon sheaths, but it also occurs in places completely unrelated to such tissue such as the neck and torso. Simple X-rays often reveal a shadow of a

in his right kidney. He has strong nausea from chemotherapy and feels terrible.

Pulse Diagnosis: Kidney deficiency

Treatment: SRT applied on KI-7, LU-5, BL-23, PC-6, and SP-4. Teishin used on LI-11, ST-36, GB-20, and GB-21. Intradermal needle retained in left PC-6. Direct moxibustion on M-LE-5 *(shitsumin/shī mián)* until heat was felt on right with three cones, on the left with five.

Progress: (2nd) Sep 20 – He reports feeling better with treatment. Spleen deficiency. Direct moxibustion on both PC-6 and SP-4.

(3rd) Oct 12 – His appetite has returned. Spleen deficiency.

Comments: The patient says he feels better after treatment. He is a senior in high school and is the captain of the soccer team. He is working hard to build himself up for soccer matches, and as his schedule doesn't match up with mine, treatments have been sporadic, but his family is very pleased that he is doing much better. The day after he received his third treatment, the local paper featured an article on his brave fight with cancer. Acu-moxa contributed greatly to his recovery, and SRT and teishin were the main modalities.

Further Progress: (4th) February 24, 2012 – He has had ascites for a month, and two to three liters of fluid were removed the first few days of treatment and about 200ml a day thereafter. Liver deficiency. SRT applied on KI-3, LR-3, and LR-8. Teishin used on BL-17, BL-18, and BL-23 in the side-lying position.

(5th) Mar 2 – There is no more fluid accumulation after the last treatment. Spleen deficiency.

(6th) Mar 10 – No more fluid accumulation.

Further Comments: Ascites or fluid accumulation in the abdomen which had continued for a month stopped with just one treatment. The patient was hospitalized, and he came for treatment the day he was discharged from the hospital. It was a very simple treatment, but the results were good and everyone was very pleased. The survival rate for synovial sarcoma is not very good but I hope that the acu-moxa treatments will extend his life as much as possible. While I had hoped for the best, the patient died several months later.

1.5 Acu-moxa in conjunction with conventional treatment for liver cancer

Finally, I had a case recently with promising results from acu-moxa treatments in conjunction with conventional medical treatment for liver cancer. The patient was a 65-year-old woman who came to me on January 4, 2012. She was diagnosed with liver cancer the year before after a check-up. The tumor was in several places, so she received

---

tumor, and in about half the cases within this shadow there are spots of calcification. Treatment generally consists of surgery. The five year survival rate is 30-50%, and the 10 year rate is even lower. (Nanzando Medical Dictionary CD-ROM, Pro Medica Version 3, 2007) chemotherapy and laparoscopic surgeries. According to the patient the strategy of this treatment at a hospital was to remove her liver after the cancer had been reduced to a certain level.

She had worked for a long time at a soy sauce factory and had even put off her retirement. This diagnosis came soon after she retired and was finally ready to take it easy, so this really made her depressed. She came back to me for treatment after an absence of about a year. Before that time she had been coming to me a few times a month. Mostly I was treating her for shoulder joint issues, and I usually did four points for root treatment and the rest was local treatment. I had done very little treatment on her abdomen.

Reviewing her charts, she had a history of duodenal ulcers and liver dysfunction. I regret that I had not treated her abdomen and back associated points more. If only I had done this and she had continued with treatments, perhaps we could have prevented this.

When I palpated her abdomen, she had quite a bit of fat and she told me her primary physician had told her to lose some weight. I pressed lightly on her abdomen to find indurations and retained needles superficially and applied small cones of direct moxibustion after removing the needles. These included points like CV-12, ST-21, ST-19, upper ST-19, right LR-14, and CV-6. At the end of each treatment I retained an intradermal needle at either right ST-19, CV-12, or left ST-21.

Her pulse indicated Liver deficiency, and in addition to root treatment points, I applied direct moxibustion on LR-3. On her back I found induration and tender points between BL-17 and BL-20 on the right. I selected the tightest point on the right and inserted the needle and rotated it a bit longer than other points. This was followed by direct moxibustion on BL-17 and the tight and tender point on the right side. I instructed the patient to apply moxibustion on LR-3, ST-36, CV-12, and left ST-21. I had her begin with the milder stick-on moxa for self-treatment. Eventually I had her treat herself with direct moxibustion.

I had this patient come twice a week for the first month, and once a week the following month. Her disturbed mental state finally settled down, and the results from the hospital started looking better and a smile returned to her face. It is hard to say how far we can get, but I am hopeful that this combination of acu-moxa and Western medical treatment will have a good outcome.

Update: This patient continues to get treatments from me twice a month and a medical exam in June 2017 showed no abnormalities.

Summary

1. Acu-moxa can also be effective for the side effects of chemotherapy.

1.6 Preventing cancer

I recommend acu-moxa treatments once a week for prevention. Getting treatments every day would be even better if one could afford it. Of course, you also need to follow general recommendations for cancer prevention. It is inevitable as the incidence of cancer increases that acupuncturists also get cancer. It is interesting to look at the incidence of cancer among acupuncturists in Japan. In the October 2006 issue of *Ido-no-Nippon (Journal of Japanese Acupuncture and Moxibustion),* the publisher Soshichiro Tobe featured a list of 156 notable acupuncturists since 1945 who had died together with the causes of death. Looking at acupuncturists who died between the ages of 50 and 80 in this list, 41 died of cancer. Especially when they are acupuncturists I respected, I am at a loss to explain this. Why did they get cancer? There are many causes of cancer including heredity, heavy drinking, smoking, excess consumption of animal food products and lack of vegetables and fruits, overwork, lack of exercise, and heavy stress. But we are acupuncturists! If we really believe in acupuncture, it makes sense that we would give ourselves acupuncture all the time. Just once a week would be enough if we are healthy. We could exchange treatments with colleagues. For me, daily self-treatments serves as the best prevention. It is a complete contradiction when an acupuncturist dies of cancer without receiving acupuncture. It may not be possible to avoid cancer entirely even as we provide acupuncture treatments. Nevertheless, at least we can find a method of acu-moxa treatment that allows us to co-exist with cancer.

When I organized the Beppu Conference of the Japan Traditional Acupuncture and Moxibustion Society in 1998, I asked Ryuji Shimada, the president at the time, to give a talk on how cancer was viewed, treated, and prevented in the classics. I will share a summary of this talk below.

Cause

"The cause of cancer is excess emotions such as grief and anger, also chilling from within and without, that is, exposure to cold and cold food and drinks. It occurs when measures are not taken in a timely manner to such imbalances."

In other words, the cause is stress and getting chilled while also not receiving preventative treatments before it produces cancer.

Prevention

1. Avoid things that cause qi stagnation.

2. When qi gets stuck, clear it as soon as possible. Both functional stasis and structural stasis are reversible. Structural pathology like cancer can be turned back into a qi stasis (which gave rise to it) with acu-moxa treatments. And the qi stasis can be resolved.

3. When there is a possibility of cancer, get treatments once a week.

   Ryuji Shimada also said that when you feel a strange sensation of cold when palpating a patient, it is probably cancer or a pre-cancerous lesion.

Summary

1. Cancer is caused by stress and chilling of the body.
2. Acu-moxa is one way to prevent cancer.
3. Release qi stasis with acupuncture, and don't allow blood (structural) stasis.

2. Dizziness

There is nothing really that compares to the discomfort of dizziness. This is true for any symptom, but only those who have experienced it understand. In the early years of practice when I hardly had any patients, I would treat anyone at any time, so even now, when I have a lot of patients, I am still in the habit of treating every patient that shows up even if I'm exhausted. Even now when I'm 80 years old, when patients plead with me to treat them that day, I try to work them in somehow. This is ostensibly because I can't stand the thought of them suffering, but the truth of it may be because of my early experience. In any case, I continue giving treatments (even if I'm tired) no matter what symptoms I myself may be experiencing. Dizziness, however, is another matter. When the room starts to swirl and waves of nausea come, I can no longer remain standing. This is why, when I can use just one needle to clear this symptom up, the passage in the first chapter of *Vital Axis* fits perfectly: "… like the wind blowing the clouds away. It becomes clear and bright as if looking into the blue sky."

Even as a child I had a tendency toward dizziness. When I had to stand for a long time in the school yard, for example, I would start to feel sick. The worst time was when I took ill as a teenager and I got dizzy at the same time as coughing up blood. The vertigo would have my head spinning, and then I would go into respiratory distress with hemoptysis. When I recovered a bit, a wave of dizziness would come over me, and this vicious cycle repeated itself. I understood then how life could be hell. While I was afraid to die, yet I sometimes thought that it might be okay if I could escape that suffering.

Even after I recovered, this tendency toward vertigo remained, so after I became an acupuncturist, I continued searching for ways to relieve this condition by trial and error. As I began to incorporate Meridian Therapy and study the classics, I started to understand the theory behind dizziness.

2.1 Dizziness is related to the Liver

There is the following passage in chapter 78 of *Basic Questions:* "The various wind [conditions with] shaking and dizziness are all associated with the Liver." Simply put, all dizziness and loss of balance are related to the Liver. Treating the Liver will cure it. 'All' means there are no exceptions. Associated with the Liver means the organ as well as the Liver meridian. Which point is used? Any point on the Liver meridian should work, but the essential points are best. This means the five-phases points and the connecting, cleft, back associated, and front alarm points.

But then there is the following passage in chapter 68 of the *Classic of Difficulties*: "Well points control fullness in the epigastrium." This can be taken to mean that using the well points is good for the symptom of tension or hardness in the pit of the stomach. The epigastrium or pit of the stomach becomes hard when a person has dizziness, headaches, or neck and shoulder tension. Objectively, tension or hardness can be palpated. Subjectively, the patient feels fullness and discomfort in the epigastrium.

Putting these two passages together, it can be surmised that the well point of the Liver meridian, LR-1, is good for dizziness. Sure enough, Okabe Sodo, one of the founders of Meridian Therapy, stated as follows: "LR-1 and LR-8 work well for symptomatic treatment [of dizziness]."[3] Using these points together, I find they work wonderfully. SRT works well, and also the needle can be retained superficially after SRT. When the dizziness is acute, when doing house calls for example, it is good to retain needles superficially and rotate them now and again. Direct moxibustion on LR-1 also works, but you must apply the moxa in a way that does not cause pain.

2.2 Points related to dizziness

Based on the reactive points that show up in patients with dizziness, the following points are closely related to this condition:

GV-22: A tender point can be found on the crown. The point is soft and indicates poor blood circulation. Pressing is painful but pleasurable at the same time. Sometimes the tender point is at GV-20. More often the reaction appears more anterior on points like GV-22. While I have done bloodletting because the point is boggy, this makes the dizziness worse. Also, inserting big needles can exacerbate the symptom. I recommend SRT or superficial retention with a very small needle (02 gauge, 0.12mm). Five small cones of direct moxibustion is also good. Moxibustion at home is also recommended.

GB-20: This point is effective when it is hardened and there is an induration. I recommend SRT and superficial retaining or retaining an intradermal needle. Avoid strong stimulation. The above two points are directly related to dizziness.

TB-17: This point seems to have some relationships to dizziness from inner ear problems.

UPPER BL-10: When I ask patients with dizziness which part of their neck is the stiffest, most often they point to GB-20, and upper BL-10 next. The trapezius gets hard with dizziness. BL-10 also should be needled superficially with a thin needle. Deep needling and strong stimulation makes the problem worse.

GV-9: Sometimes a reaction shows up between the spinous processes in this area, but this is not specific to dizziness.

There is one more important point for dizziness. It is Nogier's auricular vertigo point.

---

3. *Shinkyu Keiraku Chiryo (Acu-moxa Meridian Therapy)*, Okabe Sodo. Tokyo: Sekibundo, 1974.

At one time the auricular acupuncture of the French doctor Nogier was featured in the *Japan Journal of Acupuncture and Moxibusion*, and it became popular for a while. Nagatomo Tsugio translated Nogier's text and gave seminars on auricular acupuncture, including demonstrations. I recall that Dr. Nagatomo used an electric point locator to decide which points to treat. Dr. Ohta Rinsai in Kumamoto also used a lot of auricular acupuncture, but he decided which points to treat on the ear by pinching the ear and finding tender or hard points.

Auricular acupuncture works well when used skillfully. When there are reactive points on the ear, they can be used for many conditions. Back when I used to do house calls, I encountered a patient whose dizziness did not diminish after my acu-moxa treatment. The moment I tapped a needle into his auricular vertigo point he exclaimed, "It stopped!" Even today, 30 years later, this patient's dizziness does not resolve no matter which hospital he goes to, but my acupuncture works. It goes away after several treatments. After this experience, I started to test this method on myself. I pinch the area close to the auricular vertigo point (around the occiput area in the antitragus) between my thumb and index finger and retain a small needle in the hardest point. Otherwise, I may retain an intradermal needle. The side with the reactive point works best, but if it is unclear, I alternate between the right and the left sides. I don't treat both sides at once. I give this treatment once a week for patients with dizziness.

2.3 Diagnosis for dizziness

I have detailed the treatment for dizziness already, but what about differential diagnosis? Is all dizziness caused by the Liver? Is it Liver deficiency or Liver excess? In my experience the vast majority are Liver deficiency. There are exceptions, of course. Otherwise there is no point in determining the pattern. Revolving vertigo (where it seems the room is spinning) is Liver deficiency or Liver excess. Unsteady dizziness (where one easily loses one's balance) is usually Kidney deficiency. Dizziness with weak digestive systems, dampness, and edema is Spleen deficiency. I had almost decided that there was no Lung deficiency, but there actually is. Once I treated a male high school student whose dizziness did not improve at all after one treatment. As I will mention later, in my treatment system for dizziness, except for cases of benign positional vertigo, one acu-moxa treatment resolves dizziness. So I took this boy's pulse carefully and found that it was Lung deficiency instead of Liver deficiency. So I tonified LU-9 and SP-3. Then I did exactly the same treatment as the previous session and the dizziness resolved nicely. So it is important to determine the pattern and get the right diagnosis.

2.4 Treatment of dizziness

Let us review my standard treatment for dizziness. I begin with the patient supine and perform the root treatment. I use SRT on the following points according to the pattern:

Liver deficiency – LR-8 & KI-10

Kidney deficiency – KI-7 & LU-5

Spleen deficiency – SP-3 & PC-7

Lung deficiency – LU-9 & SP-3

In cases of Liver excess, I insert needles in LR-2 to disperse.

For the branch treatment I retain needles in the auricular vertigo point, LR-1, and the depressed point around GV-22. I apply SRT at CV-12, CV-14, and GB-20. Then I do direct moxibustion on GV-22 and LR-1 (80% moxibustion because the latter point is very sensitive). Finally, I retain an intradermal needle in the auricular vertigo point.

In acute cases, when the dizziness gets worse with movement, I move the pillow upward, off of the occipital area, and apply SRT on GB-20 without making the patient turn over. For acute cases, treatment is complete with the above. If patients can lie on their side, I perform SRT on GB-20, TB-17, and GB-21 on the top side. Patients cannot lie on the affected side when the dizziness is from inner ear problems, so just treating the affected side is enough.

Note: How to determine the affected side: this is the side with worse hearing, the side with a bigger induration at TB-17, or the side with greater reaction at the auricular vertigo point. This jibes with the diagnosis of the otolaryngologist. When the patient is lying supine and has his head turned to the left, for example, the side that is on the top (right) is the affected side. Lying on the affected side will exacerbate the dizziness, thus only the affected side is treated, but this works in our favor.

When the patient is able to lie face down, I check for reactions at GV-9 and -10, and if there is a depressed point, I apply SRT and direct moxibustion. I retain needles in depressed back associated points (such as BL-18 and BL-23 for Liver deficiency). Sometimes I also apply direct moxibustion on these points.

When the dizziness is mild, I suggest treatments once a week. If the dizziness is severe, I ask patients to come more often. Even every day is good. Dizziness resolves quickly, so once that happens you can go to once-a-week treatments. This treatment is quickly effective and usually 3-5 treatments is enough to resolve the symptom. When dizziness recurs over and over, it is good to have the patient apply moxibustion at home on GV-22 and LR-1. When moxibustion is done every day, even just doing it on the tip of the big toe is enough to bring relief. When you think about the fear and discomfort of dizziness, patients say that the pain of moxibustion is nothing. For patients with chronic dizziness, recommend treatments once a month even after their symptom of dizziness has gone.

The point that needs to be kept in mind is that hearing loss and tinnitus can remain as sequelae. I like to check their hearing all the time by rubbing my thumb and index finger together by their ears. I also scrape the nails of these fingers together (they have hearing loss if these sounds cannot be heard in one ear or another). I also lightly strike metal needle trays with a metal needle tube next to their ear for a louder sound.

Not all cases of dizziness and hearing loss can be resolved. It will resolve in one-third of the cases, be mitigated in one-third of the cases, and show no improvement in one-third of the cases. This is looking at the treatment results of 100 cases of dizziness, but it sounds like a weather report and doesn't sound right.

I first reported on the treatment of dizziness at the Japan Meridian Society conference in Fukuoka. It was my very first presentation in a conference and one of my senior colleagues suggested that I would feel less anxious if I had a shot of whiskey before I presented. I gratefully took his advice, but my anxiety only increased and it had no effect. I recall the effect of alcohol came on only after I had finished giving my presentation. Anyway, even looking through the association journals of that time, there were no reports on dizziness except for just one by Miki Kenji of Osaka on the treatment of autonomic dysregulation. In short, the perception in the profession at that time was that acupuncture was not effective for dizziness. Looking at the journals these days, there is an abundance of articles on treatment of dizziness. Times have changed, and it's a wonderful thing.

2.5 Varieties of dizziness

I find that often those who get dizzy have an overly honest and serious compulsive character from birth. They have a strong sense of responsibility, so they do their work with 120% effort and then get dizzy from the relief when the work is finished. This is fine for an employer, but it's a problem for employees. You can teach them ways to take a break or they can find their own methods. The key is not to become sleep deprived, and to get plenty of sleep whenever they are feeling really tired. When they have difficulty falling asleep, add direct moxibustion on M-LE-5 *(shitsumin/shī mián)* to the treatment. Also, such patients tend to dislike strong stimulation, so it's better to avoid needle sensation. It's best to use SRT.

What causes dizziness anyway? From the perspective of Western medicine there is inner ear vertigo, cervical vertigo, and other vertigo. The vast majority of cases are the first two. Inner ear vertigo is represented by Ménière's disease.

Dizziness from sudden hearing loss and Ramsay Hunt syndrome, which is caused by the chickenpox virus, are similar in nature. There is another inner ear vertigo called paroxysmal positional vertigo (benign positional vertigo). For a time, it was said that electron microscopes showed a misalignment of the otoliths (granules of calcium carbonate in the inner ear), but more recently it is thought that the otoliths fall into a crevice and the vertigo continues until this goes away. The symptom of this type of vertigo is dizziness when getting up from bed and going to bed for only a few seconds to less than a minute. The rest of the time there is no problem. The acu-moxa treatment for benign positional vertigo, unlike for other types of vertigo, does not have an immediate effect. The symptom remains unchanged for the first treatment or two. I used to get worried about it, but the reason for this slow response is obvious from the latest studies on this condition. As I treated more cases of this type of vertigo, I realized that the response was slow, but it could be completely cured with acu-moxa. I explain to these patients that it can be cured with weekly treatments for at least a month and at most three months, or from four to 12 treatments. This condition is actually quite common among people with dizziness, but you won't find out about it unless you question the patient in detail. The diagnosis for vertigo has become very accurate in Western medicine these days. So it is best to refer patients to specialists when the dizziness requires more than a few treatments, as this will also rule out serious diseases like brain tumors and auditory nerve tumors that are beyond the scope of acupuncture. Once the Western diagnosis is made, acu-moxa can do wonders in the arena of treatment.

The next most common type of vertigo after inner ear vertigo is cervical vertigo. This is dizziness that is caused by problems in the neck or the cervical vertebrae. It is usually caused by cervical syndrome or arteriosclerosis in the vertebral artery associated with aging. It can also be caused by muscular tension. Use X-ray, CT scans, and MRI findings from hospitals for reference and perform orthopedic tests like the Jackson and Spurling tests (compression tests for cervical foramina) to get a sense of the degree of cervical pathology. The treatment is pretty much the same as for inner ear vertigo, but take time to carefully palpate and treat tension in and around the neck. One must be careful, however, not to overdo finger pressure and needle stimulation on occipital points like GB-20. This can aggravate the problem. Orthopedic tests can also exacerbate the symptoms. Perform the tests and palpation gently, just enough to get a sense of where and what the problem is.

Vertigo other than inner ear vertigo and cervical vertigo include that caused by abnormal blood pressure, anemia, autonomic dysregulation, and eye problems. When the patient's complexion and palpebral conjunctiva indicate anemia, refer the patient to an internist for a Western diagnosis. If the anemia has a cause, this must be treated first. I have had patients with excessive menstruation during menopause or due to fibroids that got dizziness from anemia, whose vertigo resolved after an operation.

2.6 Dizziness from the perspective of East Asian medicine

The cause of dizziness in East Asian medicine is internal wind, which is attributed to Liver qi stasis or Liver blood stasis *(oketsu)*. In modern terms, some cases are due to stress. Those with the tendency to get dizzy become unsteady under a bit of stress. I myself would become unsteady on my feet when I worked in the clinic for a while. When I attended association meetings in this state, I would be asked, "Are you alright?" I attended one party hosted by an association at which there was a certain acupuncturist. As soon as Ogawa Harumichi from Tokyo, who was known for his sharp tongue, approached my table, he rebuked me saying, "What kind of complexion is that you have? It is fine to help others, but you better do something about that face." I was suffering from vertigo, unsteady on my feet, and my complexion looked terrible. I can't say that my complexion is any better these days, what with my old age, but I don't get dizzy any more. Have I become tougher, or more obstinate? The answer is aging. I don't have the energy, I'm too dried up to get dizzy.

When the pulse indicates Liver excess, LR-2 needs to be dispersed. I insert the needle about 5mm and apply minute sparrow-pecking motions four or five times. I like to measure the blood pressure of Liver excess patients to make sure that it is not high. The treatment is a success when the hardness in the pulse at the left middle position softens.

Once another acupuncturist consulted me about a case of dizziness that just wouldn't improve with acu-moxa treatments. My advice was to treat according to the pattern, as I detailed above, and not to use any other points. After that, the patient improved right away. The acupuncturist called me back and said that he may have been using too many needles, thinking it would help. When too many needles are inserted, it can become excessive stimulation. If you are using SRT, you can needle a few more points, but even then, the simpler the treatment, the better it works.

Far more people suffer from dizziness than we realize. Those who make the rounds of hospitals and clinics and get no relief become psychologically unstable. They even start to think that they have some serious disease that remains undiscovered. Since they tend to be overly serious to begin with, they become distrustful. When you tell them flat out, "it can be cured," just saying that is the same as getting 50 percent better. Then the treatment works, so they become 100 percent better in both mind and body. One patient told me that he passes my clinic on the way to work every day and thinks, "I am still alive and well." And just thinking that, he relaxes and doesn't have any dizziness. I understand that there are other patients of mine who feel the same way.

2.7 About "dizziness syndrome"

The symptoms that accompany dizziness are provisionally termed "dizziness syndrome." These symptoms include physical fatigue, neck and shoulder tension, headache, heaviness in the head, loss of appetite, nausea, loss of strength in legs, and a blocked feeling in the ears. These are all symptoms associated with dizziness, and my acu-moxa treatment for dizziness will alleviate these. Cases of dizziness syndrome that don't really involve dizziness per se make some patients worry if that they have a disease in an organ such as the liver. Medical exams typically reveal no abnormality, so they become even more concerned. When I explain to them how symptoms like motion sickness can occur, patients then understand that they have this syndrome rather than some organic disease. Or should I say, they feel much better after my treatment so they understand from their body that there is nothing seriously wrong.

2.7.1 Prevention of dizziness

When patients receive the acu-moxa treatment for dizziness, it eventually stops happening completely. When conditions get worse, however, a syndrome can occur that does not include what is called "dizzy vision" (目眩 *mokugen/mùxuān)* in the classics, which refers to blurred vision accompanied by dizziness. So even though there is no dizziness, there are symptoms like headaches, fatigue felt over the whole body, and loss of taste in food. All these symptoms will go away quickly with acu-moxa treatments. This must be explained to patients with vertigo. Some patients discontinue treatments once the dizziness is gone, but often the dizziness returns. It is fine to give more treatments each time the dizziness returns, but it is better to get treatments once or twice a month. Every patient has a weak link, and treatment before the appearance of symptoms serves as prevention or "treatment before the disease manifests."

Other than acu-moxa treatments, light exercise is good. It is even better if they are exercises that prevent neck and shoulder tension. It is best if one does not spend too much time on the computer or listening to music with earphones.

Summary

1. Acu-moxa is ideal for treating dizziness.
2. Liver deficiency is most common.
3. Use LR-1, GV-22, and the auricular vertigo point.

Case Study 139

Patient: Female, 40 years old

FOC: February 3, 2007

Main Complaint: Headaches

Symptoms and Condition: Along with headaches, she has flushing, eye strain, neck stiffness, anxiety, shoulder pain, numbness in the arms, low back pain, numbness in the legs, and heaviness over the whole body. Her sleep and bowel movements are good. Her appetite is off when she is not feeling good.

Examinations: Orthopedic test for the neck and shoulders were negative.

Pulse Diagnosis: Liver deficiency

Treatment: Root treatment – SRT on LR-8, KI-10, LI-11 and BL-23.

Branch treatment – SRT on CV-12, BL-2, Yanagiya's GB-20, Upper BL-10, GB-21, SI-11, BL-43, Iliac point, and BL-58. Direct moxibustion on GB-21, SP-6, and BL-52.

Progress: (2nd) May 28 – She was a bit better after the last treatment.

(6th) June 25 – A ENT specialist diagnosed her as benign positional vertigo.

(10th) Aug 4 – Lung deficiency. She feels unsteady on her feet.

(11th) Sept 1 – Liver deficiency. Intradermal needle retained in left auricular vertigo point.

(13th) Oct 13 – She feels like she is floating.

(18th) Jan 26 – Liver deficiency. It feels like there is something stuck in her stomach.

Comments: Benign positional vertigo takes time to cure even with acu-moxa. Having said that, this patient took longer than usual as they commonly get better within three months. The point selection of LR-8 and KI-10 is correct, but the other points are not good. It may have taken less time if I would have treated points like GV-22, LR-1, and the auricular vertigo point, but it's hard to say. The next case study is closer to the mark.

Case Study 140

Patient: Female, 74 years old

Symptoms and Condition: Severe headaches and dizziness. An examination at the neurologist shows no abnormalities. A month after that exam she began to feel dizzy every time she moved her head. Someone referred her to me, telling her that I could cure dizziness in three treatments.

Pulse Diagnosis: Liver deficiency

Treatment: (Same point selection as case 140.) Root treatment – SRT on LR-8, KI-10, LI-11, and BL-23. Branch treatment – SRT on CV-12, BL-2, Yanagiya's GB-20, Upper BL-10, GB-21, SI-11, BL-43, Iliac point, and BL-58. Direct moxibustion on GB-21, SP-6, and BL-52.

Progress: Her dizziness resolved completely in just three treatments.

Comments: The effect in this case came almost too fast. It could be due to the patient's personal conviction. There is often a strong psychological component in cases of vertigo.

Case Study 141

Patient: Female, 58 years old

FOC: April 30, 2011

Main Complaint: Dizziness

Symptoms and Condition: She has had dizziness for the last two years. She gets dizzy when lying on her left side. She cannot lie on her back or stomach either. Cannot hear the rubbing of fingers together on the left, but can hear the scraping of nails.

History: Thyroid disease

Pulse Diagnosis: Liver deficiency

Treatment: (Same point selection as cases 140 & 141.) Root treatment – SRT on LR-8, KI-10, LI-11, and BL-23. Branch treatment – SRT on CV-12, BL-2, Yanagiya's GB-20, Upper BL-10, GB-21, SI-11, BL-43, Iliac point, and BL-58. Direct moxibustion on GB-21, SP-6, and BL-52. In addition, intradermal needle was retained in left auricular vertigo point and LR-1 and left TB-17 were additional moxibustion points.

Progress: (2nd) May 11 – The dizziness is better. Lung deficiency. I asked her to lie on her left side, and she had no trouble doing so.

(3rd) May 22 – All symptoms are gone. No dizziness in any position.

Comments: This patient had dizziness for two years and she could only sleep on her right side. During the first treatment she was able to lie on her back without dizziness, and her symptoms resolved soon thereafter. It was almost too easy.

In my article "Acu-moxa Treatment for Vertigo" featured in the November 1976 (No. 387) and February 1977 (No. 390) issues of the *Japan Journal of Acupuncture and Moxibustion,* there were cases of acute dizziness that I treated when I used to make house calls. I think these cases are instructive, so I have included them below.

Case Study 142

Patient: Female, 72 years old

FOC: June 6, 1975

Situation and Symptoms: I got a call one evening asking that I make a house call because the grandmother was experiencing discomfort in her chest. Due to her age and symptoms, I suspected angina pectoris and instructed them to take her to a hospital for an exam. I don't know what they were thinking, but the next day this elderly woman was brought to my clinic. She threw up several times. She was pale and dizzy.

Blood Pressure: 195/90

Pulse Diagnosis: Rapid, hard; Liver deficiency

Treatment: This treatment was before I started using SRT. Needles were inserted superficially and retained in auricular vertigo point, auricular hypertension point (Fig. 14-1), GV-22 (needle rotated from time to time), TB-20, LR-8, KI-9, and GB-21. With the patient still in the supine position, I moved her pillow upward off the occipital area and palpated indurations at GB-20 and retained needles. I asked her to open her eyes and she no longer had dizziness or nausea. I left all the needles in about 20 minutes and had her sit up after that. She didn't have any dizziness. I retained an intradermal needle in the auricular vertigo point.

Progress: (2nd) June 7 – Blood pressure: 162/75. Pulse slow and with Liver deficiency. Her complexion was better and she was free of dizziness. She had had a good night's sleep.

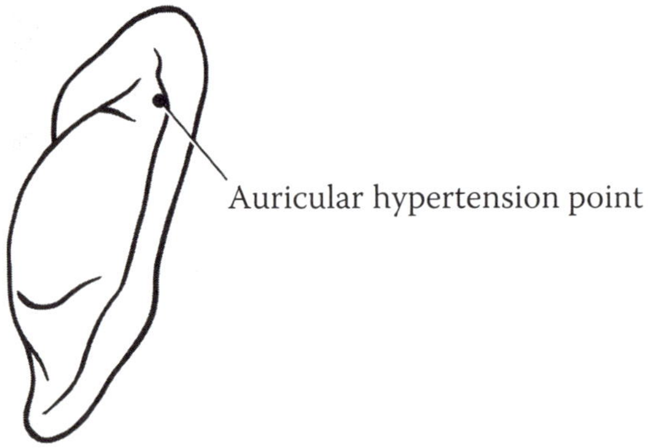

Fig 14-1 Auricular hypertension point

(3RD) Blood pressure: 160/75. She has had no more dizziness or nausea.

COMMENTS: This patient still has hearing loss, aural discharge, neck and shoulder stiffness, and a constant feeling of heaviness in her head. This must have been a case of auricular vertigo.

Case Study 143

PATIENT: Female, 62 years old

FOC: April 7, 1976

SYMPTOMS AND CONDITION: She had nausea and dizziness from the night before. She feels dizzy when she lies on her back and looks upward toward her forehead.

PULSE DIAGNOSIS: Floating, slow, and tight; Liver deficiency

TREATMENT: Needles inserted superficially and retained in auricular vertigo point, GV-22, LR-8, KI-10. Her dizziness persisted. The needle in GV-22 was inserted a little deeper and rotated a few minutes and retained for another 10 minutes. After that the patient sat up and looked upward, but had no dizziness. I retained an intradermal needle in the auricular vertigo point and concluded the treatment with superficial insertion in Upper BL-10, GB-20, GB-21, and BL-43.

PROGRESS: The dizziness resolved in one treatment and did not recur.

Case Study 144

PATIENT: Female, 49 years old

FOC: June 4, 1974

SYMPTOMS AND SITUATION: She had Ménière's disease 10 years ago and has continued to have dizziness and considerable hearing impairment. She requested a moxibustion treatment because she had been to many acupuncture clinics, but it did not work. I convinced her to let me give her a treatment consisting primarily of acupuncture.

BLOOD PRESSURE: 115/70

PULSE DIAGNOSIS: Sunken, thin, and slow; Liver deficiency

TREATMENT: Needles inserted superficially and retained in auricular vertigo point, GV-22, LR-8, KI-10, GB-20, GB-21, and Upper BL-10. Direct moxibustion on GB-2, GV-22, and KI-9.

PROGRESS: (4th) June 16 – Her dizziness that had persisted for 10 years resolved, but the hearing loss remained.

Summary

1. Many people don't believe that acupuncture works for dizziness.
2. Acupuncture does not have much effect on hearing loss.

Case Study 145

Patient: Female, 30 years old

FOC: May 1, 1975

Main Complaints: Fatigue over the whole body, nausea, and dizziness. Loss of hearing in left ear.

Pulse Diagnosis: Liver deficiency

Treatment: Needles inserted superficially and retained in auricular vertigo point, TB-20, GV-22, Upper BL-10, GB-20, and GB-21. Simple insertion in LR-8, KI-10, KI-9, and BL-43.

Progress: All her symptoms resolved in six treatments.

Comments: When a person gets Ménière's disease, a heaviness and fatigue comes over the whole body such that it feels like you are going to collapse on the ground. It is mysterious how just a few needles in the head and ear makes you feel strong and upright. Nausea also goes away.

Case Study 146

Patient: Female, 75 years old

FOC: March 16, 2011

Symptoms and Situation: Dizziness from one week ago. She does not experience spinning but feels somewhat unsteady. Her head feels heavy. She received an exam at a hospital and was told there was nothing really wrong, but she should remain in bed.

She had surgery for breast cancer on the right side, and the right arm has edema. Her doctor told her that she must not have acupuncture for this reason. She has neck and shoulder tension, so she wanted to get acupuncture but had refrained. I explained that I could give her a safe treatment using just a gold teishin, and she agreed. Finger rubbing sound was audible (so her hearing is normal).

Pulse Diagnosis: Liver deficiency

Treatment: Rotation of teishin on LR-1, LR-8, and KI-10. Rechecking the pulses, they had balanced. I continued with rotation of teishin on left auricular vertigo point, LI-11, TB-5, TB-17, TB-16 (induration and tenderness), and GB-21. Direct moxibustion on LR-1.

Progress: The heaviness in her head was gone after the treatment. She called after getting home and cheerfully reported that she felt much better.

Case Study 147

Patient: Female, 75 years old

FOC: April 15, 2005

Main Complaint: She woke up feeling dizzy about 2 a.m. last night. It continues to the present (10 a.m.).

Blood Pressure: 125/75

Pulse Diagnosis: The patient insisted on lying on her right side. Her pulse pattern seemed to be Liver deficiency in this position.

Treatment: Needles inserted superficially and retained on the left side in auricular vertigo point, GB-20, Upper BL-10, LR-1. Then she was able to lie on her back. I confirmed that the pulses were Liver deficiency and performed simple insertion at LR-8. Then I inserted needles superficially and retained them in GV-22, right auricular vertigo point, and LR-1. Direct moxibustion on GV-22, LR-1, and CV-12. The patient opened her eyes and reported that the dizziness was gone. The treatment was concluded with retaining an intradermal needle in the left auricular vertigo point and direct moxibustion on GV-11, which was tender.

Case Study 148

Patient: Female, 59 years old

FOC: June 22, 2001

Symptoms and Situation: She suddenly experienced vertigo on May 27. The ENT doctor said it was not Ménière's disease. She has continued to experience dizziness when first going to bed and first getting up. She also has neck and shoulder stiffness, headaches, and heaviness of the head and leg pain.

Blood Pressure: 134/84, pulse rate 54

Pulse Diagnosis: Spleen deficiency

Treatment: SRT on CV-12, SP-3, LI-11, BL-58, BL-32, and GB-20.

Needle inserted superficially in left ST-12. Needles retained superficially in GV-22 and Upper BL-10. Direct moxibustion on LR-1, GB-21, GV-11, and left BL-15. In addition, intradermal needle was retained in left auricular vertigo point.

Progress: (6th) July 23 – Kidney deficiency. Dizziness is much better. Left occipital pain and left knee pain.

(8th) Sept 1 – No more dizziness.

Case Study 149

Patient: Male, 18 years old (high school student)

FOC: June 16, 2007

Main Complaints: Ménière's disease. He has had dizziness every day for two years and his neck and shoulders are stiff.

Pulse Diagnosis: Liver deficiency

Examination: Nail scraping sounds inaudible on left. GV-9, GV-10, and GV-11 tender.

Direct moxibustion on LR-1, GB-21, GV-11.

Treatment: Direct moxibustion on GV-22, left TB-17, LR-1, M-LE-5 *(shitsumin/shī mián)*, GV-9, GV-10, and GV-11. Needles retained superficially in GV-22, auricular vertigo point, and LR-1.

Intradermal needle retained in left auricular vertigo point. SRT on LR-8, KI-10, GB-20, GB-2, ST-36, BL-23, and BL-58.

Progress: (2nd) June 30 – He still has dizziness every day. Lung deficiency.

(3rd) July 7 – No more dizziness. Lung deficiency.

3. Insomnia

Insomnia is a problem that has affected people across the ages. There is even a book titled, *For Sleepless Nights*, by Carl Hilty.[4] Insomnia must be really difficult. It is hard to imagine for a guy like me who loves to sleep, but as I become older, my sleep is no longer as deep as it used to be. I never miss the late night radio program. I think this is really a good program, and every night I think that I'm going to really listen, but I'm usually asleep before I know it.

Speaking of insomnia, I remember one patient very well. He was the president of a mid-sized company and was extremely hard working. He started reducing his sleeping hours and finally he stopped sleeping at all. Even when people say they are not sleeping at all, actually they are getting in some sleep. But this man insisted that he didn't sleep even one minute. That's impossible! You die if you don't sleep at all. Then he told me that once a month he went to a hospital where they administered an anesthetic (for surgery) and he finally went to sleep. Of course, one would do such a thing if there was no other way to get any sleep.

I started treating this man once a week but could not get a good effect. He was not upset at all, saying that the insomnia he had for over 10 years was of course not about to go away that easily. But gradually he began to sleep, and two hours became three, and

4. Carl Hilty: A Swiss writer, philosopher, and lawyer (1833-1909). Author of many books including *For Sleepless Nights* (*Für schlaflose Nächte*).

eventually he started to sleep normally again. After about one year of treatments, he invited me to a New Year's Party at his company. He gave me a formal introduction to everyone there, but it was a bit strange. Not quite right. The next year he invited me to the party again, but this time his introduction sounded more normal. This means it took him two years to recover from his insomnia. This was a very unusual case.

3.1 Treatment of insomnia

I find that many people with insomnia have Spleen deficiency. The production of qi and blood is insufficient when there is a weakness in the Spleen. In this sense (of qi deficiency) Lung deficiency is also common. In both cases it happens when one is feeling low or depressed. When Liver deficiency patients have insomnia, they respond rather well to treatment. When a patient is Liver excessive, there is extreme irritability.

Liver deficiency: SRT on LR-3, LR-8, KI-10, LI-11, and ST-36. Retain needles superficially in BL-18 and BL-23. Direct moxibustion on back associated points after removing needles.

Spleen deficiency: SRT on PC-7, and retain LR-3, retain needles superficially in SP-3, BL-15, and BL-20. Direct moxibustion on back associated points after removing needles.

Liver excess: Dispersing needles in LR-2 and BL-18, followed by direct moxibustion.

Points common to all patterns: Retain needles superficially in CV-6 and CV-12. SRT on BL-2, GV-22, GB-20 (or Yanagiya's GB-20), and GB-21. Check GV-9, GV-10, and GV-11 for reaction; insert needle and follow up with direct moxibustion when there is a clear reaction. Direct moxibustion on M-LE-5 *(shitsumin/shī mián)* until a burning sensation is felt. If there is a sensation from the first cone, apply a total of five cones. Have the patient apply direct moxibustion on M-LE-5 *(shitsumin/shī mián)* at home.

Key areas for treatment:

❶ Carefully needle points in the upper abdomen like CV-12, CV-14, and left ST-21 when tight or tender.

❷ Upper back points including GV-9 to GV-11, and BL13, BL-14, and BL-15 on the left side. Back associated points that are depressed or indurated can be treated.

❸ Be careful not to over-treat the occipital area.

Case Study 150

Patient: Female, 78 years old

FOC: July 23, 2010

Main Complaints: Insomnia, neck and shoulder tension, low back pain and cold feet. Her appetite, urination, and bowel movements are normal.

History: Sarcoidosis, heart disease, glaucoma with normal ocular pressure, and gallstones

Pulse Diagnosis: Liver deficiency

Treatment: SRT on LR-8, KI-10, CV-6, CV-12, LI-11, BL-2, Yanagiya's GB-20, GB-20, GB-21, GV-10, GV-11, BL-18, BL-23, and BL-58. Direct moxibustion on GV-10, GV-11, and M-LE-5 *(shitsumin/shī mián).*

Progress:

(2nd) July 31 – She is doing a little better.

(4th) Aug 23 – She sleeps well when she takes medications.

(8th) Oct 5 – Treatments concluded for time being.

Comments: She started to sleep better after treatments, but she wanted to be able to sleep without medications if she could. Unfortunately, she lived far away and didn't have transportation to my clinic and had to terminate treatment. I think she could have come at least once a month. In any case, it gets complicated when you try to get involved with a patient's medications, which is something that acupuncturists should avoid. That the patient was elderly and had side effects from medication was not the point. I had the patient apply moxibustion on M-LE-5 *(shitsumin/shī mián)* at home. I did moxibustion on GV-10 and GV-11 because they were reactive. I don't treat these points unless there is a reaction. Her sleep is still good according to reports from another patient who lives in her neighborhood.

Case Study 151

Patient: Female, 65 years old

FOC: September 27, 2011

Symptom and Situation: She doesn't have any other physical problem, but she has difficulty sleeping. Her affect is flat. Medical exams show no abnormality and she is taking sleep medications. Her appetite and bowel movements are normal.

Pulse Diagnosis: Liver deficiency

Examination: I looked for reactive points, but all I found was a bit of tension between CV-12 and 14, and there's nothing that stands out.

Treatment: SRT on LR-8, KI-10, CV-6, CV-12, ST-36, LI-11, BL-2, Yanagiya's GB-20, GB-21, BL-18, BL-23, and BL-58. Direct moxibustion on CV-12, LR-3, and M-LE-5 *(shitsumin/shī mián)* (heat felt after 15 cones).

Progress: (2nd) Her head feels heavy and her chest feels full.

(3rd) Insomnia continues.

(5TH) Sleep is a little better.

(6TH) Nov 2 – She can sleep much better. Her mood is also better and she feels happy. We reduced treatments to every other week.

COMMENTS: After that, this patient's sleep has remained good, but she comes in from time to time saying she doesn't feel so good. She asks me, "Do you think I need to come in once or twice a month for maintenance?" That is good. She must feel the difference when she gets regular treatments.

4. Diabetes

During the Second World War when I was growing up, there was a scarcity of everything, including food, and it wasn't unusual to miss a meal. It's been more than 65 years since then, and now all kinds of delicacies from all over the world are shipped to Japan, especially Tokyo, and luxury and gluttony have become common for the first time in Japanese history. In addition, the modern trend is to avoid physical labor like farming and 3D occupations.[5] Not making much physical effort, lack of exercise, and excess intake of high fat foods results in contracting diabetes while still young. We have entered an age of excess. There is a disconnect for people of my generation who lived with deprivation. There was one politician who called it a punishment from God, and this view isn't difficult to understand.

The incidence of disease changes with the era. Diabetes is clearly on the rise. If we are not careful, we may treat patients without knowing about their diabetes. Ask about it, and if the patient doesn't know, have them get a check-up, persuade them to get a more accurate picture of their physical condition. These days I am always asking questions that patients do not expect from an acupuncturist: Do you have diabetes? What about high blood pressure? There are patients who know they have sugar in their urine but have not been seen by a doctor. They are careless because the symptoms have yet to manifest, but we must inform them that they will surely suffer five to ten years down the line. Basic medical knowledge about diabetes is essential for an acupuncturist, and it's necessary also for communicating with patients and their doctors. A quick review here could be helpful.

4.1 Basic facts related to diabetes

TYPES OF DIABETES

TYPE 1 DIABETES: Beta cells in the pancreas are damaged and insulin cannot be produced so life-long insulin shots are required.

TYPE 2 DIABETES: This is the more common type of diabetes, with insulin resistance,

5. 3D occupations: Those occupations that are dirty, dangerous, and difficult and are therefore considered less desirable.

or a failure to respond to insulin adequately. Causes include heredity, over-eating, lack of exercise, obesity, and stress.

Blood values for diabetes

HbA1C (glycated hemoglobin): less than 6.1% (conventional Japanese JDS standard); less than 6.5% (international standard since April 2012)

Fasting plasma glucose: 110mg/dl to 125mg/dl is borderline diabetes. Caution needed.

Complications of Diabetes (The three primary complications)

1. Nerve damage (peripheral neuropathy)
2. Retinal damage (diabetic retinopathy), vitreous hemorrhage, retinal detachment, blindness
3. Kidney damage (diabetic nephropathy), kidney dialysis

4.2 Treatment of diabetes

Before treating diabetes you must decide if the diabetes is to be the main focus of treatment or if the patient has come in for something like low back pain and their diabetes is to be treated along with everything else. In either case, find out if the patient is receiving medical treatment. You must ask them if they are on any medications or giving themselves insulin shots, and whether they have been hospitalized.

The basic health guidelines for diabetics are as follows:

1. Diet: Eat only 80% of satiety. Reduce calories and chew well.
2. Exercise: Make a habit of walking 50 minutes to one hour a day. Make sure their legs and knees are capable of long walks.
3. Weight reduction: As much as possible, bring weight down to standard level. Do not restrict the diet too much, however, because being too strict makes it hard to stick to it.

Acu-moxa treatment

Root treatment: Treat KI-7, LU-5, BL-13, and BL-23 in cases of Kidney deficiency. Treat SP-3, PC-7, BL-15, and BL-20 in cases of Spleen deficiency.

Branch treatment: (local treatment for the pancreas) CV-12, left ST-21 (only when there is sensitivity to pinching, tenderness, or induration), GV-6 (only when there is depression and tenderness between spinous processes), and left BL-20. Retain needles superficially in above points for about five minutes and apply five small cones of moxibustion afterward.

Moxibustion: Instruct the patient to apply direct moxibustion on the four points above that are active. The results will be good when the patient receives moxibustion at home. Be sure that the patient pays close attention to the condition of the skin and avoid blistering because there is a susceptibility to infections with advanced cases of diabetes.

When we compare the organs in East Asian medicine to those in Western medicine, the Lungs, Heart, Liver, and Kidneys match up well. The Spleen, however, doesn't correspond well. In the translation of Dutch anatomy texts, which took place in 18th century Japan, they had to create a name for the pancreas that didn't exist in Chinese. Clinically speaking, I feel more and more that the Spleen points to the function of the pancreas. In my thinking, CV-12 and left ST-21 are the treatment areas for the pancreas. According to the physician and classical scholar Iemoto Sei-ichi, the Spleen of Chinese medicine is actually the pancreas. So the connection between the pancreas and diabetes is related to the Spleen of classical medicine. Thus, it makes sense to treat the Spleen and Spleen meridian for diseases of the pancreas. There is a passage in the third-century book *Systematic Classic of Acupuncture and Moxibustion (Zhēn jiǔ jiǎ yǐ jīng)* that mentions a condition that sounds like a mixture of jaundice and diabetes. The treatment points GV-6, BL-20, BL-49, LR-4, KI-3, and KI-2 are listed.

Case Study 152

Patient: Female, 64 years old

FOC: February 25, 2011

Main Complaints: She has bad constipation and pain in the left eye. She has type 1 diabetes.

Pulse Diagnosis: Liver deficiency

Treatment: SRT on LR-8, KI-10, ST-36, LI-11, BL-2, CV-6, CV-12, left ST-21, and GB-21. Needles retained superficially in GV-6, BL-18, and BL-23. Needle inserted but not retained (simple insertion) in Yanagiya's GB-20.

Direct moxibustion on CV-12, left ST-21, LR-3, GV-6, BL-18, and Fukaya's LI-14 (located two finger-widths inferior to LI-15).

Progress: (2nd) Kidney deficiency.

(11th) July 4 – Blood sugar level fell to 93. HbA1c: 5.4. Kidney deficiency.

(16th) She stopped taking her medications.

(18th) Nov 8 – Her bowel movements are so easy she can't believe it. Insertion into left SP-14 in the 17th treatment was effective for this.

Comments: This patient did not come to my clinic expecting treatment for diabetes, but her blood sugar level returned to normal and she reported this with joy. Her charts show she has received 13 treatments this year (2012). There is a note that her physician was pleased that her blood tests showed improvement. This patient is not taking any medications now. I have advised her to see her ophthalmologist at least once a year, and her internist quarterly, to stay on top of her condition. Even if there are no symptoms of diabetes as such, it is a terrible disease and one must not be careless about it. I advised her also to get dietary therapy, exercise, and periodic acu-moxa treatments. It is up to her now.

Case Study 153

Patient: Female, 76 years old

FOC: January 17, 2011

Main Complaints: She was told that her blood sugar was high in December.

Pulse Diagnosis: Liver deficiency

Treatment: SRT on LR-8, KI-10, LI-11, ST-36, GB-20, GB-21, BL-23

Needles retained superficially in CV-12, BL-18, GV-6, and left ST-21. Needles inserted 2cm and retained in Onodera's points.

Direct moxibustion on CV-12, left ST-21, ST-36, LI-11, GV-6, left BL-20, and Onodera's points.

Progress: March 28 – Blood sugar level 116, HbA1c: 6.7.

(10th) Oct 11 – Blood sugar level 100, HbA1c: 6.1.

Comments: This patient continues to receive monthly treatments. She doesn't do moxibustion at home, but the results are good. This demonstrates that occasional acu-moxa treatments can be sufficient.

4.3 Treating complications of diabetes

(1) **Glaucoma:** The treatment points for glaucoma are LR-8, BL-18, LI-11, LI-14, Yanagiya's GB-20, GB-21, and points around the eye such as BL-2, GB-14, and M-HN-9 *(tài yáng)*. Use the above points in combination with the branch treatment points listed for acu-moxa treatment in section 4.2 "Treatment of diabetes" above.

(2) **Fundal hemorrhage:** I had a patient who could not see at all out of one eye and her ophthalmologist told her it couldn't be operated on because the area of hemorrhage was too large. Acu-moxa treatments brought her vision back to where she can read with glasses.

(3) **Extraocular muscle paresis (external ophthalmoplegia):** Once a patient came in with the main complaint being unable to move her right eye. The diagnosis at a medical university in Tokyo was that there were no abnormalities, and thus there was no treatment. I had never seen a case of ocular muscle paresis, but the problem resolved with three months of acu-moxa. Later on, she was told that she had diabetes, so the eye problem was neuropathy secondary to diabetes. After that, I've seen a few more cases of ocular muscle paresis, and in most cases the cause was

diabetes. Diabetes is associated with neuropathy, neuritis, and paresis.

(4) **From diabetes to dialysis:** I had a patient who was ready to begin kidney dialysis in one week but was able to avoid dialysis with acu-moxa treatments.[6] She is still alive and well 20 years later. Later on, she had a rapid decline in liver function and hospitalization was advised, but her liver function quickly normalized after acu-moxa treatments. These days she comes for treatment occasionally, saying that her blood sugar is high. She does moxibustion at home and seems to have an affinity for acu-moxa treatments. I don't have any cases of treating kidney damage from diabetes yet, but it seems like there would be great benefit.

4.4 Conclusion

I believe acu-moxa treatments are effective for patients with high blood sugar and could be used much more. Home moxibustion treatment is good, but one has to be careful about infections. This is a condition that will need to be researched more by acupuncturists because not only do we have to advise patients about good medical treatments, there is also the difficulty of having to actively intervene in their lifestyle issues.[7]

5. Rheumatoid arthritis

Arthritis with polyarthropathy is a difficult disease to deal with indeed. Is acu-moxa even indicated? Multiple joints are in pain at the same time. One does not move them due to the pain, and then they harden into contracture. Once it reaches this stage, no matter what kind of amazing acupuncture techniques you apply, it is pointless. The patient must make efforts to keep moving the joints despite the pain so that they do not reach this stage. Acu-moxa is indicated in the early stages of rheumatoid arthritis. Actually, pretty good results can be obtained. Sometimes, however, nothing we do has any effect. It is not good to keep asking patients to endure the pain. Refer difficult cases to arthritis specialists. Continue with the acu-moxa treatments even as they undergo medical treatment. This will bring satisfactory results. The outcome will be better than medical treatment alone. It is important, however, that the physician is not against acupuncture and that the patient is willing to undergo both treatments. This requires a great deal of trust.

5.1 Treatment of rheumatoid arthritis

The following are the main points in treating rheumatoid arthritis in the early stage:

---

6. See section 5.1 "A case in which dialysis was avoided" under Kidney diseases in Chapter 12.

7. "Because many become fat by eating sweets and delicacies, their qi ascends and overflows, and then transforms into wasting and thirsting disorder. Acupuncture CV-12 and KI-19; moxibustion on ST-36." From the Japanese acupuncture classic, *Rule of Acupuncture and Moxibustion (Shinkyu-Soku)*, by Suganuma Shukei, published in 1766.

1. Determine the pattern. Spleen deficiency is likely.
2. When joints in the upper half of the body are affected, find indurations around BL-13 on the affected side. When joints in the lower half of the body are affected, find indurations around BL-25 on the affected side. Applying many cones of moxibustion on these indurations is effective.
3. One must be selective about which points at which inflamed joints to treat.

Determining the pattern and performing a root treatment has a profound effect on the body, like shaking the whole body up. The root treatment creates a foundation for the rest of the treatment.

Direct moxibustion on indurations around BL-13 and/or BL-25 on the affected side is a very effective method that I adapted from Fukaya style moxibustion. Be that as it may, some people these days are adverse to direct moxibustion. When patients are unwilling or unable to receive moxibustion at home, that means they get moxibustion only when they come for treatment. (This means the effect will not be as good.)

When a patient has rheumatic joint pain in the upper extremities, there is always an induration at BL-13 or adjacent points. Most often the induration is tender. This induration appears with any arthritis in the upper half of the body and corresponds in size and extent to the degree of arthritis. Think about this induration whenever a patient has upper body joint pain including jaw pain, shoulder pain, and elbow pain. When the swelling in the hand begins to diminish from the application of direct moxibustion on the induration around BL-13, you will also find that the induration also starts to diminish.

The induration around BL-13 can also be used to differentiate frozen shoulder when a patient presents with shoulder pain. When there is an induration around BL-13 on the affected side, you can assume there is arthritis, and it is not frozen shoulder. Even if there is a diagnosis such as frozen shoulder or adhesive capsulitis, inappropriate treatment (such a mobilization) will always make it worse. (The inflammatory process of arthritis requires more conservative treatment and less local stimulation.)

In the case of indurations between BL-25 and BL-27 for arthritis in the lower half of the body, the effect of treatment on the induration is not as good as that around BL-13. Nevertheless, if you find an induration, it is better to use it.

Be sure to carefully inspect the condition of each of the affected joints. Is it swollen, is it warm, or is it cold? Gently move them to examine the range of motion. Next look for tender points on the joint, such as on the palmar surface of the metacarpophalangeal joint of the thumb. Be careful not to press too hard. If you practice palpation on a daily basis, you won't even have to ask patients about tenderness. I apply SRT on the most reactive point of the joint. When many joints are affected, the number of points needled increases. To keep the number of treatment points down, you have to reduce the number of reactive points you select. One or two points per joint is enough.

The root treatment and direct moxibustion on indurations around BL-13 and/or BL-25 are also important for the purpose of reducing the number of points and avoiding over-treatment. Once you gain some experience, you can quickly stroke over the joints and tell which one is the most painful without the patient even telling you. Continuing SRT with special emphasis on those joints will enable you to perform treatments quickly. When you do many needles in many joints, it becomes over-treatment, so keep paying attention to avoid this.

Also pay attention to the patient's positioning and comfort, to avoid unnecessary stress. Patients need to avoid bathing during the acute phase. Of course, patients don't usually feel like bathing when they are in pain. They do want to take a bath, however, when they feel a little better. Japanese love to take baths. Ask your patients to take showers instead. Alcohol should also be avoided. A drink should only come as a toast after the pain resolves. I also advise patients with arthritis to avoid meat and raw vegetables in their diet. I recommend a lot of cooked vegetables instead.

5.2 Treatment of different joints

Finger joints: Treatment points increase when many fingers are involved, so apply just one cone of moxibustion on the most reactive point of each finger. For acupuncture, just do contact needling by holding the body of the needle and placing it on the reactive point.

Wrist joint: This is often the first place affected in rheumatoid arthritis. Reactions tend to appear near LU-9, TB-4, SI-6, Sawada's HT-7. This is a difficult joint to heal.

Elbow joint: The reaction appears on the lateral epicondyle of the humerus or around HT-3 or more toward PC-3 on the medial side. (The medial side is also affected with repetitive stress injuries like baseball elbow.) Also use LI-11 for treatment.

Shoulder joint: To treat arthritis in the shoulder joint, use M-UE-48 *(mae kengū/jiān qián),* SI-9, and SI-10. Sometimes the anterior reactive point is at LI-15 or two finger-widths below it. Also find and treat an induration around SI-11 to treat shoulder pain.

Sternoclavicular joint: Arthritis in this joint is rarely felt by the patient, so we must palpate the joint. The treatment point is around KI-27.

Hip joint: Arthritis in the hip cannot be determined by palpation. Use the Patrick test. For treatment, use GB-29, Onodera's point, and reactive points around the greater trochanter palpated in the side-lying position. If there is an induration or tender point around the greater trochanter, it makes a good treatment point.

Knee joint: Treat reactive points around the knee including M-LE-16 *(shitsugan/xī yǎn),* ST-34, ST-36, BL-40, SP-9, and SP-10.

Ankle joint: Treat reactive points around the ankle including GB-40, LR-4, KI-6, and BL-39. Also direct moxibustion on M-LE-5 *(shitsumin/shī mián)* has the effect of alleviating rheumatoid arthritis. Apply as many cones as it takes until the patient feels a burning sensation.

When the inflammation is bad, put extra effort into the root treatment and direct moxibustion on the indurations around BL-13 and BL-25. Just do SRT on the joints that are inflamed. Any direct moxibustion on the joints must be burned just 80%. Absolutely avoid having the patient feel a burning sensation on inflamed joints. You can also use an intradermal needle on inflamed joints. When a treatment like this is given 2-3 times a week, the acute symptoms usually resolve in three treatments. When the symptoms do not improve with this treatment, we feel the limits to what we can do. It's time to refer the patient to a specialist. You can find a specialist on the internet who is a member of the arthritis association.

When the patient is able to get over the acute stage in this way, things begin to get a bit more relaxed. The pain diminishes and the heat in the joints decreases. Treatments can be reduced to once a week, but it is ideal if patients can also receive moxibustion at home. Have them apply five cones each on the induration around BL-13 and BL-25. It actually works better when the moxa cones on these points are bigger and hotter. The points on the affected joints get 1-3 smaller cones. It is enough for just the heat to be felt (*chinetsu-kyu*/heat-sensing moxibustion). Just remember that the indurations around BL-13 and BL-25 sometimes move. Be sure to check these points at each treatment and correct them if necessary.

When treatments like this are continued once a week, the inflammation subsides and swelling in the joints diminishes. This also increases the range of motion. As the patient continues with the treatments, the pain gradually goes away. Sometimes the serum RF (rheumatoid factor) even becomes negative. Even if the symptoms are alleviated or go away completely, it is desirable to continue treatments a few times a month, or at least once a month. It is ideal if moxibustion is continued at home on indurated back associated points, but this is not required. You can see how things are coming along by palpating each of the affected joints each time the patient comes in for treatment. When things don't look right, you can get right on it to fix it.

There is no such word as cure for rheumatoid arthritis. The word they use is alleviation. This means it goes into remission and the disease lies dormant. When the physical condition deteriorates, the symptoms show their face again. I tell these patients there are countless rogue genes that have been inside of us for hundreds and thousands of years, and when the conditions are not right, one or two of them act out. I tell them you need to be careful and take care of yourself so that the conditions stay good. Then patients seem to understand what I'm talking about. It is common for those who face a misfortune to become distraught and think, "Why me, why do I have to suffer?" How do we answer such a question? One can seek answers in various paradigms like medicine, genetics, philosophy, and religion. The answer is an eternal mystery.

5.3 Case studies of rheumatoid arthritis

5.3.1 CASE 1 (ARTHRITIS IN SHOULDER AND KNEE)

This is a story that began four years ago. A 67-year-old woman came to me complaining of pain in the right shoulder and knee joints that made it difficult to sleep. She was told she had rheumatoid arthritis after an exam at a hospital. Palpating her right shoulder and knees, I could feel heat in the shoulder and right knee. Checking her pulse, it was Liver deficient, but not rapid. This meant that the heat was localized, not all over her body. She began a course of weekly treatments.

The treatments consisted of SRT on LR-8, KI-10, ST-36, CV-12, GB-20, GB-21, BL-18, and BL-23. Also SRT was used on the local areas: ST-35, M-LE-16 *(shitsugan/xī yǎn),* and BL-39 (painful and tender point) on the knees; M-UE-48 *(mae kengū/jiān qián),* SI-11, and SI-9 on the right shoulder. Direct moxibustion was applied on M-UE-48 *(mae kengū/jiān qián,* SI-11, SI-9, and BL-13 on the right, and on LI-11, ST-36, ST-35, and M-LE-16 *(shitsugan/xī yǎn).*

The patient did moxibustion at home and her pain diminished. Two months later the heat felt on the joints became negligible. In four months there was no more heat at the joints, and the swelling had been reduced. All symptoms disappeared in six months, but the patient continued with treatments 2-3 times a month. After two years of treatment the serum RF became negative and the patient returned to work. She works in an inn helping serve food. When she works, she often strains herself, and she once developed a bad case of low back pain. It was probably rheumatic. More treatments took care of the pain, but try as we may, her stooped posture did not improve much and she quit her work.

Currently she comes once or twice a month for treatment. She doesn't do moxibustion at home, but her condition is satisfactory. She does moxibustion when the pain recurs, but now she says moxibustion is too hot. As far as the pattern, it became Spleen deficiency after a month, but sometimes it is Lung or Kidney deficiency.

5.3.2 CASE 2 (ARTHRITIS IN ARMS)

An 83-year-old farmer's wife developed right shoulder pain after pulling weeds. There hadn't been much rain and the ground was dry, so she must have had to work hard pulling up the weeds. Her shoulder is swollen and warm to the touch. She can flex the arm, but extension, lateral rotation, and getting the arm behind her back is difficult. I treat her for Liver deficiency.

The treatments consisted of SRT on LR-8, KI-10, CV-12, CV-6, ST-36, LI-11, GB-20, GB-21, BL-18, and BL-23. SRT was also used on the right M-UE-48 *(mae kengū/jiān qián),* SI-9, and SI-11. Direct moxibustion was applied on the right at M-UE-48 *(mae kengū/jiān qián),* LI-11, SI-9, SI-11, and BL-13.

Ten days later, on the fourth treatment, I treated her for Lung deficiency. She had indurations at BL-13, BL-14, and BL-15 on the right side. Direct moxibustion was applied on these three points. BL-14, which had the hardest induration, received 20 cones.

She came in three months later with pain in both wrist joints. They are swollen and warm. I found reactions at TB-4 and LU-9. One month later she came in with swelling and pain in her palms, which was worse on her right hand. This patient does not apply moxibustion at home, but it is unusual for the arthritis to move around like this.

Summary

1. Find out if the RF (rheumatoid factor) is positive.
2. Direct moxibustion on indurations at BL-13 and BL-25, especially in the early stages.
3. Keep treatment of affected joints to a minimum.
4. Continue with periodic treatments once the condition stabilizes.

6. Shingles (herpes zoster)

Herpes viruses are everywhere. They can grow when our resistance goes down. People whose nerve cells have an affinity for herpes viruses tend to get shingles. It seems to have something to do with genetics. This is how I explain it to my patients, but I am at risk myself. Now that I've lived for 80 years, I was thinking I could relax and live out my days on accrued interest. But the joke was on me, because I was hospitalized for shingles on the day of my 52nd wedding anniversary. I got a cold and sore throat early in the New Year, and I thought that I would be able to stop it at that, as usual. That was what I had expected, but that's not how it turned out. From January 6th I started to run a fever of 37.5 °C. From the evening of the 8th I started to feel a crawling sensation between my left temple and top of my head. I touched it and found what seemed like herpes. It was an unusual kind of pain. I've experienced all kinds of pain, but this was different. In my case, I can describe it as an electric pain along with heaviness. When I went to the hospital for an examination, I was told this was clearly a case of herpes zoster. I was advised to stay in the hospital and receive treatment.

Acu-moxa can be very effective for shingles, but the situation is different when herpes occurs in the face or on the scalp. When it is in the face it can also cause corneal inflammation or iritis and becomes complicated to treat. When it occurs on the scalp it could cause herpes encephalitis (myelitis or meningitis) which can be life-threatening. It is best to receive treatment in a hospital. Since this is how I advise my patients, I took my own advice and stayed in the hospital.

As far as acupuncture, I gave myself three STR treatments as is my habit, but I used a teishin instead of a needle on points above my shoulders. I was impressed by the effect of the antiviral drugs I received in the hospital, but my quick recovery was probably due to the combined effect of this and my SRT self-treatments. So why did I get shingles in the first place? It could have been lack of exercise, reading late into the night, or drinking too much. I could reduce these activities a little, but my understanding and behavior are not always in line.

6.1 The warning signs of herpes zoster

It is difficult to detect signs of herpes zoster before the vesicles breaks out.

Spontaneous pain (pain at rest) usually improves at least a little with acu-moxa treatments. There is something wrong when such pain does not get any better, or becomes even worse. Suspect herpes zoster when you encounter pain like this. Orthopedic tests will be negative. The source of the pain is nerve plexuses, so considering the location of the pain, press and strike the spine in the same dermatome. Usually you will find tender points, but sometime there is no reaction. Refer the patient to a hospital if your doubts about the pain are not resolved. Antibodies can be found from blood tests, so the answer will be immediate. Once an elderly woman came in with occipital neuralgia that did not improve with one treatment, so I referred her to a hospital. The tests determined that she had herpes zoster and she was hospitalized right away. The very next day she had a herpes outbreak.

The next issue is whether herpes zoster can be identified right away after the herpes appear. Things are simple when there is a dense cluster of herpes, but it's not easy to recognize them when there are only a few.

6.2 Case in which shingles was predicted

A 79-year-old male patient came in with spontaneous pain in the right low back that started five days ago. Looking at his chart, I saw that he came in eight years ago with similar symptoms. Eight years ago, however, the spontaneous pain was on the left low back and he was limping. He had recovered after a few treatments.

The orthopedic tests were negative this time also. Examining his low back, I found a few skin lesions. He had put pain-relieving plasters on his back, so it was hard to tell if he had developed a rash or if he was getting herpes zoster. I told the patient to get an examination at a hospital if the acupuncture treatment didn't work or if the pain got worse. He needed to get an injection of antiviral drugs if it was found that he had herpes zoster. Acu-moxa in addition to medical treatment may seem unwarranted, but it is my opinion, after treating the sequelae of patients with shingles, that the chance of suffering from the sequelae of post-herpetic neuralgia is reduced when they receive acu-moxa treatments.

This patient did not exhibit any tenderness or percussion pain on the Governing vessel in the low back. I treated him for Liver deficiency and gave him my sciatica treatment. I didn't insert any needles except for one, using only SRT and moxibustion. The treatment consisted of SRT on LR-8, KI-10, CV-12, CV-6, ST-36, LI-11, BL-18, BL-23, and BL-25. SRT was also performed on the right side on BL-37, BL-58, and BL-59. I inserted the needle 1cm in the right Ischial point, applying minute sparrow-pecking motion five times. Direct moxibustion was applied on ST-36, and on just the right side, BL-25, Ischial point, BL-58, and BL-59.

This patient returned two days later and told me that the pain was almost gone. The day after his first treatment he got an exam at a dermatologist and was diagnosed with herpes zoster. Earlier in the day he came for his second treatment, a large number of herpes lesions broke out in his low back, hip, and the anterior, medial and posterior aspect of his leg. It makes sense to warn patients about what might happen, and you gain the patient's trust when your predictions come true.

6.3 Case of post-herpetic neuralgia

A 79-year-old woman came to me with pain in her left upper back that had persisted for nine months. This was the sequelae of herpes zoster, and she was told flatly at the hospital that this would not improve. Because she is elderly, she thought that maybe it couldn't be helped, but living with pain was no fun at all. She wanted the pain to be alleviated if at all possible.

She had a large scar in her left axilla which was from surgery for breast cancer. She had marked hardness in the left upper back from BL-13 down to BL-17. There were no findings on the right side, so the pain must have been caused by the herpes zoster. I treated her for Lung deficiency and performed SRT on LU-9, SP-3, LI-11, ST-36, CV-12, GB-2, GB-21, BL-13, BL-15, and SI-3 and BL-62 on the left. Direct moxibustion was applied on SI-3, BL-62, and BL-15 on the left side only.

She reported that the pain was somewhat alleviated after the first treatment. She came for treatments once every week or two after that, but the pain on the left side of her back was stubborn. In the course of treatment, other symptoms came and went like left pectoral pain (SRT on KI-23), left axillary pain (intradermal needle in axillary point), and insomnia (moxibustion on M-LE-5 *[shitsumin/shī mián]*), and the back pain gradually diminished.

In about three months (10 treatments) only a little pain remained in her back. Since she had almost given up, the patient was beside herself with joy. People around her told her she looked happier. It is natural that one would become depressed with constant pain. The patient told me herself that life was becoming fun. By this time, the hardness on the left side of her back had become softer, and the size of the induration also diminished. Her musculature is soft, so the boundary of the induration became quite clear. It seemed to be tender now, and the patient is amazed that my hand would go to places that hurt. I believe that the extent of this induration and the patient's symptoms are directly correlated.

The pattern for this patient shifted between Lung and Liver deficiency, and she feels better when she is Liver deficient. After five months (18 treatments) the pain is almost all gone, but the induration in her right upper back remains to a lesser degree. The patient seems to understand this and said she will continue with treatments until it goes away. In this way, when there is a marked change in the painful area such as in an induration, the results are good.

I will present one more case history below.

Case Study 154

Patient: Female, 73 years old

FOC: June 21, 2011

Main Complaint: Pain in the right pectoral and upper back region as well as the medial upper arm due to herpes zoster

Questioning: Herpes outbreak began on June 9. She received intravenous drip and medications. The lesions are large and spread over a large area, but she says the pain is not as bad as it looks.

Palpation: Indurations at BL-12 and 13 on the right. Slight tenderness found at GV-11.

Pulse Diagnosis: Liver deficiency

Treatment: SRT on LR-8, KI-10, LI-11, SI-11, and HT-7 as well as the reactive points on the upper back on the right. Teishin used on reactive points along the upper Kidney meridian on the chest. The herpes are still wet. The pain on movement is reduced after acupuncture. Direct moxibustion was applied on LI-11, HT-7, SI-11, and BL-12 and -13 on the right.

Progress: (5th) Feb 21 – She is 100% better. Treatments concluded.

Summary

1. Acu-moxa is effective for shingles or herpes zoster.
2. If herpes zoster is suspected early on, recommend getting antiviral drugs.
3. Treat and soften any indurations in the area of the lesions.

Once, shortly after I opened my practice, I saw a patient with herpes lesions all over his front and back. He claimed that they had been there for a whole year. It was unbelievable! This young man didn't have much money, so I recommended that he have moxibustion done at home. Soon thereafter, he told me the lesions had all disappeared. I still really don't know what happened!

7. Skin diseases

It is said in Japan that "a clear complexion hides seven defects." My mother had a dark complexion, but she always told me that a wife with lighter complexion was preferable. When I was first formally introduced to my wife when my marriage was being arranged (the traditional way), the room was dark so I wasn't really able to judge her complexion. It turned out that she had a lighter complexion.

A lighter complexion is fine, but weak or sensitive skin is a problem. This is largely a matter of heredity, but those with sensitive skin get hives (urticaria) and skin reactions to medications. Also, after receiving direct moxibustion, the skin itches around the point. Some even have what's called geriatric pruritus. This is what my body is like. My mother, and her mother, both had sensitive skin. I recall how bad my heat rashes used to be in the summer.

7.1 Urticaria

It is common in Japan to get urticaria from eating raw mackerel. Getting urticaria from eating raw squid, however, is unusual and I must have been pretty exhausted. Once, the morning after I gave a lecture at an acupuncture conference, raw squid was served for breakfast. I started feeling itchy all over soon afterward and my skin broke out. On my 30-minute ride to the airport that morning, I did some acupuncture on myself sitting in the back of the car. I inserted a needle in right ST-19 and continued rotating it. By the time I got to the airport, the itching and skin rash were gone. I must have been rotating the needle for about 20 minutes. There is a reason I selected ST-19 on the right.

Once a 33-year old man came to me who had been having urticaria outbreaks every night for six months. He was taking medications but not getting much relief. Palpating his abdomen I found he had tenderness and sensitivity to pinching at right ST-24. His pulse indicated Spleen deficiency. I inserted needles in right ST-24, CV-12, SP-2, PC-4, LI-11, GB-20, and GB-21 and retained them for 15 minutes. I did direct moxibustion on M-LE-1 *(uranaitei/lǐ nèi tíng)* and he felt heat after 10 cones. When he came in the next day, his pulses indicated Liver deficiency. His urticaria had not occurred at all, and it had gone away, never to return.

Ever since this treatment, I have come to believe that the secret to treating urticaria lies in the abdomen. I find that reactions at right ST-24 indicate some abnormality in the duodenum. I suspect it's caused by stress. So I started to pay attention to the upper abdomen not just in cases of urticaria, but on everyone with skin disease. I often find reactions on the right upper abdomen in these cases around ST-19, ST-21, and ST-25. This may be jumping to conclusions, but it seems like it's related to the liver. It is rare for the liver function tests to reveal an abnormality in such cases, but I suspect there is some relationship.

Things turned out well in the above treatment and the patient's urticaria resolved completely in just two treatments. Yet there was an issue about retaining needles in the abdomen. I used to insert needles more deeply. I used #1 gauge (0.16mm), 40mm needles and inserted them until they were right up against the rectus abdominis. I would retain these needles after rotating them for a while. Thinking about it now, it seems unnecessarily deep. All you need to do is to tap the needle in (4mm). Also, the needle only needs to be retained about five minutes. The way I approach it today is to regulate the whole body with Meridian Therapy and briefly retain needles in a few tight points on the upper abdomen. I follow this up with an intradermal needle in the tightest point. This basic approach applies not only to urticaria, but skin diseases in general. Sometimes this does the trick, and sometimes it doesn't work at all. There are many causes of urticaria, and it's hard to pin-point, but this approach is worth trying out in both chronic and acute cases.

Case Study 155

Patient: Male, 72 years old

FOC: September 4, 1976

Main Complaint: Itching after bathing for two years. He cannot take a bath. He has been diagnosed with urticaria.

Pulse Diagnosis: Liver deficiency

Palpation: There were no clear reactions on abdominal points.

Treatment: Needles inserted and retained in CV-14 and ST-19, ST-21, and ST-24 on the right. Needles also retained in LR-8, LI-11, BL-18, BL-23, and GB-20.

Progress: (2nd) Sept 9 – No effect. Kidney deficiency.

(3rd) Sept 21 – He does not have any more itching when he bathes. Ten months later, this patient had a little itching after bathing, but this symptom went away after one treatment.

In cases of cold urticaria, the itching occurs when exposed to cold. Often patients have a liver dysfunction. I once treated a patient with urticaria who was receiving treatment for the liver at a hospital. The urticaria resolved with three acu-moxa treatments.

7.2 Atopic dermatitis

This is a skin condition that has become very common in Japan in recent years, but the results from acu-moxa are not so good. According to the papers published by some acupuncturists in Japan, some are getting good results. It must be that I just don't hang in there long enough. It is difficult when a young woman's face breaks out with atopic dermatitis. I have had a case where a treatment like the ones discussed above cleared up a woman's face. I thought this would work, but it hasn't always worked as well. Yet acu-moxa is not completely without effect, so it is worth a try.

Give a root treatment for Lung or Liver deficiency. Insert needles and retain superficially in reactive abdominal points, and retain an intradermal needle in the most reactive point. Light skin needling (see Fig. 1-9 on p. 47) is good for affected areas other than the face.

7.3 Eczema of infants (miliaria)

To treat eczema or miliaria for infants, retain an intradermal needle in the right subcostal area around ST-19. (If the baby is able to lie supine, look for an induration.) This works well to make the eczema clear up. Have the parent remove the intradermal needle in three days to avoid a rash. I recommend the above treatment combined with gentle skin needling.

Summary

1. Treat for Lung or Liver deficiency.
2. Retain needle in reactive point in upper abdomen and afterward place an intradermal needle in the most reactive point.

8. Alopecia areata

Once a woman who was almost 80 years old came for treatment of her knees. She complained in a whining voice that her hair had been getting very thin recently. So I said let's get the hair growing, and applied direct moxibustion on one of my favorite head points, CV-22, to see what would happen. Before I knew it, her hair began growing and furthermore, it was dark black. Of course, the patient was overjoyed, but I was the one who was surprised. It would be great if this worked so well for every patient with hair loss.

Our hair and mind have a close relationship. There is a Japanese saying, "ease hair, trouble nail." It means your nails grow fast when you are going through hard times, and if life is easy, your hair grows fast. Sometimes, after going through a stressful experience, I have noticed a lot of hair coming out when I wash my hair. These days my hair is thinning even without any stress. Of course, that is only natural. The condition of hair loss in specific areas, known as alopecia areata, is often detected by the barber or hairdresser. The more you worry about it, the worse it gets. Considerable improvement is possible when acu-moxa treatments are undertaken with the view that there is a dysregulation of the autonomic nervous system.

As far as treatment strategy, I follow the protocol for psychological issues. The root treatment is important. I pay attention to reactions on the top of the head, the posterior neck, and the upper Governing vessel. For the areas of hair loss, I retain needles at appropriate intervals, apply direct moxibustion, or otherwise apply skin needling (see Fig. 1-9 on p. 47). When the hair loss extends over the entire scalp and includes even the eyebrows and body hair, however, the situation is more serious. I haven't treated any cases like this, but I feel that there will be an effect if the patient patiently receives treatments over a long period. Milder cases can be taken on with less commitment.

Case Study 156

Patient: Female, 42 years old

FOC: July 12, 2011

Main Complaint: Loss of hair to the left of the crown in an area about 5cm in diameter

Pulse Diagnosis: Liver deficiency

Treatment: SRT on LR-8, KI-10, CV-6, CV-12, ST-36, LI-11, BL-2, GB-21, BL-18, BL-23, and BL-58. Needles retained superficially in Upper BL-10. Needles inserted in Yanagiya's GB-20. Direct moxibustion on GV-9, at GV-10, and GV-11.

Also three needles inserted 1mm and retained in the area of hair loss—one in the center and two on the perimeter. After retaining needles for 20 minutes, direct moxibustion was applied to each point.

Progress:

(**4th**) Aug 5 – Baby hair begins to grow in bald spot.

(**5th**) Aug 12 – She notices a lot of hair loss when washing her hair.

(**6th**) Aug 19 – A lot of hair is growing in the bald spot.

(**7th**) Sept 16 – The hair has grown to about 1cm. It is getting harder to tell where the bald spot was.

(**8th**) Oct 14 – The bald area now looks normal. There is hair loss on the exact opposite side. Coming for treatment once a month may not be enough.

(**15th**) Dec 19 – The previously bald area is indistinguishable.

Comments: This was a mild case so I thought it would resolve in a short time, but it took longer than I thought. It seemed like her hair growth was slow in general, and it required more patience and long-term treatment.

9. Tic syndrome

People with tics make sounds or shake their body; they happen suddenly and the movements are quick. Those who don't know about this are surprised and look askance at people with tics. Since they are not conscious of these tics, it is all the more embarrassing. Acu-moxa works very well for tics when the patient is a child.

9.1 Treatment of tic syndrome

The pattern is often Liver deficiency. This makes sense from the symptom of spasmodic movements. The most effective technique is SRT. I think contact needling and superficial insertion works well also. It is just my supposition, but I believe that the more superficial the insertion, the greater the effect of releasing neurotransmitters in the brain.

The standard points are LR-8, KI-10, GV-22, LI-11, and ST-36. Additional points could include BL-2, CV-12, CV-6, GB-21, GB-20, Yanagiya's GB-20, BL-18, and BL-23. Otherwise, reactive points on the Governing vessel from GV-9 to -11, and Bladder meridian points on the leg can be included. Use SRT on the standard points for patient of elementary school age or younger, and the rest of the points can be treated quickly like pediatric acupuncture. Applying rotations with a teishin is also good. Moxibustion at home on points like GV-22 (or GV-20) and reactive points on the Governing vessel (GV-9 to -11) is also good. On-going monthly treatments are highly recommended.

Case Study 157

Patient: Male, 9 years old (3rd grader)

FOC: January 24, 2003

Main Complaint: Tic syndrome

Situation and Symptoms: He has recently started to have motor tics and vocal tics. It comes in a series but varies by the day. Often the tic is a neck flexion movement. He was given the diagnosis of Tourette syndrome at the university hospital. His mother explained that they were told drug therapy was possible, but they wanted to try another kind of treatment if there was one. The patient has normal sleep, appetite, and bowel movements.

Pulse Diagnosis: Liver deficiency

Treatment: SRT on LR-8, KI-10, ST-36, LI-11, GV-22, Upper BL-10, GB-20, GB-21, BL-43, BL-18, BL-23, and BL-58. Direct moxibustion on GV-12 and GV-22.

Progress:

(2nd) Jan 29 – The neck movement tics are almost gone. He still stutters.

(3rd) Feb 4 – He caught a cold. SRT on LU-5.

(4th) Occasional neck movements.

(6th) Treatment frequency reduced to once every two weeks.

(8th) Occasional vocal tics.

He received 23 treatments in 2004; six treatments in 2005; three treatments in 2006; two treatments in 2007, and nine treatments in 2008. Currently, in 2009, he is a freshman in high school (9th grade) and busy on the baseball team.

Comments: He contracted Osgood-Schlatter disease by working out too hard, and this treatment is detailed in Case Study 73, in Chapter 5 (Leg Problems). His tic is not completely cured as of yet, but acu-moxa treatments alleviate the problem.

Case Study 158

Patient: Female, 10 years old

FOC: May 30, 2009

Main Complaint: Tic syndrome

Pulse Diagnosis: Liver deficiency

Treatment: She is very afraid of acupuncture. SRT on just LR-8 on the left. I used a teishin on the rest of the points: ST-36, LI-11, GB-20, GB-21, BL-18, and BL-23. Intradermal needle (Pyonex[8]) retained in GV-12.

Progress: She received my acupuncture treatment with a smile from the second treatment on. Her symptoms went away after the third treatment. I continue to treat her 5-6 times a year.

8. Pyonex: Color coded press tacks of Seirin Corporation, which come in five lengths. I generally use the yellow Pyonex (0.16mm x 0.6mm).

Comments: The treatment for this girl is nothing special. I lightly stimulate points on the skin surface, much like pediatric acupuncture. Light, non-point-specific pediatric treatments would probably be just as effective for children.

Summary

1. Acu-moxa works well for tic syndrome in young patients.
2. Use SRT, teishin, and skin needling.
3. Use points like LR-8, GV-12, and GV-22.

10. Pediatric diseases

Pediatric acupuncture, which is called *shoni-shin* in Japan, seems to have become popular among the common people in the Osaka region of western Japan. This must have been the fruit of the hard work of acupuncturists of an earlier generation. In Ohita, where I live, pediatric acupuncture is known by the name of *mushi-bari* (which means colic acupuncture). There was an acupuncturist in Ohita named Ono who specialized in the treatment of children, and when a child came for treatment, he practically ignored his adult patients to treat the child. His results were so good that he received the support of the community. It seems that he soaked his needles in the juice of a certain plant, so his needles were not painful at all. The rumor was that little children felt no pain with his acupuncture so they gladly received his treatment. I don't know whether this rumor is true or not because I never asked this acupuncturist myself. Nevertheless, he made an impact and even now after he has passed away, I hear talk about his pediatric treatments.

10.1 Treatment of infants and children

My technique is to hold three Chinese needles together between my thumb and index finger. It is better if the needle tips are not too sharp. It is important to avoid a pricking sensation. (It may be better to use other pediatric needles.) I tap the skin surface gently and rhythmically so that it doesn't hit the skin too hard. (See Fig. 1-9 on p. 47.) Instead of making the needles penetrate into the skin, the idea is to lightly and rapidly tap the skin surface with the needle tips.

Except for those children who are already used to pediatric acupuncture, most children are full of fear. The key to treatment is how to get them to relax. Keep talking to them about familiar things like food, animals, and their family members and keep them distracted so they don't start to cry. For infants especially, seat the mother down on a chair to hold the child during the treatment. The practitioner also sits opposite the mother and child on a chair to give the treatment.

I like to begin the treatment on the abdomen. I do thorough skin needling on the abdomen. I work all around the navel. Next I work on the four limbs. On the arms I do skin needling from the elbow down to the wrist over both the yin and yang meridians, half stroking, half tapping. On the legs I needle from the knee down to the ankle, mostly along the Stomach meridian.

Then the mother turns the child around so I can treat the back. I treat by stroking and tapping the Governing vessel and the Bladder meridian from top to bottom down to the low back. Next I tap the needles over the scalp. When I press on the shoulders around GB-21, I often feel tension. Pediatric patients from a few months old to older kindergarteners (5 years old) tend to have tension at GB-21, especially on the left side. Some may laugh to hear that babies have shoulder tension, but little children may be sensitively responding to their parent's stress.

I may just start to needle GB-21 by tapping the needle part-way in with a tube. Sometimes I retain a Pyonex intradermal needle on the tight side. When colic (level of irritability) is especially bad, I will do superficial needling (barely in the skin) on Upper BL-10 or GB-20. When there are specific symptoms (such as digestive or respiratory issues), I could also do SRT on one root treatment point. The whole treatment takes about five minutes.

The children who are brought in for *mushi-bari* (abdominal acupuncture) typically have trouble sleeping at night, or stay up crying, or bite their parents, but usually they improve with just one treatment. When this is not sufficient, all you have to do is repeat the treatment several times.

10.2 Additional pediatric strategies

When infants or children show up with special symptoms, I give additional treatment as follows:

Asthmatic coughing: Teishin on LU-9 and one small cone of direct moxa on GV-12. Place an intradermal needle on the axillary point. Leave the intradermal needle in for three days. Have the parent remove the intradermal needle after three days to prevent the development of a rash.

Nasal congestion: One to three small cones of direct moxa on GV-23.

Spasms: Insert needles superficially in LI-4, ST-36, and GV-22. This usually wakes them up, so follow this with skin needling all over and by tapping the needle part-way in at GB-20 and -21.

Diarrhea: It is better not to force the diarrhea to stop. When it goes on for a while, use a teishin or SRT on CV-6, BL-23, and BL-32.

Sweat rash (miliaria): Place an intradermal needle at right ST-19. This also works for skin diseases.

Ear infection (otitis media): Place an intradermal needle at TB-17 after doing SRT there.

CHAPTER 15

Conditions Helped by Acupuncture

1. Motion sickness

There is nothing quite as unpleasant as nausea. When it gets worse, you throw up. It's fine when you feel better after throwing up, but sometimes a vicious cycle of nausea and vomiting continues even when there is nothing left to throw up. It feels like you will vomit blood. Sometimes this isn't just a thought, but you actually start to vomit blood. This is hell on earth. Nausea can be caused by dizziness, hangovers, and food poisoning. Motion sickness is also a cause of nausea.

1.1 How to prevent motion sickness

Two men came into my clinic to prevent motion sickness on their upcoming company pleasure trip on a bus. Their co-workers laughed when they heard about this. Perhaps they thought there was no way acupuncture would work for that, or that they could just use over-the-counter medications for motion sickness. In any case, the result was that the two men who got treatments to prevent motion sickness had no problem at all, while all of their co-workers had motion sickness. These two men got the last laugh over that incident. The treatment to prevent motion sickness is simple, and its almost 100% effective. The basic components of the treatment are as follows:

1. Retain an intradermal needle in KI-9 (the cleft point of the Yin Heel vessel) on the left side. I use a variation of KI-9, which is quite a bit different from the standard location. It is at the hardest point in the medial aspect of the gastrocnemius muscle, about one-third the distance down from the crease of the knee to the medial malleolus. (See discussion in *Finding Effective Acupuncture Points*, p. 198.)

2. Perform a root treatment.

3. Examine the whole body and treat anything that needs treatment. The upper abdomen is of particular importance. Check points like CV-12, left ST-21, and right ST-19. Also, people tend to get motion sickness when they have tension in their neck, shoulders, and upper back. Check for reactions in the Governing vessel between GV-9 and -11. Retain an intradermal needle in the auricular vertigo point for those who have dizziness or poor balance. Retain only on one side based on which auricular vertigo point is harder, or on which TB-17 has an induration, or on which GB-21 is tighter.

In my long years of clinical experience, no case has been ineffective. This is unusual because typically, the more cases you see, the more ineffective cases accumulate. It seems to me that the intradermal needle at left KI-9 is the most effective. Does that mean we only need to treat this point? I told an elementary school teacher about this once and applied just the intradermal needle at KI-9 on some children before a school trip. I was told that a few of these kids had motion sickness, so this means that a whole-body treatment is necessary.

In any case, an intradermal needle at KI-9 is simple and amazingly effective. This is something that we need to widely inform the public about, like treating SP-6 and BL-67 for fetal malpresentation.

Case Study 159

Patient: Male, 70 years old

FOC: March 24, 2010

Main Complaint: He wants to prevent motion sickness.

Examination: Tenderness at GV-10 and slight induration at GB-20 and 21

Pulse Diagnosis: Liver deficiency

Treatment: SRT on LR-8, KI-10, LI-11, CV-6, GV-10, GB-20, and GB-21. Intradermal needle retained at KI-9 variation. Direct moxibustion on GV-10 and ST-36.

Comments: This patient only comes for treatment before a trip to prevent motion sickness. He has been coming to me now for several decades. Usually, when people get several treatments and don't experience any motion sickness, they become confident and don't need any more treatment. This patient says that he still gets motion sickness if he doesn't get preventive treatments.

1.2 Treatment after getting motion sickness

So how do we treat someone who is actually experiencing motion sickness? Usually the discomfort subsides after lying down for a while, but the effect of treatment for nausea is fantastic. Often the patient becomes hungry after the treatment and wants to eat something. Refer to the treatment for dizziness in Chapter 14. That's right, the symptoms for dizziness and motion sickness are identical, so the treatment is also the same.

Patterns: Liver or Spleen deficiency

Treatment: The nausea will go away as you perform the root treatment. Then retain needles superficially at GV-22, auricular vertigo point, and LR-1. Also apply SRT at GB-20 and -21.

1.3 Example of treating myself for motion sickness

I had a good breakfast before a trip and was on my flight for about an hour. I got tired of reading and was beginning to get sleepy when all of a sudden I felt a heavy stifling sensation come over the pit of my stomach. I started to feel nauseous and began sweating. I tend to get cold so I was dressed warmly and the inside of the airplane was warm. Checking my own pulse, it was deep and beating weakly. The plane was already descending for landing and I couldn't get to the toilet. I got myself ready with the emesis bag and bore the discomfort. It must be motion sickness; it was extremely uncomfortable.

As soon as we landed and disembarked, I sat down in the waiting area and inserted a needle in left LR-1. My pulses quickly became bigger (normal) and my nausea subsided. I felt completely better after I did SRT on LR-8, KI-10, and SP-1. That night I became drunk at the banquet. So I ended up feeling sick twice in one day! I had been tired from writing for many days, and lack of sleep is a cause for getting sick. Acupuncture is an ideal treatment for feeling nauseous or sick to the stomach. I prove this all the time by treating myself.

When you feel sick, you feel much better just lying down on your back. Root treatment is the best way to treat nausea. When the pattern is Liver deficiency, use LR-8 and LR-1. When the pattern is Spleen deficiency, use SP-3 and SP-1. The well points are effective for fullness and distention in the epigastrium. In addition, points like the auricular vertigo point, GV-22, GB-20, GB-21, CV-14, BL-17, and BL-18 are useful. Use SRT on all of these points. A light treatment with the intention of relieving fatigue serves best for treatment and prevention. This is the best treatment for motion sickness.

Summary

1. Motion sickness can be prevented with an intradermal needle at KI-9.
2. Whole-body treatment is also necessary.
3. When feeling nauseous, use well points like LR-1.

2. Hiccoughs

This is a story about a patient who had been coming to me for treatment of his shoulder. He had been hiccoughing for two days. He hiccoughed regularly—once every five seconds. I examined his abdomen. There was no abnormality in his subcostal region. Checking his pulses, I found he had Spleen deficiency. His tongue had a thin grayish-yellow coating.

So I began treatment by retaining needles in PC-6, but this didn't change anything. I started SRT on left SP-3 and rotated the needle for 30 seconds and this stopped his hiccoughs. I retained the needle superficially and did SRT on right SP-3 and also retained a needle superficially. After about 10 minutes, I had him turn over and examined his back associated points. BL-20 was depressed. I performed SRT on these points followed by direct moxibustion. I looked for changes at BL-17, but there was no depression or induration.

This treatment was given on October 10, 2008. The second treatment was October 21, about 10 days later. He had been fine, but the hiccoughs started again three hours before he came to see me. His pulse was rapid. His temperature was 37.8°C. He had Lung deficiency. I tonified LU-9 and SP-3. I retained a needle in his right axillary point. This time his hiccoughs didn't stop.

He came in again on October 28 and told me that his hiccoughs stopped three hours after the last treatment and his slight fever subsided. He has had no hiccoughs since. I gave him another treatment for Lung deficiency. I asked him if he had any idea what might be causing his hiccoughs. He said it could be because he had over-eaten.

For me, treating hiccoughs is a rare thing. I recall treating a case 30 years ago. The hiccoughs did not stop after several treatments. An examination at the hospital revealed a gallstone, and his hiccoughs stopped after its surgical removal. So the above case was my second, and I felt I might be able to help this time. Spleen deficiency makes sense for hiccoughs and in fact he turned out to have Spleen deficiency.

I had read somewhere that SP-6 was effective, so I tried it but to no avail. So I just followed the principle of treating the Spleen meridian. Points like SP-2, SP-2, SP-3, and SP-8 come to mind, but I just selected the standard point, SP-3. The desired results were obtained with SRT.

> **Hiccoughs:** A phenomenon in which the muscle groups of the diaphragm repeat irregular sudden contractions. It can occur when the bilateral phrenic nerves, which innervate the diaphragm, and the afferent nerve fibers going to the respiratory center by way of the vagus nerve are stimulated in some way. Therefore, it is often a one-sided phenomenon, and the hiccough is suppressed if the afferent impulse is blocked at the throat. As for pathologies that give rise to hiccoughs, there is esophageal or gastric disease, inflammation in the abdominal cavity, diaphragm or cardiac disease, hepatic disease, and cerebral or meningeal disease. Usually, hiccoughs are harmless and stop on their own, but when they occur repeatedly, or continue over a long period, they interfere with ingestion of fluids and food as well as sleep. So on occasion, unremitting hiccoughs can cause fatigue and threaten life. Hiccoughs can be suppressed by swallowing, drinking cold water, holding the breath, and great surprise. Some treat them by applying pressure on the eyes or administering tranquilizers.
>
> —Nanzando Medical Dictionary CD-ROM, Pro Medica Version 3, 2007

As stated above in the medical dictionary, there doesn't seem to be a definitive way to stop hiccoughs. For those of us born in Japan before the Second World War, there is the famous old medical reference book for laymen known as the Red Book, or *Secrets of Practical Nursing Care in the Home.*[1] In this book it says to boil the calyx (outermost envelope of a flower or fruit) of bitter persimmons and have the hiccoughing person drink this brew. I once told a neighbor who had the hiccoughs about this and he told me it worked. But it would be better if we can cure hiccoughs with acupuncture.

In *Precious Record of Acupuncture and Moxibustion*[2] it says, "Needle LR-14 and apply [direct] moxibustion on BL-20, CV-12, and ST-18." LR-14 is for treating diseases of the diaphragm, and BL-20, CV-12, and ST-18 are aimed at the Spleen, but I'm not sure about their efficacy for hiccoughs. In the *Systematic Classic*[3] it says that hiccoughs are caused by the grain qi rising up to the Lungs after a meal and getting in a battle with cold qi. It also says that since hiccoughs are in the domain of the Lungs, the Lung meridian must be tonified and the Spleen meridian should be dispersed. It goes on to offer remedies like stuffing grass in the nasal cavities to cause sneezing, holding the breath, or surprising the person. The fact that such remedies are prescribed 2000 years later in Western medical references means that hiccoughs are a symptom that doesn't have a single solution. This is illustrated in the following case.

2.1 Case where hiccoughs continued for eight days

This was a 74-year-old man. Sometimes you can land in a hospital even when you are healthy. It's hard to avoid injury when a car runs into you, and this is what happened. He fractured his right radius and had surgery a week later. The hiccoughing started right after that and did not stop for eight days. They occurred every few seconds without letup. He tried medicines and even the above-mentioned brew of persimmon calyx, but it didn't work. He called me (on Oct. 15, 2011) and requested a treatment while still in the hospital. So I paid him a visit in the hospital and gave him a treatment.

I decided he had Liver deficiency and started with SRT on LR-8 and LR-1. Then I retained needles in LR-14. The hiccoughs did not stop. I checked his pulses again and this time the Spleen position was weak. Great! I needled SP-3 to see how this would work, but there was no change. I continued with SRT on PC-7, left PC-6, right SP-4. Then I had him sit up and did SRT on BL-20. I followed this with five small cones of direct moxa and then retained intradermal needles. I then left, telling him to wait and see how he responded to this treatment. That night the sake I drank didn't taste right. It must have been my regrets over what I should have done.

I got a call the next morning and was told the hiccoughs diminished sometimes, but it still continued. This patient was a doctor, his son was also a doctor, and his daughter

---

1. Chikuta Takichi, *Secrets of Practical Nursing Care in the Home (Katei-ni-okeru jissai kango-no-hiketsu).* Sanjuen-sha, revised edition, 1954.

2. Hongo Masatoyo, *Precious Record of Acupuncture and Moxibustion (Shinkyu chohoki)*, 1718. Reprinted in 1982 by the Japan Meridian Therapy Association.

3. Huang-Fu Mi, *Systematic Classic of Acupuncture and Moxibustion (Zhēn jiǔ jiǎ yǐ jīng)*, c. 282.

was an acupuncturist. Naturally, he had an understanding of East Asian medicine. At one time he had acupuncturists working for him. He even knew about and supported Gensai Jyuku, the monthly study group for acupuncturists that I was leading. So the results of my treatment were all the more disappointing. In any case, I got a call from him the second day after the treatment that his hiccoughs stopped. And of course his speech was normal. So why did the hiccoughs stop? There wasn't a direct effect, but I do believe the acupuncture treatment helped.

Murata Morihiro, one of my disciples who attends Gensai Jyuku, told me about one case of hiccoughs he treated successfully as Spleen deficiency. I would like readers to put this to the test. If we can assemble many successful cases of treating hiccoughs with SP-3, that would be very useful.

Summary

1. Acupuncture is sometimes effective in stopping hiccoughs.
2. The first choice is to treat for Spleen deficiency and use SP-3.

3. Stress (performance anxiety)

The London Olympics were held in the summer of 2012. Japan captured a record number of medals. I wanted to support our athletes. There were those who won as expected, and those who unexpectedly lost in the very first round. Even though they say that victory and defeat depend on luck and timing, there must be a way to secure victory. Or rather, there has to be a way to draw out the maximum capacity of an athlete in competition. This is something that I have given some thought to as an acupuncturist. During the Olympics, I felt something as I saw the expressions and listened to the interviews of athletes who had been unexpectedly defeated. So I submitted the following piece for a local newspaper column:

> Uchimura Kohei [a gymnast representing Japan] who had been confident of winning a gold medal made a fatal mistake in his performance. There must be a way to make four years of hard work bear fruit every time.
>
> I believe a person is healthy in body and mind when the five yin organs are in balance. How can we determine imbalances? By observation and pulse diagnosis. When Uchimura was asked how he made that mistake, he says he doesn't know. Looking at his face in the interview, it looks like there might be a problem in his Lungs or Kidneys. If the Lungs are the problem, the cause is dryness, and if the Kidneys are the problem, the cause is coldness. It isn't plausible that an athlete who is the picture of health would be influenced that easily by climate. The idea in acupuncture and moxibustion is that disease cannot occur unless there is an internal cause. Internal cause refers to psychological issues, that is, stress. When the Lungs have a problem, it is sadness or depression. When the Kidneys have a problem, it is fear or surprise.
>
> In other words, what I am saying is that Uchimura probably had something that was bothering him. The solution is to take the pulse, and when the func-

> tion of the Lungs is weak, for example, acupuncture is done on the point LU-9 on the wrist. This adjusts the imbalance among the five yin organs. When an athlete enters competition in a balanced state, he can perform up to his potential.
>
> So my practical suggestion is why not have an acupuncturist who does pulse diagnosis accompany athletes to their competition? Then he could check the pulses right before the competition begins and place just one needle. When the athletes are able to give their best performance, then they can be satisfied however the results turn out. The inability to perform up to one's potential is often a psychological issue, and this can be resolved with acupuncture. I would like the Japan Olympic Committee, the Ministry of Education, and the Ministry of Health and Welfare to give this idea some careful consideration. This is not a dream. It is an idea that can make dreams come true.

I thought this was a great idea, but the piece was summarily rejected. I suppose it went against common sense, or they thought it was preposterous. Or it could have been that they already featured my piece in July titled, "The Rainy Season is Alright: It's a Matter of Attitude."

Let me explain my point of view a little. When the five yin organs are in harmony, the mind and body are healthy. There are many people who don't have any abnormality in their body but are not psychologically stable. The psychological state can be determined by pulse diagnosis. Find the yin organ that is deficient (in a weakened state) by six position pulse diagnosis. Then we can tonify the meridian of that organ with acupuncture. If the Liver is weak, LR-8 can be tonified. The best technique is SRT. It is enough when the deficiency in the Liver position goes away and balance in the five yin organs is confirmed. This is very simple. It only takes 30 seconds.

When an athlete goes into the event balanced in mind and body, he will be able to perform up to his potential. If things go really well, he might even be able to perform beyond his potential. If he loses after performing up to his potential, that means the other competitor had greater potential, and there is nothing to cry about.

So this is my practical suggestion. An athlete must be accompanied by a qualified acupuncturist. What do I mean by a qualified acupuncturist?

- One who can perform six position pulse diagnosis. One who can determine that the pulses have balanced after performing acupuncture.
- One who can perform SRT (super-rotation technique).

The issue is finding acupuncturists who meet the first criterion. It is pointless unless one is able to tell changes in the pulse after one needle. So students and beginners are out. It would be challenging physically for older, accomplished acupuncturists to accompany athletes, so we need to have the experienced younger acupuncturists do the work. Fortunately, Japan is working to have the Olympics in Tokyo. If this comes true, acupuncturists can volunteer. Massage practitioners who volunteer to work on athletes are welcomed. Then why not acupuncturists? We could try to explain about harmony of the five yin organs to the organizers, but they probably wouldn't understand.

The ideal thing would be if athletes maintained their mind-body balance with acumoxa. Then ideally it would take just one needle before they went into competition. One acupuncturist could be in charge of 10 athletes, or a whole team. It would be wonderful if this idea could be implemented while I am still alive. It would be great if our profession and association worked together to realize this dream.

4. Chilblains

It is not too bad when the hands and feet begin to itch when exposed to cold, but it is hard to imagine the pain when the skin turns red, swells, and breaks. I use Fukaya-style moxibustion to treat chilblains and the results are excellent. People who get chilblains not only have poor circulation of qi and blood in their hands and feet, but also all over their body. This is why they need whole-body treatment including root treatment as well as moxibustion every day on the points listed below. I recommend five cones of direct moxibustion. Those who don't want to do moxibustion at home just have to come into the clinic often to receive moxibustion.

One hesitates to cause large moxa scars on the skin of young women. These days people are not very good at applying direct moxibustion. When I was young, it was commonplace for people to apply direct moxibustion on parents and family members, so even amateurs were good at it. I would like to see a revival of direct moxibustion. Japanese-style moxibustion therapy is beginning to take hold in North America and Europe in recent years due in part to the efforts of Junji Mizutani, the director of the NAJOM *(North American Journal of Oriental Medicine).*

The moxibustion points for chilblain are LI-10, LI-11, Sawada's TB-9, ST-36, SP-6, and LV-3. Treat both sides. Look for reactions because the points that work best are tender or indurated. Sawada's TB-9 is located ulnar to LI-10 in the brachioradialis muscle.

Q&A

QUESTION AND ANSWER NO. 8

Treatment beyond knowledge or logic

A young American acupuncturist in Washington State, Mr. T, sent a question to me. He came to Japan and observed in my clinic with an Australian colleague, Mr. TJ. He has some experience with Zen meditation and has written articles about acupuncture and heart/mind for the *North American Journal of Oriental Medicine*.

His question was as follows: "I would like to know about the role of intuition in practice, or treatment beyond the level of logic. In other words, I would like some advice on how young acupuncturists can leverage their clinical experience into developing intuition. I would be grateful if you could answer when you have some free time."

I answered as follows: When I observe acupuncturists who have reached a certain level, I sometimes feel that there is something (in their treatment) that is beyond knowledge or logic. It seems like it's a special talent—something that can't be copied by ordinary people. I don't know about others, so I will speak about myself.

Actually, there are patients and acupuncturists who look upon me as someone with special abilities. I myself sometimes fall under the illusion that I have abilities that are extraordinary. Does this mean that I am a genius? The answer is no.

When I entered the profession of acupuncture, I was awed by the skill of my own teacher and was pessimistic about ever reaching his level. But I had no other work and decided to continue making efforts to improve even if I was slow and unintelligent. Fifty years have passed, and now, somehow, I've reached a level where I can give treatments beyond logic or reason. Conditions that can't be figured out in hospitals somehow seem manageable, and quite often these conditions are resolved by my treatments. Seemingly difficult cases resolve, but often I myself don't know how it happened. What is going on? It is rather mysterious, but I will explain how I arrived at this place.

- Recognizing that I am stupid (the limitations of my own mind)
  - This means I must make twice as much effort as others. Good results cannot be expected when I neglect the work of acquiring the knowledge and techniques required in our work. It is necessary to study and practice over and over on a daily basis.
  - Also, I had to make an effort and find creative ways to develop my sensitivity.
  - After this we get into the realm of religion or spirit. I recite the sutras and meditate. I leave the rest up to God or Buddha.
- Cultivate an attitude of "forget oneself and serve others." We go astray when we are driven by self-interest.

This doesn't really explain how to get beyond the mind in practice, but I don't think it's anything extraordinary. I think that treatments beyond the mind only become possible when you do all you can to improve your knowledge and skill and then leave the rest up to God or Buddha.

CHAPTER 16

Special Considerations in Practice

1. Treating elderly patients

The percentage of elderly persons in Japan has now reached 24%, and it is certain that this rate will only increase in the future. The trend toward fewer children reduces the number of young people. There is not going to be enough younger adults to look after the elderly. This is why the elderly must become more independent and able to help themselves. Acu-moxa must assist this process. I would like to discuss this important topic in this section.

1.1 The characteristics of elderly patients

It is rare for elderly patients to have just one problem or disease. Often they have multiple diseases and diagnoses. Many not only have physical problems but psychological issues as well. In extreme cases there are cognitive deficits. How do we deal with multiple diseases in treating the elderly? It requires that we keep in mind the various diseases from the beginning of the treatment to the end. If we are not careful, it is easy to over-treat or over-stimulate elderly patients.

1.2 Elderly patients and acu-moxa treatments

Acu-moxa, shiatsu (acupressure), and massage are very popular forms for treatment among senior citizens. When done skillfully, these are ideal forms of treatment for elderly patients.

1.3 The psychological state of elderly patients

Elderly patients tend to get depressed. It is natural because there is a decrease in the necessary neurotransmitters. Some people withdraw and don't get out much, while others get out for activities seeking social contact. Light exercise like golf, croquet, and Taiji (Tai Chi) is highly beneficial.

The way to treat depression with acupuncture is to use SRT, contact needling, and teishin. Deep insertion is risky. It makes sense from the perspective of the spirits in the five yin organs that balancing the meridians and thus the organs will improve the psychological state.

1.4 Considerations about the bodies of elderly patients

I recommend giving the root treatment as the foundation. When the pattern is unclear, just treat them for Kidney deficiency. The decline of the Kidneys is common to all elderly patients. Is it possible to give symptomatic treatment for all their complaints? Of course, the patient wants all of them treated and we want to comply. But there is no point if we over-treat them and they can't move. I reduce the treatment points in the affected local areas. This makes the accurate location of reactive points all the more important. This is where your experience and professionalism come into play.

1.5 Treatment position for elderly patients

Is the patient able to lie on his/her back? What about face down? Some patients are bent forward with excess kyphosis, and they can only be treated in the side-lying position. It is important that they are treated in positions that are comfortable. We must decide quickly based on the looking assessment, and direct the patient to assume a suitable position. Even in the side-lying position, some patients need extra pillows or a bolster pillow between their knees.

1.6 Conditions common to elderly patients

Knee joint problems: We need to judge whether it can be cured with acu-moxa or will require surgery and advise accordingly. Treat for Spleen deficiency when there is heat and swelling. Treat for Liver deficiency when there is no inflammation, just deformity. Outcome depends on whether the patient can do direct moxibustion at home. Three to five moxibustion points is sustainable for home treatments.

Low back pain: Elderly patients must avoid electric massage devices and strong traction. Be very careful with elderly thin female patients with spinal deformities who cannot lie on their back or their stomach. There is a possibility of osteoporosis. It can be difficult to locate the places that are the source of the pain. Do not press to palpate the points. Even light pressure can exacerbate the pain. Palpate with stroking motions. The pain resolves unexpectedly soon when you give light treatments with the idea of not making them worse. Think in terms of three months. Elderly female patients especially tend to have fractures, so refer them to an orthopedic specialist when they don't get any better.

You are sure to make a mistake if you try to cure them in one or two treatments. If the patient has been coming to you for decades, sometimes they say that you used to cure them with just one treatment, but don't get suckered by that. Emphasize strengthening the legs. Direct moxibustion on ST-36 is good. Exercising the legs also serves to strengthen the internal organs, stimulate the brain, and prevent dementia.

General advice: Suggest mental exercises like calculations and reading out loud to prevent aging of the brain. Reading out loud is especially good. Moving and exercising the hands and feet each stimulate about a quarter of the cerebral cortex. Exercising the jaws stimulates about half of the brain. Advise chewing each bite 50 times. This produces neurotransmitters in addition to the digestive enzymes in saliva. What if the patient doesn't have the teeth to chew? My grandmother had no teeth at all when she was 94. She used to chew pickles with her gums. Dental care is very important. Regular brushing and treatment of periodontal diseases also prevents arteriosclerosis.

Ear problems: Tinnitus and loss of hearing are difficult to treat, but there can be some effect. Treat the Triple Burner and Gallbladder meridians.

Diabetes: Direct moxibustion works well, but one has to be very careful to avoid burns and infections.

Respiratory System: Many elderly people die of pneumonia. Often it is aspiration pneumonia due to food "going down the wrong way." I experience this from time to time when spicy foods like curry or horse radish stimulates my throat and I inadvertently inhale. Acupuncture around the throat, chest, occiput, and shoulders can prevent the tendency of nerve paralysis (swallowing reflex).

Circulatory system: When there is chest pain or discomfort, there is risk of sudden death. Be sure to have the patient see a cardiac specialist. Also provide moxibustion on points like PC-6, SP-4, LI-11, and BL-15.

Digestive system: Elderly patients must avoid overeating, especially of sweet foods. Eating to about 80% of full is best. One must also not go to the other extreme and eat less than necessary.

Eye problems: Cataracts can be fixed with surgery. Glaucoma is helped by acu-moxa.

Things to avoid:

- Thick needles, deep needles, and too many needles.
- Painful moxibustion.
- Strong pressure with palpation, especially for acute low back pain in elderly women with spinal abnormalities.
- Percussion, strong massage, forceful chiropractic, and forced exercises.

How to please elderly patients: Don't exaggerate too much. Praise them a little.

1.7 Ideal treatment for elderly patients

The ideal is to treat them every week. How does that work for them financially? There are many ways to look at it, but it seems wise to invest in one's health in old age. It is difficult to completely cure elderly patients. It is enough to alleviate symptoms. The secret is to constantly continue working on correcting issues that come up all over the body. The effect of direct moxibustion at home is also substantial. Does the elderly patient express pleasure at the end of treatment? When they tell you, "Please don't die," they are counting on you to take care of them. So that means we need to take good care of ourselves as well.

1.8 Conclusion about elderly patients

Acu-moxa, shiatsu, and massage are ideal forms of treatment for elderly patients. Because the tools and techniques seem simple, however, it is actually very difficult to get good results. This is why we must maintain a professional attitude. These methods can be used to treat patients right up until they die, and they generally feel good, and patients can die with a smile on their face. It is the ultimate treatment modality, but can we gain the patient's confidence? It takes knowledge, skill, character, and common sense.

The mother of one of my students died of lung cancer. She received treatments until the very end and died with little suffering. I was told it was a delicate transition from regular acupuncture to the use of teishin at the end.

2. Patients who are afraid of needles

Sometimes I get patients who just want moxibustion. They absolutely refuse acupuncture. The following case is about one such patient. I really wanted to do acupuncture. But there is no point in forcing the patient to submit to something they don't want. Having said that, as an acupuncturist, we want to use needles to help the patient.

No matter how I tried to explain to this patient that my acupuncture was absolutely painless, she was in no mood to listen. I could tell that it was pointless from her strained look. She didn't have any experience of acupuncture, but she had received massage before. It is understandable how lacking any experience, the idea of inserting steel needles inside the body was anxiety-provoking. Furthermore, she has watched acupuncture on TV, and it appeared invasive and painful. Her apprehension was no laughing matter since I can be quite spineless myself.

This patient was 73 years old. Her main complaints were dizziness, neck and shoulder stiffness, low back pain, and sores in her mouth. The Wright's test was positive. (Hyper abduction of the arm caused a decrease in radial pulse.) She didn't object to my taking her pulses. The pulses were sunken, slow, and deficient. I determined she had Lung deficiency.

I gently pressed LU-9 and SP-3 with the tip of my middle finger and took her pulses again, and they seemed to improve quite a bit. I told her to let me examine some points and placed a 4cm gold teishin on them in a way that the patient couldn't see what I was doing. I gently touched and rotated the teishin on LU-9, SP-3, ST-36, CV-12, LU-1, and GV-22. When I checked the pulse again, the quality had improved nicely. After that we applied direct moxibustion on ST-36 and LI-11.

Then the patient turned over onto her stomach and I continued treatment with the gold teishin on BL-13, BL-20, BL-53, BL-25, and BL-58. This was followed up with direct moxibustion on BL-13, BL-20, and BL-53. Then I had her sit up and used the teishin on GB-20, GB-21, and ST-12. I concluded with direct moxibustion on GB-21. The patient said she felt good and seemed satisfied.

This first office call was on December 21, 2007. I didn't think she would need another treatment if she did moxibustion at home as advised, but she came in again two months later on February 16, 2008. When I asked her if she had any dizziness, she said no. She told me she had visited her daughter in America for 40 days and was exhausted. Her pulse quality was pretty good, and the pattern was Liver deficiency. She told me she wasn't able to do moxibustion. I gave her a similar treatment using teishin. This patient thought that both of these treatments were moxibustion treatments. I didn't say anything because she was happy with the treatment and a detailed explanation didn't seem necessary.

2.1 The use of teishin and healing hands

A lot of moxibustion is used in the Sawada-style. For the above-mentioned case, for example, aside from the points I listed, additional points like CV-12, CV-6, left TB-4, KI-6, GV-12, BL-18, BL-20, BL-23, and BL-32 would receive direct moxibustion. This type of treatment brings the pulse up quite a bit, but I like to adjust qi with needles. If I have to use only moxibustion, I am not quite satisfied. As an acupuncturist we want to insert needles. It's just like a surgeon wanting to make an incision (operate).

Actually, when it comes to adjusting the qi, it works better the more superficial the needle. I say this from long years of experience. There are a variety of techniques from superficial insertion, to SRT, to contact needling, to teishin. Qi can be adjusted when performed skillfully. The pulse becomes vibrant and balanced.

What if we used our fingertip instead of a needle? Sometimes it works, like in the above-mentioned case. As long as the diagnosis, point selection, and location are accurate, the pulse improves surprisingly well. Does that mean finger pressure works also, and that diseases can be cured with finger pressure?

I think that the fingers of seasoned practitioners have the power to heal people. The places that energy can be emitted from people include the tip of the middle finger, the center of the palm (PC-7), and the point between the eyebrows (M-HN-3 *[yìn táng]*). These are places from which qi can be radiated most strongly. This is the pose of pressing the hands together and bringing them up to the face, as if in prayer. There is one theory that the strongest qi is generated when the above three points are brought together. I am not sure about the truth of this idea, but in recent years I have come to believe that when a person gives treatments over many years, they begin to emit qi that heals people. The hands of masters are in this category. Also, the fingers go right to the place that has a problem. The fingers go there without thinking. Sometimes the pain eases just by their touch.

When my mother was still alive, there was a young man who suffered from pain all over his body for unknown reasons. Unlike today, the diagnosis and treatment were unclear. When my mother would stroke his body where it hurt, the pain would go away miraculously. After receiving my mother's ministrations for several months, his pain resolved completely. This happened back when I was still a child, and I barely remember it. But this man moved to Tokyo and whenever he came back home, he always came to visit my mother and repeated his story. He must have really been helped. Thinking about it today, it might have been a symptom of depression or something, but it also points to the effect of treatment with gifted hands.

How can we develop such gifted hands? I cannot say for sure, but the following points come to mind.

- Train your fingers. In my case I have developed the sensitivity of my middle fingers, especially the right.
- The desire to help patients is important.
- Training in mental concentration like meditation and reciting the sutras.

Speaking of the subject of special hands, there is the term "bad hands" (惡手 *è shǒu*) in the 73rd chapter of *Vital Axis*. "When those with poison in their hands press down on a vessel with a turtle inside, the turtle will die in 50 days. When those with sweetness in their hands press on the same vessel, the turtle will come back to life." Since our hands have such a huge role in giving acu-moxa treatments, we cannot be careful enough with them.

POINT INDEX

Boldface entries appear in illustrations.

CONCEPTION VESSEL

EMPIRICAL POINTS

Extra / Miscellaneous points

Gallbladder meridian

Governing vessel

Heart meridian

Kidney meridian

Large Intestine meridian

Liver meridian

Lung meridian

Pericardium meridian

Small Intestine meridian

Spleen meridian

Stomach Meridian

Triple Burner meridian

GENERAL INDEX

Boldface entries appear in illustrations.

B

D

F

G

L

M

N

Q

R

S

T

U